Oral Health Essentials

Oral Health Essentials

Editor: Patrick Hall

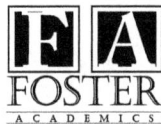

FOSTER
ACADEMICS

www.fosteracademics.com

www.fosteracademics.com

FA
FOSTER
ACADEMICS

Cataloging-in-Publication Data

Oral health essentials / edited by Patrick Hall.
    p. cm.
Includes bibliographical references and index.
ISBN 978-1-63242-933-9
1. Mouth--Care and hygiene. 2. Oral medicine. 3. Dental care. 4. Oral hygiene products. I. Hall, Patrick.
RK60.7 .O73 2020
617.601--dc23

Foster Academics,
118-35 Queens Blvd., Suite 400,
Forest Hills, NY 11375, USA

ISBN 978-1-63242-933-9 (Hardback)

Contents

Preface

The main aim of this book is to educate learners and enhance their research focus by presenting diverse topics covering this vast field. This is an advanced book which compiles significant studies by distinguished experts in the area of analysis. This book addresses successive solutions to the challenges arising in the area of application, along with it; the book provides scope for future developments.

Dental and oral medicine is a field of medicine, which is concerned with the diagnosis, treatment and prevention of diseases and disorders of the oral cavity. It encompasses the study of the dentition, the temporomandibular joint, and supporting muscular, nervous, lymphatic, vascular and anatomical structures. Dental caries and periodontal disease are two of the most common oral diseases. Dental caries or tooth decay is the breakdown of the teeth due to acids produced by bacteria. The inflammation of the tissues surrounding the teeth is referred to as periodontal disease. Scaling and root planing, teeth restoration, surgical extraction of teeth and endodontic root canal treatment are certain dental treatments that may be performed for the maintenance of oral health. Oral diseases can be largely prevented by maintaining proper hygiene and with regular professional cleaning and evaluation. The aim of this book is to present researches that have transformed the discipline of oral health and dentistry and aided its advancement. It strives to provide a fair idea about this discipline and to help develop a better understanding of the latest advances within this field. With state-of-the-art inputs by acclaimed experts of this field, this book targets students and professionals.

It was a great honour to edit this book, though there were challenges, as it involved a lot of communication and networking between me and the editorial team. However, the end result was this all-inclusive book covering diverse themes in the field.

Finally, it is important to acknowledge the efforts of the contributors for their excellent chapters, through which a wide variety of issues have been addressed. I would also like to thank my colleagues for their valuable feedback during the making of this book.

Editor

Cone beam computed tomography in implant dentistry

Reinhilde Jacobs[1,2,3]* (iD), Benjamin Salmon[4,5], Marina Codari[6], Bassam Hassan[7] and Michael M. Bornstein[1,8]

Abstract

Background: In implant dentistry, three-dimensional (3D) imaging can be realised by dental cone beam computed tomography (CBCT), offering volumetric data on jaw bones and teeth with relatively low radiation doses and costs. The latter may explain why the market has been steadily growing since the first dental CBCT system appeared two decades ago. More than 85 different CBCT devices are currently available and this exponential growth has created a gap between scientific evidence and existing CBCT machines. Indeed, research for one CBCT machine cannot be automatically applied to other systems.

Methods: Supported by a narrative review, recommendations for justified and optimized CBCT imaging in oral implant dentistry are provided.

Results: The huge range in dose and diagnostic image quality requires further optimization and justification prior to clinical use. Yet, indications in implant dentistry may go beyond diagnostics. In fact, the inherent 3D datasets may further allow surgical planning and transfer to surgery via 3D printing or navigation. Nonetheless, effective radiation doses of distinct dental CBCT machines and protocols may largely vary with equivalent doses ranging between 2 to 200 panoramic radiographs, even for similar indications. Likewise, such variation is also noticed for diagnostic image quality, which reveals a massive variability amongst CBCT technologies and exposure protocols. For anatomical model making, the so-called segmentation accuracy may reach up to 200 μm, but considering wide variations in machine performance, larger inaccuracies may apply. This also holds true for linear measures, with accuracies of 200 μm being feasible, while sometimes fivefold inaccuracy levels may be reached. Diagnostic image quality may also be dramatically hampered by patient factors, such as motion and metal artefacts. Apart from radiodiagnostic possibilities, CBCT may offer a huge therapeutic potential, related to surgical guides and further prosthetic rehabilitation. Those additional opportunities may surely clarify part of the success of using CBCT for presurgical implant planning and its transfer to surgery and prosthetic solutions.

Conclusions: Hence, dental CBCT could be justified for presurgical diagnosis, preoperative planning and peroperative transfer for oral implant rehabilitation, whilst striving for optimisation of CBCT based machine-dependent, patient-specific and indication-oriented variables.

Keywords: Cone beam computed tomography, Dental implants, Presurgical planning, Guidelines, Radiation dose, Virtual patient

* Correspondence: reinhilde.jacobs@uzleuven.be
[1]OMFS IMPATH Research Group, Department of Imaging and Pathology, Faculty of Medicine, University of Leuven, Kapucijnenvoer 33, 3000 Leuven, Belgium
[2]Department of Oral and Maxillofacial Surgery, University Hospitals Leuven, Leuven, Belgium
Full list of author information is available at the end of the article

Background

Radiography is considered the most frequent diagnostic tool in daily dental practice, with more than one quarter of all medical radiographs in Europe being made by dentists. Since the discovery of x-rays 120 years ago, dental radiographs have been the predominant source of diagnostic information in the oral and maxillofacial complex. Yet, two-dimensional (2D) imaging techniques are unable to depict complicated three-dimensional (3D) anatomical structures and related pathologies.

In the nineties, there was a growing tendency in using 3D information as an aid for dentomaxillofacial diagnosis and treatment, while in the nillies, cone beam computed tomography (CBCT) imaging started to offer a solution for this growth by being made available in specialty clinics [1], These developments went hand in hand with the increasing use of 3D imaging applications for presurgical planning and transfer of oral implant treatment [2–4]. While the required 3D acquisition for dental applications was initially realized by medical computed tomography (CT), dental CBCT rapidly took over [1, 5]. The main reasons for the triumph of CBCT are its capabilities of volumetric jaw bone imaging at reasonable costs and doses, with a relative advantage of having a compact, affordable, and nearby or in-house equipment. For the clinicians involved in implant rehabilitation, the power of a dental 3D dataset is not only situated in the diagnostic field, but also in the potential of gathering integrated patient information for presurgical and treatment applications related to oral implant placement. Nowadays, rapid advances of digital technology and computer-aided design/computer-aided manufacturing (CAD/CAM) systems are indeed creating challenging opportunities for diagnosis, surgical implant planning and delivery of implant-supported prostheses. While there is still a huge demand for maximised integration of 3D datasets acquired from various imaging sources, there is also a call for simplified solutions. Yet, when striving for optimized patient-specific implant rehabilitation, the ultimate goal remains to fully integrate the available 3D imaging data thus creating the virtual patient, aiding presurgical simulation and peroperative transfer to the surgical field with further prosthetic rehabilitation [1, 5].

The aim of the present state-of-the-art paper is to present a narrative review providing support for the hypothesis on using CBCT for oral implant planning and to attempt formulating recommendations for justified and optimized CBCT imaging. Requirements for optimized use of CBCT and the related limitations are presented including a maximized use of available 3D CBCT data.

Methods

In order to find the relevant literature included in this article, an electronic search of MEDLINE (PubMed) database was performed. This literature search included studies published in English language or with an English language abstract published prior to November 30th, 2016.

To classify the available literature, specific search queries were used (Table 1). In particular, these queries were combined in order to divide the available literature by specific topics. Figures 1 and 2 show the results of the searches and classification processes.

The performed electronic search was complemented by hand-searching, and the final selection of publications was performed after consultation of the working group, consisting of all coauthors of this paper. Disagreements regarding study inclusion were discussed by the investigators. The results of the search process were then summarized in 12 focused questions that identify different areas on the use of CBCT in implant dentistry:

1. *Why to use CBCT in implant dentistry?*
2. *What is the radiation dose level of dental CBCT?*
3. *Which parameters influence image quality in CBCT?*
4. *When to use CBCT in implant dentistry: existing guidelines?*
5. *How to apply CBCT guidelines for the individual patient?*
6. *How to optimize scanning during presurgical use of CBCT?*
7. *How to use dental CBCT beyond radiodiagnostics?*
8. *What are the requirements for creating a virtual patient?*
9. *What are the requirements for 3D model making?*

Table 1 Search queries combined in order to classify the available peer-reviewed literature, in MEDLINE (PubMed) database, on the use of CBCT in implant dentistry

ID	Related topic	Search query
#1	CBCT use	cbct OR cone beam computed tomography OR cone beam computer tomography
#2	Implant oriented application	jaw OR teeth OR dental OR dento*
#3	Presurgical imaging	planning or presurgical OR preoperative OR planning or drill guide OR drilling guide OR template
#4	Postsurgical imaging	radiological follow-up OR follow-up or postsurgical* OR postoperative* OR post-operative* OR after surgery
#5	Image quality	image quality OR artifact* OR noise OR accuracy
#6	Dose evaluation	dose OR radiation dos* OR dosi*
#7	Implant planning	planning OR (planning AND (accuracy or accurate or validate or validation or evaluation))
#8	Postsurgical complication	complica* OR nerve OR iatrogenic OR damage OR neuro* OR vascular OR neural

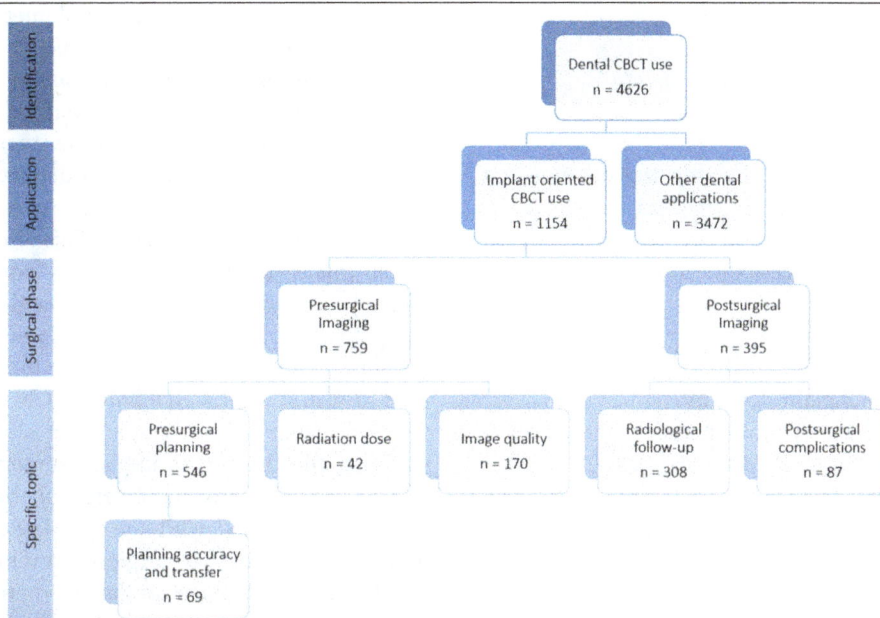

Fig. 1 Availability of peer-reviewed articles on the use of CBCT is dentistry and more specifically in the pre- and postsurgical phases of implant dentistry (PubMed output up till November 30 2016). Roughly, every fourth article published on CBCT is related to the use of CBCT in implant dentistry, with two out of three on the presurgical use of CBCT, with a vast majority on the application of CBCT for presurgical planning and transfer to implant placement

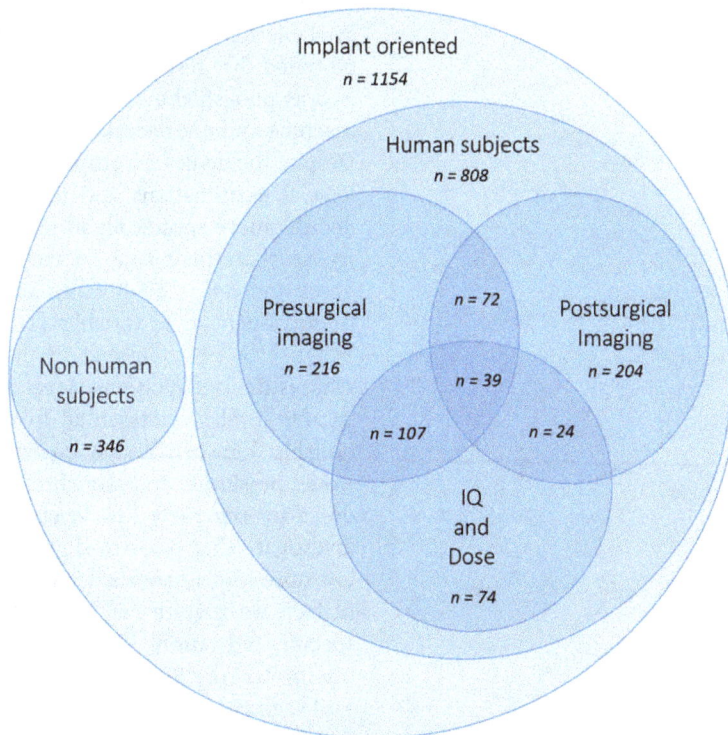

Fig. 2 Availability of peer-reviewed articles on the use of CBCT dentistry in implant dentistry, focused on studies performed on human subjects (PubMed output up till November 30 2016). The articles are then divided in three main areas of application: Presurgical and postsurgical imaging and image quality (IQ) and dose evaluation. A Venn diagram was used to highlight the intersections of these research areas

10. *What should we know about metal artefacts in CBCT?*
11. *How to export and transfer image data?*
12. *When to use CBCT postsurgically?*

These questions trace step by step the decision path that clinicians face in daily practice, see Fig. 3. All together, they represent a series of recommendations that try to integrate the evidence found in the literature with the needs of the clinician.

Results & Discussion
Why to use CBCT in implant dentistry?
The first CBCT device was introduced in the late nineties (NewTom 9000, QR, Verona) with the initial scientific reports dating back from 1998 [6]. The overall advantage of using CBCT in implant dentistry is related

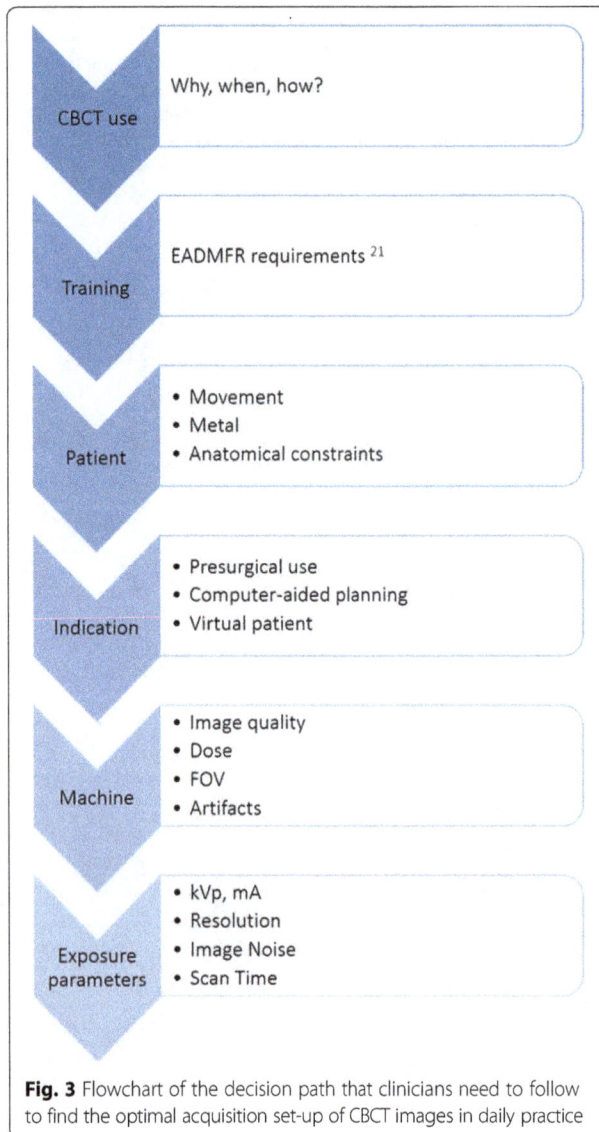

Fig. 3 Flowchart of the decision path that clinicians need to follow to find the optimal acquisition set-up of CBCT images in daily practice

to its ability to acquire detailed volumetric image data of the maxillofacial region for diagnostic and presurgical planning purposes. Yet, the accessibility of dental CBCT, due to its compact size, reasonable dose, low cost and ease-of-use is probably the prime contributor to its growing success. Since its introduction, the market has been exponentially growing with more than 85 distinct CBCT models readily available. This also includes hybrid or so-called multimodal systems for combined 2D (panoramic and/or cephalometric) and 3D (CBCT) imaging apart from less expensive and primary panoramic machines with a small detector size for scanning narrow field-of-views with a 3D button. CBCT machines are used for diagnostic indications, yet also for presurgical planning and transfer to implant surgery and rehabilitation [1, 5]. The growing interest in dental CBCT use went hand in hand with the growing market for third party software for 3D surgical planning and guidance [2–4]. This is evidenced in Fig. 6, where it becomes obvious that since the introduction of CBCT, there has been a significant increase in publishing scientific papers in relation to dental applications, with roughly a fourth of these studies on CBCT in implant dentistry, following the same upward tendency. Unfortunately, and disregarding the positive trend in publications, a direct consequence of this CBCT revolution and the exponential rise in equipment remains the creation of a clinically significant gap between the existing scientific literature and available hardware and software [7]. It should therefore be stated that research findings cannot simply be generalised as published evidence may often refer to one CBCT machine and not necessarily apply to other equipment [5]. Despite the dedicated properties of CBCT for dentomaxillofacial examinations and its growing use over the last decade, more specifically in implant dentistry, one should realise that there is a enormous variation in radiation doses and image quality and attributed to machine- and protocol-dependent variables [1, 5, 8].

What is the radiation dose level of dental CBCT?
At this level, it is essential to recognise the close relationship between image quality and radiation dose. It would be simple and straightforward to reduce radiation doses to extremely low levels, but one has to properly investigate that prior to doing so. Indeed, such extreme low dose levels may render images diagnostically useless. In fact, we require diagnostically adequate images for a specific indication. This has evolved in adapting the traditional ALARA principle toward ALADAIP (As Low as Diagnostically Acceptable being Indication-oriented and Patient-specific), as position statement of the Dimitra Research Group [9].

Effective radiation doses for CBCT should be typically far below the levels of spiral CT, thus being considered as a true advantage. It should preferably be an equivalent of 2 to maximally 10 panoramic radiographs (20–100 μSv) [1, 5, 8]. Unfortunately, commercially available CBCT systems seem to vary enormously. Radiation dose levels differ according to the CBCT device being assessed, from around 10 μSv to 1000 μSv (which is an equivalent of 2–200 panoramic radiographs) (Fig. 4). It is noteworthy that even one CBCT may present with a huge range in parameter settings, likewise creating an enormous variation in dose and image quality output [1, 5, 8].

Low dose protocols have been recommended to assist practitioners in optimisation [7, 8]. This has been picked up by manufacturers of CBCT equipment, who introduced low-dose protocols that might even get into the dose ranges of panoramic images. Nevertheless, there is still a need to design studies defining the required image quality in relation to implant dentistry, meanwhile fully balancing the radiation dose output of such image quality requirements [9]. Furthermore, medical imaging is constantly on the move, and thus it should be realised that the dose advantage frequently cited for CBCT compared with mulitslice CT is relative. Depending on the CT generation and the applied exposure protocol, radiation levels for multislice CTs may even be lower than for CBCT scans [8, 10]. This progress in dose optimisation for 2D and 3D technologies demonstrates clearly that radiation dose and related risks are dynamic entities, that need to be frequently monitored and reconsidered.

Furthermore, radiation dose levels should be regarded as indication-oriented and patient-specific. Only when respecting the strategy of time-dependent monitoring of indication-oriented and patient-specific radiation doses, a dental practitioner may really comply to ALADIP principles for optimisation and radiation protection in daily practice (Fig. 5) [9].

Which parameters influence image quality in CBCT?

Image quality performance of CBCT devices may vary widely, similar to, but not only related to exposure protocols and radiation dose ranges [1, 7, 8]. CBCT images are usually considered offering a high spatial resolution with voxel sizes of reconstructed CBCT datasets ranging between 0.08 and 0.4 mm [1]. Small voxel sizes could be diagnostically useful for cases in which small structures such as root canals and periodontal tissues need to be depicted. Variation is also observed when it comes to segmentation accuracy. The latter is a crucial factor when going for an integrated virtual planning including jaw bone models, fabrication of radiographic and surgical guides as well as further prosthetic models. Depending on the CBCT and the parameter settings, a 200 μm accuracy level should be feasible [1, 5]. However, larger inaccuracies may apply (up to 1000 μm and above) [1, 5]. Multi-slice CT often has a better contrast resolution, aiding segmentation and bringing error rates down as compared to CBCT.

Another shortcoming of CBCT is the lack of diagnostically distinct soft tissue contrast, narrowing down the diagnostic potential and hampering applications for soft tissue integration in the presurgical planning. Furthermore, Hounsfield units do not apply to CBCT images, yielding it impossible to compare grey values among or within patients over time [11]. This lack of standardized grey value distribution is complicating the use of CBCT for clinical bone density assessment and follow-up of bone density changes. Hounsfield units (HU) have been designed for medical CT, but do not apply for CBCT [11]. Compared to HU units for medical CT, the reliability of CBCT-based jaw bone density assessment has been found unreliable over time and with significant variations influenced by CBCT devices, imaging parameters and positioning [11]. This lack of HU standardization is a major

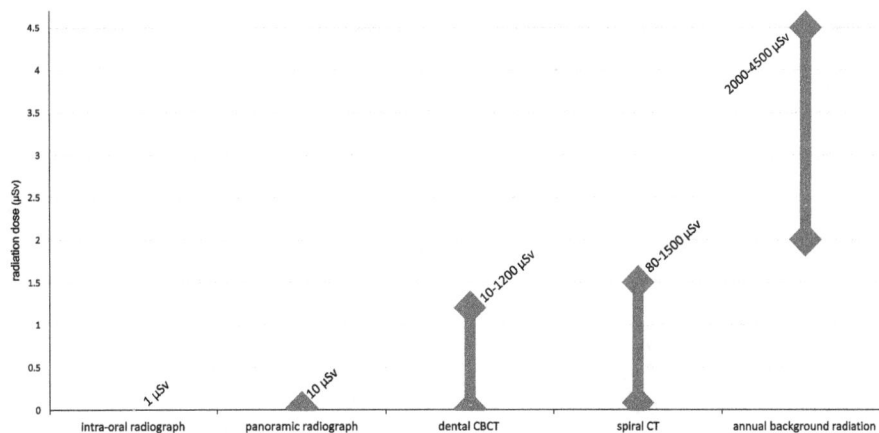

Fig. 4 Variation in radiation doses of dental CBCT in relation to dose ranges of other orofacial imaging modalities and natural background radiation

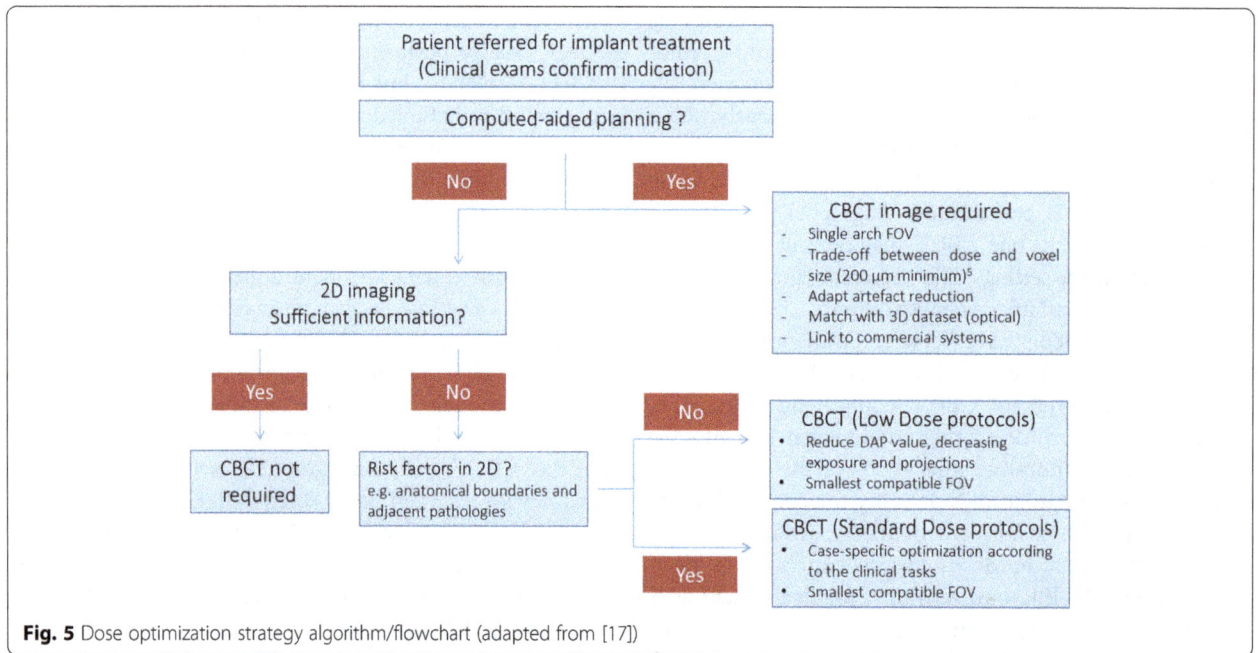

Fig. 5 Dose optimization strategy algorithm/flowchart (adapted from [17])

problem for most CBCT devices. Hitherto, one may question the relevance of this problem when it comes to actual implant dentistry, considering that nowadays a healthy vascularized bone may be more beneficial for implant placement than a sclerotic dense and poorly vascularized bone. What one might thus need instead is a structural bone analysis, like that available in dedicated μCT software. Such structural analysis has already been validated to be used for CBCT imaging, and thus might even have clinical potential for presurgical assessment of bone quality [12]. Also, CBCT images are generally hampered by varying degrees of artefacts expression, mostly deriving from patient motion and from dense restorative materials or a combination of both [1, 8, 13–15].

When to use CBCT in implant dentistry: existing guidelines?

Guidelines are either consensus-based or derived from a limited methodological approach [8]. One recent systematic review on CBCT guidelines for use in implant dentistry presents an overview of all published guidelines including indications and limitations of CBCT use in implant dentistry [8]. Crucial and still valid are the set of 20 basic principles published in 2009 by the European Academy of Dental and Maxillofacial Radiology (EADMFR) [16]. The set of principles was formulated to act as core standards, useful for reference and adoption to national procedures within European countries and elsewhere. While statements one to eight relate principally to CBCT justification, statements nine to fifteen broadly deal with dose optimisation in relation to image requirements. The last four statements discuss the need for adequate

training and competence levels for CBCT use. For diagnostic viewing, a distinction is made between diagnosis in the area of teeth and jaw bones and larger or other anatomical areas. Teeth and jaws may be diagnosed by general practitioners who received adequate training, while specialist training is required for evaluation of larger or other anatomical areas [7, 16].

A more recent publication [17] is based on the sedentexCT guidelines [7] with a further elaboration on the principles for justification and optimization strategies for CBCT use, when dealing with oral implant placement. This document represents the current EAO guidelines for the use of diagnostic imaging in implant dentistry based on a consensus workshop organized by the European Association for Osseointegration in 2011 [17], and contains a revision of the initial EAO guidelines from 2002 [18]. Likewise, a position paper with specific reference to oral implant placement and the potential use of CBCT prepared by the American Academy of Oral and Maxillofacial Radiology was published around the same time [19], being also a revision of the 2000 AAOMR guidelines [20]. Once more, the main reason for both revisions is to be found in the growing role that CBCT started to play over the last decade, particularly in implant dentistry. The main difference in these guidelines is probably the fact that EAO is stressing the needs for adequate and specialist training in relation to the use of CBCT in dental practice, even if simply referring the patient for CBCT. This issue was already eleborated in an additional two documents, namely the sedentexCT guidelines [7] and the EADMFR position paper on training requirements for CBCT use [21].

How to apply CBCT guidelines for the individual patient?

In general, when benefits outweigh the risks, CBCT is justified [8, 17]. Since the appearance of dental CBCT, there has been an exponential growth in scientific publications in relation to dental applications, with a fourth of the studies on CBCT in implant dentistry, following the same growth tendency (see Fig. 6). This trend and proportional use of CBCT in implant-related research is matching well with the clinical indications for CBCT use in private practice. Roughly, every fourth article published on CBCT is related to the use of CBCT in implant dentistry, with two out of three on the presurgical use of CBCT, primarily for presurgical planning and transfer to implant placement (Fig. 1). The justification for CBCT use during the preoperative planning phase is based on the need for specific anatomic considerations (identification of anatomic boundaries and morphology, proximity of vital anatomic structures; Fig. 7), esthetic challenges in the anterior maxilla, insufficient bone volume, shape and quality, the use of more advanced surgical techniques (grafting, distraction, zygomatic implants) and the integrated presurgical planning and virtual patient approach (Table 2) [2, 4, 5, 8, 17, 19, 22, 23].

One of the most frequent applications of presurgical use of CBCT is the computer-aided planning and transfer for oral implant placement. This approach inevitably requires 3D datasets for further planning in a dedicated software and potential transfer to the surgical field [2, 4, 5, 8, 17, 19, 22, 23]. The advantage of such a digital planning is expected to be an integrated approach of biomechanical, functional, and esthetic aspects to strive for a more predictable outcome, meanwhile avoiding complications [2–4]. Most often, such planning and transfer is realised based on surgical planning and related static drill guides. Fewer surgeons use a dynamic transfer of the planning via a navigaton system. Whilst the latter may be considered somewhat more time-efficient during the presurgical phase, with an additional advantage of real-time visualisation and thus some potential added intra-operative degrees of freedom, its widespread use in clinical practice might be self-limiting. This is mainly related to the complex set-up during surgery, the need for an additional and sophisticated peroperative tracking system, requiring calibration of the surgical field and recalibration upon jaw motion, while being restricted by the mouth opening (surely for posterior implants), with additional bounds to accessibility of the surgical field caused by the added appliances of the tracking system [3]. A meta-analysis on the accuracy of computer-aided implant planning and transfer revealed implant placement with a mean error of 1 mm (up till 6.5 mm) at entry and 1.2 mm (up till 7 mm) apically with an average angular deviation of 3.8° (up to 25°). Less deviation was found when using static surgical guidance, preferrably with a single surgical template and more fixation pins. Overall, computer-guided implant placement can be considered accurate, if carefully performed. Errors during CBCT imaging, planning and surgical transfer may however lead to significant and clinically unacceptable deviations [3].

Postoperative use of CBCT in implant dentistry represents a minority of the applications (see Fig. 1) and will be discussed later.

How to optimize scanning during presurgical use of CBCT?

CBCT images are composed of isotropic and high resolution voxels (from 0.08 to 0.4 mm depending on device and acquisition parameters), providing the essential prerequisites for image resolution and high signal to noise ratio for presurgical planning of implant placement [5].

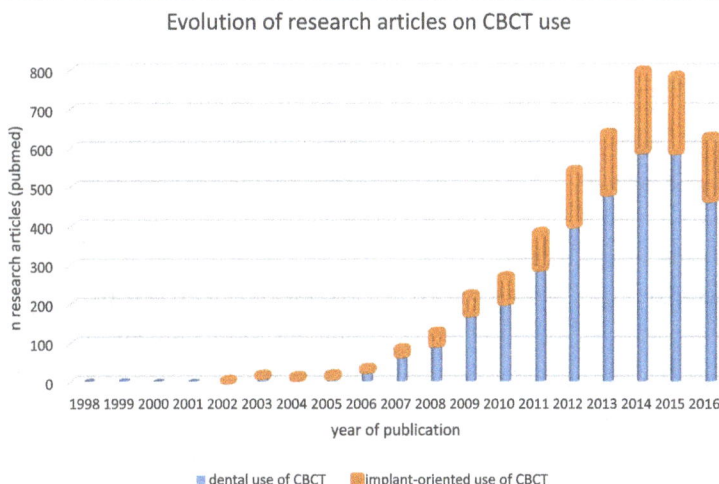

Fig. 6 Exponential growth in publishing scientific papers in relation to dental applications, since its first appearance in 1998, with a fourth of the studies on CBCT in implant dentistry, following the same growth tendency (pubmed output up to 2016)

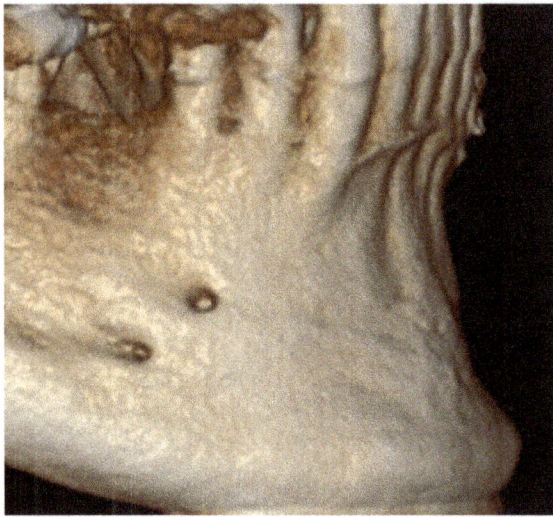

Fig. 7 Double mental foramen visible via volumetric imaging of the jaw bone, presenting a risk for nerve damage, if left undetected

However, small voxel sizes may cause a reduction in contrast-to-noise ratio, meanwhile requiring higher radiation exposure levels to the patient [1, 13]. This implies a need for optimization, by balancing patient-specific requirements with indication-oriented settings and machine-dependent parameters (ALADA). Yet, the lack of standardization among CBCT systems leads to a wide difference in acquisition parameters and performances among different devices, making it extremely difficult to generalize research finding and standardize imaging requirements for computer aided surgical planning [1].

Considering that there may still be room for optimization (See Fig. 5), this paragraph lists some clinical tips and tricks optimizing CBCT scanning for presurgical planning rendering its transfer to surgery more predictable. CBCT imaging should always be carried out while maintaining the correct balance between cost and radiation

Table 2 Presurgical use of CBCT: indications described in guidelines and other scientific reports

Indications for presurgical use of CBCT in literature
Identification of critical anatomic boundaries [8, 17, 19]
Prevention of neurovascular trauma [8, 17, 19]
Specific challenges for the anterior esthetic zones [8, 17, 19]
Borderline cases related to inadequate bone morphology, volume and quality [8, 17, 19]
Augmentation procedures [8, 17, 19]
Special techniques (grafting, distraction, zygoma implants) [8, 17, 19, 22]
Suspected trauma history of jaws and teeth [8, 17, 19]
Doubtful prognosis of neighboring teeth [5, 8, 17]
Presurgical planning and transfer [2, 4, 5, 8, 17, 19, 22, 23]
The virtual patient [23]

dose on one hand and required clinical information on the other hand. Protocols should be patient-specific and indication-oriented [1, 5, 8, 9, 16, 17]. This strategy is heavily influencing the radiation dose output as no machine is producing one standard dose for all patients and all indications. Depending on patient age and anatomy as well as the requirements for the specific diagnostic tasks, the field of view should be individualized, the required resolution adapted and the patient conditions carefully observed.

A stressed or easily moving patient might be advised closing the eyes to avoid motion artefacts. The presence of restorations, implants, metal posts and endodontic obturations may significantly hamper the image quality and thus the segmentation procedure during model making for presurgical planning and transfer. The negative impact of artefacts on segmentation may be reduced by adjusting the field of view during scout viewing prior to actual CBCT scanning to avoid image acquisition of metal-containing diagnostically unuseful areas (e.g. by deselecting the clinical crown level; by removing a prosthetic structure not rigidly fixed in the mouth; by strictly limiting the field of view area to the jaw bone involved). Further reference to the factors causing metal artefacts and their clinical applications are listed below in a separate paragraph.

For surgical guide fabrication, scanning at 200 μm resolution may be sufficient [1, 5]. Selecting a higher resolution scan may lead to more noise and sometimes even more scattering hampering the segmentation process of the anatomic jaw bone and the registration of a 3D impression scan on top of the 3D jaw model. During CBCT scanning with a radiographic scanning template, it is required to check for perfect fit at the occlusal level or on the soft tissues of edentulous jaws. Scanning templates should not be fabricated from a high-density material and/or not be too thick. The same applies for the occlusal splints which may be very useful separating upper and lower jaw models when there is a need for distinct jaw bone segmentation. Cotton wools are easy-to-use solutions for keeping lips and cheeks away from the gingiva when there is a need for assessing gingival thickness at the vestibular bone site [24].

Presurgical planning and transfer is often a multistep approach, with each step contributing to the resulting discrepancy between the original presurgical planning and the final outcome result following implant placement. When opting for such a procedure, it is necessary to take into consideration the proper time for optimised CBCT image acquisition, diagnostic interpretation, data manipulation, volume segmentation, registration or fusion of distinct 3D datasets, integrated planning and further accurate transfer to enable a predictable outcome, meanwhile avoiding complications. There is an urgent call for simplification of this complex and lengthy procedure, involving less steps as this may lower the threshold for clinicians to opt for such a digital approach, meanwhile decreasing the number of potential errors inherent to each of these individual steps [25].

How to use dental CBCT beyond radiodiagnostics?

Apart from its radiodiagnostic potential, dental CBCT may present a further treatment potential, such as the potential for surgical guides and prosthetic rehabilitation via CAD/CAM procedures [23, 26–31]. The large variations within CBCT units may lead to variable degrees of linear, diagnostic and 3D model accuracy, which are all needed to refine diagnostic tasks, surgical planning and CAD/CAM transfer. Nowadays, studies are focusing on overcoming technological shortcomings by assessing optimisation of exposure protocols or by registration of CBCT scans with optical datasets to eliminate the drawback of CBCT-derived metal artefacts [26, 30]. These optical datasets are derived from 3D optical cameras, which may offer the possibility to avoid traditional impression-taking. This may help to eliminate the necessity of intra-oral impression materials and subsequent fabrication of dental casts, meanwhile reducing time and handling errors inherent to these procedures. The available intraoral 3D scanners may offer excellent accuracy (up to 10 times better than CBCT), while being more comfortable for the patient than conventional impression-taking and far more efficient for the daily workflow [23, 26, 30]. By image-fusion with basic CBCT data, a digital cast with an accurate surface would thus enable further treatment using integrated 3D dataset for patient-specific CAD/CAM procedures [23, 30, 31].

This semi-automation may eliminate manual steps and inevitable human errors when producing dental restorations [32–34]. Continuous developments may evolve to further simplification and automation, with less chair-side time and fewer recall visits for the patient at an expense of more computer time for the practitioner. This may then result in virtual model creation to allow for patient-specific customization of oral implant rehabilitation [29].

Meanwhile, it should also be mentioned that integrated 3D facial scanning has become available for various CBCT units. The latter implies a concomitant 3D laser acquisition of facial soft tissues during CBCT scanning. This may then allow for a fully integrated planning with the 3D facial tissue scan registered onto the bony skull image, which may contribute to enhancing planning efficiency and prediction of the treatment outcome [28, 32, 35]. It may also create opportunities for surgical case follow-up, free of ionising radiation.

What are the requirements for creating a virtual patient?

The aforementioned evolution towards the concept of a virtual patient for dental implant surgery, creates new challenges for appropriate CBCT scanning. The virtual patient is a digital record that is used to plan the ideal implant position with respect to aesthetic, prosthetic and surgical requirements. It integrates information (datasets) obtained from facial scanning technology, digital intra-oral impressions and CBCT imaging in one virtual coordinate system [23, 28, 31, 32]. The virtual teeth arrangement is planned with regards to aesthetic and prosthetic functional requirements so that the ideal prospective implant position can be identified [29, 33]. Subsequently, a surgical guide is fabricated for fully guided implant insertion, and the treatment can then proceed with creating the provisional and final prosthesis using the same pre-operatively planned prosthetic setup [29, 30, 32, 33]. There are several imaging requirements to achieve this functional prosthetically oriented surgical goal, which are related to the accuracy of each scanning modality as well as to the fidelity of the image integration procedure.

Three-dimensional (3D) facial scanning provides information regarding the external soft tissue profile in three dimensions, and it can be of tremendous aid during the 3D digital smile design phase of the treatment [28]. In prosthodontics, facial scanning needs to provide high resolution 3D mesh data and photorealistic texture rendering in order to permit a virtual clinical evaluation phase. Several facial scans in neutral head position, maximum smile and using cheek retractors need to be obtained and merged together and the labial surfaces of the anterior teeth should be clearly depicted to allow registration with the digital dental model scans [28, 33, 35, 36]. In order to integrate facial scanning with CBCT, the forehead region needs to be clearly visible in both scans. This approach has been previously validated and the accuracy was found within clinically acceptable limits [35]. Recent studies demonstrated the applicability of the virtual patient approach to preoperatively plan the surgical placement of dental implants and to CAD-CAM design and fabricate screw retained prosthesis in partially and completely edentulous patients [31, 35, 36].

Several factors influence the accuracy of guided surgery systems related to CBCT image accuracy such as type of tissue support, flap approach, free or full guided implant insertion [36–40]. In partially edentulous cases, the surgical guide is fitted onto the teeth (tooth-supported). The imaging requirements of CBCT in these cases include high fidelity depiction of the dental arches including both teeth and alveolar process. However, CBCT limited spatial and contrast resolution impede accurate 3D reconstruction of the teeth to allow for the fabrication of a surgical guide [3, 27]. Therefore, CBCT 3D models are integrated with digital teeth models obtained using digital intraoral impressions at a spatial resolution of around 50 μm [39]. Recent research in this area demonstrated that this approach is valid and can be applied in the daily routine although the accuracy of CBCT 3D models of the teeth remains largely influenced by scan field of view and resolution in addition to the presence of artefacts originating from metal or zirconia structures [41]. The presence of pre-existing metal or zirconia prosthetic work largely deteriorates the visibility of the teeth on CBCT scans, thereby impeding accurate integration (registration) with teeth models obtained from digital intraoral impression. A significant negative influence of metal artefacts on the 3D teeth visibility in CBCT, and therefore on the overall accuracy of guided surgery planning was recently reported [40, 42]. As has been previously suggested in orthognathic surgery literature, a workaround to solve this imaging requirement is to artificially install landmarks in a radiographic template or directly on the gingiva to act as a common fiducial reference for the registration procedure [43]. Currently, radiographic templates could also be CAD designed using the information obtained from intraoral scanning and can be 3D milled or printed thereby eliminating the need for a conventional impression [44].

In complete edentulism, the situation is drastically different due to the absence of teeth as a fixed common reference. Typically, a radiographic template containing the ideal prosthetic setup would be CBCT scanned together with the patient and the resulting surgical guide would be either bone or gingiva supported. Beside the general requirements for CBCT image quality to visualize vital anatomical structures, the scan data should also be able to provide good visibility for the radiopaque fiducial markers in the radiographic template and preferably, the outer contour of the gingiva should also be made visible to facilitate accurate implant planning [45]. Perhaps the most promising development in recent years is the mini-implants supported surgical guide placement in completely edentulous patients. Using this approach, the guide is screw retained on mini-implants thereby eliminating the inaccuracies incurred from bony and gingival support [46]. In addition, the mini-implants can be used to fabricate a radiographic template, which can also be employed for creating a virtual teeth try-in. However, studies on this approach are still lacking.

Another important element in the surgical implant virtual patient approach is the virtual articulator, which is used to simulate the dynamics of the patient's jaw movement during chewing, swallowing, breathing, bruxing and speech. Several techniques are currently available to virtually mount the upper cast in the correct coordinate system with reference to the skull base using the kinematic or hinge axis of the temporomandibular joint (TMJ) as a neutral zero position [47, 48]. An important requirement here is the Euclidean dimensional correspondence between the starting point of the jaw motion tracing device and the virtual articulator. More development on this front is necessary. Towards the future, reconstructions from MRI might potentially get integrated in the virtual patient model, which could be particularly interesting for dynamic TMJ evaluation.

What are the requirements for 3D model making?

The accuracy of templates strictly depends on virtual 3D model accuracy. Poor image resolution may result in insufficient image quality. The latter is the main cause of 3D model inaccuracy, since it amplifies the effects of all image processing approximations [49].

As for teeth, occlusal surfaces require a five to tenfold better image resolution than the lowest voxel size levels of CBCT. On top of that, tooth restorations may increase the inaccuracy level by artefact formation. To overcome this limit, recent studies try to compensate the lack of information on teeth morphology by fusing the CBCT surface model with a digitalized dental model acquired with optical systems [26–28, 30].

Surface accuracy is also related to the Field of View (FOV) used during the acquisition step. Different studies concluded that images acquired with medium and small FOV allow to obtain more accurate models compared to those acquired with a large FOV [50, 51]. Nevertheless, small FOVs show more pronounced artefacts and wider grey level variability compared to larger FOV scans [50]. Model accuracy is also depending on the segmentation process. Currently, in dentomaxillofacial applications, segmentation is mainly performed by expert operators using manual thresholding [50, 52]. This approach is very subjective and strictly related to operator experience. In addition, anatomical structural variations in the craniofacial region require to develop specific segmentation approaches [50, 53, 54]. To reduce operator dependency and improve segmentation accuracy, some fully or semi-automatic segmentation approaches were developed [52, 55].

In conclusion, image segmentation, can deeply affect 3D model accuracy, even if generated from high-resolution image data. For this reason, surgeons that use virtual planning must have a deep knowledge of the imaging techniques involved in the presurgical work-up [49]. Only adequate training will allow them to set the optimal acquisition parameters and post-processing steps to improve model accuracy and consequently patient treatment.

What should we know about metal artefacts in CBCT?

CBCT images are often corrupted by artefacts, which are defined as visualized structures in the reconstructed data that are not present in the scanned object [41]. In particular, the presence of dense materials, such as metals, causes different kind of artefacts in CBCT images. Among these the most common are: beam hardening, extinction and exponential edge gradient effect artieacts [56].

The presence of these artefacts affects image quality in several ways, ranging from bright streaks radiating from the metallic object, dark areas near it to the complete loss of information between adjacent dense objects [13, 14]. This group of artefacts represents the so called "metal artefacts".

The presence of such artefacts in CBCT compromises diagnosis and surgical planning. Material density and exposure parameters play a key role in artefact expression. Pauwels et al. quantified the impact of different CBCT devices and exposure protocols on the expression of metal artefact induced by titanium implants, with an advice to develop optimized exposure protocols adequate for metal artefact reduction [14]. Material density, design and composition yield a variable radio-opacity, with a strong effect on the amount of artefacts, due to the inability of the X-ray beam to pass through the imaged object and the consequent insufficient number of photons that reach the detector [41]. Based on the increased material density as compared to titanium, zirconium dioxide implants might thus generate stronger artefacts as compared to other materials.

Due to the clinical relevance of this matter, several efforts were made to reduce metal artefacts in CBCT images. A recent study conducted by Kuusisto et al. demonstrated that composite materials give less artefacts, finding the cut-off point of artefacts at 20% radio-opaque filling material in composite implants [56].

Another approach to reduce metal artefact is to implement specific metal artefact reduction (MAR) algorithms, which allow improving image quality. These correction algorithms can be classified in three different groups: interpolation-based methods, iterative reconstruction approaches and adaptive filtering algorithms [57]. In the last years, specific MAR algorithms for CBCT images were developed [45, 46, 57–61], and now MAR solutions are available in most of the commercial devices. Bechara et al. evaluated the performance of some MAR commercial solutions measuring image quality parameter such as contrast-to-noise ratio and the gray value variation concluding that the tested MAR solution were able to improve image quality [62, 63].

However, only a few studies evaluate the clinical applicability of these artefact reduction methods. The presence of metal artefacts can affect the visualisation of the periimplant bone. This may lead to a biased and/or erroneous diagnosis and therefore also to inappropriate treatment decisions [64].

Unfortunately, as mentioned before, the lack of standardization among CBCT device settings makes it difficult to generalize these findings. Nevertheless, it seems that right now MAR solution do not add diagnostic information, even if image quality parameters are improved.

How to export and transfer image data?

DICOM (Digital Imaging and Communication in Medicine) was originally developed to create a worldwide norm for digital image acquisition, storage, and display in medicine, and also to have a standardized method for transmission of medical images and related information on patient and technical image parameters. "Digitization" is increasingly widespread in dental medicine in terms of radiographic image acquisition (2D and 3D), optical surface scanning (intra- and extraoral), CAD/CAM systems, and the electronic charting of patient records. Unfortunately, the DICOM standard is not really fully implemented in oral health care, with primarily hospital and dental school settings complying with the standard [65].

Picture archiving and communication systems (PACS) software act to integrate image acquisition, storage, retrieval, and viewing based on the DICOM standard. In dentistry, the use of PACS is often limited to hospital facilities, larger dental clinics and academic centers [66]. Newer standard dental digital imaging devices including intraoral digital radiographic systems, panoramic views, and CBCT scanners in large part are mostly DICOM compliant. Nevertheless, standards for DICOM compliance for some devices including CBCT and CAD/CAM systems and their interoperability with respect to PACS have not yet been fully established. To facilitate standard communication, accurate image data exchange and 3D data integration into a virtual model, radiographic devices and third-party dental implant software applications should be forced to offer fully compliant DICOM data export [8, 67]. The huge data volume of CBCT DICOM images requires high storage capacity. To save storage space, DICOM viewers usually compress DICOM imges into smaller files during file export [68]. This compression is done using specialized algorithms and can be performed using both lossy or lossless methods [69]. Lossy compression permanently eliminates redundant information, but can result in eccessive image degradation [68]. In order to avoid loss of information, it is advised to use the original data or data compressed with lossless compression algorithms when transferring information to a third-part software. Unfortunately, in literature there is a lack of studies validating the process of image conversion from a proprietary format into DICOM format. Further studies are needed to quantify the amount of information lost during DICOM export, in order to make clinicians aware of this source of error, on top of all other possible sources of inaccuracy during computer aided surgical planning. It is clear that for most CBCT systems there is a diagnostic data loss upon DICOM export and potentially even a further loss when imported into a PACS system or third party software. Indeed, most third party softwares have some additional filtering (e.g. smoothening) at the import phase, which may result in additional information loss. It is therefore recommended to do presurgical diagnostics in the dedicated CBCT-software of the imaging device, prior to export for presurgical planning purposes.

Other challenges in the digital data flow include the fact that there is a growing availability of non-DICOM 3D imaging data formats required to be used for an integrated virtual patient dataset [23, 28, 38, 39]. Examples include STL and OBJ formats, respectively, used for digital intraoral impressions and printing as well as for facial scanning. Transferring those datasets to PACS systems is actually not possible, as such that the power of the integrated virtual patient information is lost at this level.

When to use CBCT postsurgically?

Postoperatively, CBCT is used for evaluation of graft healing, to assess complications mostly related to neurovascular trauma and when implant retrieval is anticipated, as shown in Table 3 [5, 8, 17]. More than a fifth of the articles (22%) dealing with postsurgical CBCT scanning are related to postsurgical complications (see Fig. 1). While implant placement accounts for only 3% of cases with neurosensory disturbances, when focusing on cases with a permanent neurosensory deficit, implant placement is responsible for a four-fold number of cases (12% of all iatrogenic permanent trigeminal injuries) [70] (see Fig. 8). Besides, implant surgery carries a risk to cause severe intraoral hemorrhage. For mandibular implant placement specifically, multiple reports have been documenting life-threatening upper airway obstruction after postoperative bleeding in the mouth floor [71]. According to a recent study of Yilmaz et al. [72], an inadequate radiological assessment is the most common reason for postsurgical neural injury. This finding supports the need for proper training on CBCT use and its

diagnostic interpretation, even when being a simple referrer for CBCT imaging [21].

For mere follow-up of implant placement, CBCT seems not be the ideal diagnostic tool. Up till now two-dimensional intra-oral radiographs are still considered the prime tool when there is a clinical need for postsurgical implant monitoring [73]. In contrast to continuously moving concepts and revolutionary changes in implant dentistry, no consensus conference has ever questioned the 2D intra-oral peri-implant bone level measures [8, 17]. Yet, considering that we are nowadays more and more focussed on bone grafting for defect fill up and sinus augmentation, vestibular bone in the esthetic zone, severe peri-implant bone loss (e.g. peri-implantitis), alternative implant and abutment designs, we should question the traditional two-dimensional imaging diagnostics. Realising that we need to evaluate three-dimensional bone healing, including morphological, volumetric and trabecular remodelling, one could wonder what could be observed and diagnosed by merely looking to 2D approximal peri-implant bone. We should admit that marginal bone levels only reflect a few μm of observation along a peri-implant circumference between 6 and 13 mm long. The only way to fully grasp the peri-implant tissues, is indeed to obtain a true 3D view of the clinical situation, which brings us back to three-dimensional imaging of the peri-implant bone [74, 75]. It is hoped that towards the future, CBCT hardware and software may overcome the current limitations and as such to allow for clinically realistic peri-implant diagnostics.

Although the CBCT market has been rapidly growing, few companies seem to have paid enough attention to the huge problem of metal artefacts, surely when it comes to presurgical implant planning and peri-implant follow-up [13, 14, 40]. Artefacts are even worse with denser material and thus more pronounced with implants in zirconium than in titanium [76]. In general, such materials cause blooming of the implant with enlargements easily reaching a third of the implant diameter, apart from other artefacts such as streaks and black bands [76]. In areas where the thin vestibular bone plate needs to be observed, blooming artefacts may bias

Table 3 Postsurgical use of CBCT: indications described in guidelines and other scientific reports

Indications for postsurgical use of CBCT in literature	Needed 3D info	Drawback CBCT
Postsurgical complications (e.g. neurovascular trauma) [8, 17, 19]	Evaluate location and severity of problem and how to approach	Artefact by implant may mask neurovascular bundle CBCT fails to visualize neurovascular bundle
Healing follow-up of complex surgical procedures [8, 17, 19]	Check bone healing and volumetric outcome	Detrimental artefacts of implants in borderline case (pneumatised maxillary sinus with inadequate bone)
Maxillofacial trauma with suspected complications at the implant level [8, 17, 19, 22]	Check mechanical failure implant or superstructure	Diagnostic failure to spot trauma caused by metal artefacts
Retrieval of osseointegrated implants (infectious or mechanical failure etiology) [8, 17, 19]		Blooming of implant masking neurovascular structures

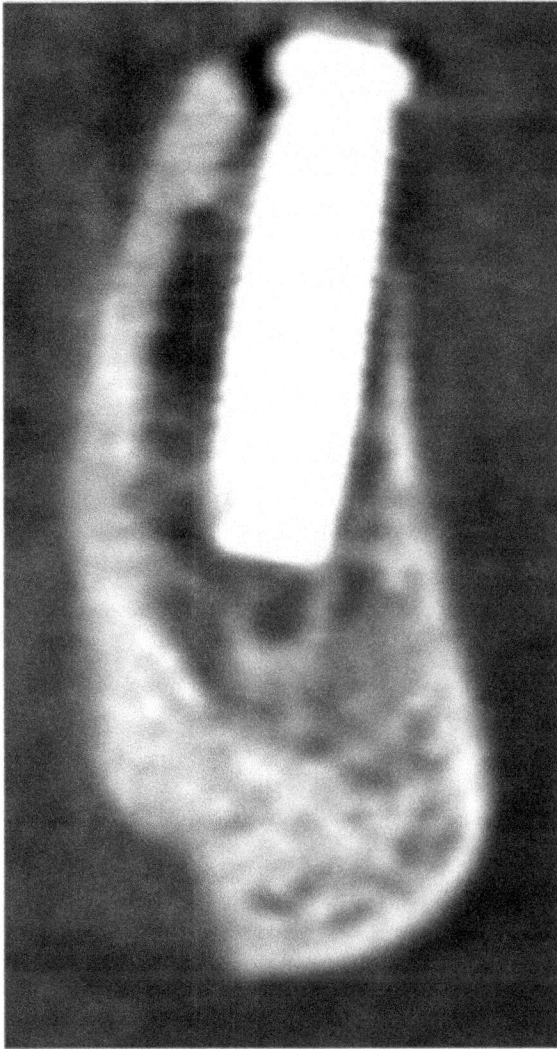

Fig. 8 Implant in the mandible showing some beam hardening artefact, and in addition a position at the roof of the incisive canal, causing neurosensory disturbances

diagnosis. Only a few CBCTs and specific protocols seem to allow a reasonably improved peri-implant depiction [76], but still with some patient-specificity. Another point of attention with CBCT use is the lack of standardised grey level calibration or hounsfield scoring, making the comparative follow-up of bone healing, grafting and implant placement rather difficult and quite unreliable [11]. Monitoring pathological changes or quantification of bony healing is possible, yet at the moment, not always possible considering artefact expression and often too complicated for widespread use in clinical practice. Thus and as for now, we need to remain with peri-implant 2D bone level measures using strictly paralleling intra-oral radiographs, even when realising that we may only visualise and measure a glimpse of the entire defect.

Conclusions

CBCT imaging is a well-established radiographic modality in treatment planning for dental implants, becoming increasingly popular and globally used in oral health care. This is partially due to new insights into anatomic landmarks, and structures at risk during implant placement such as neurovascular structures. Another reason for the growing use of CBCT scanning is the increasing popularity of computer-guided surgery that relies on digital planning based on high-quality CBCT images [38], but may also include the superimposition of intraoral scans and extraoral face scans to create a 3D virtual dental patient [36, 37]. The virtual patient concept is actually demonstrating again the need for standardisation of image data formats enabling a smooth integration of all available datasets (DICOM, STL, and OBJ files) into a craniofacial virtual reality model.

The use of CBCT imaging following insertion of dental implants should be restricted to specific postoperative complications (such as iatrogenic neurovascular trauma), required implant retrieval and follow-up of complex surgical procedures. While to fully grap the peri-implant tissues, is to obtain a three-dimensional view or the peri-implant tissues. And that brings us back to the clinical and the potential means for three-dimensional evaluation For long-term maintenance and follow-up of dental implants, we are still forced to remain with peri-implant bi-dimensional bone level measures on correctly taken periapical radiographs, even if had has no true prognostic value and considering that only the proverbial tip of the iceberg of the actual size and morphology of a defect seen.

The variation in CBCT performances related to radiation doses and image quality, emphasizes the need for more research to establish proper solutions for three-dimensional imaging following the ALADA principle, whilst focussing on artefact reduction caused by motion and metal. A further standardisation is needed for the grey level output as such to be able to assess bone healing, follow-up and evolution of pathological processes. Finally, lossless standard image communication as well as smooth and accurate integration of multiple image datasets, beyond the borders of CBCT, is another point of attention for future developments towards digital dentistry and the creation of an integrated virtual patient.

Acknowledgements
The authors acknowledge the Digital Dental Society (DDS) allowing the working group consisting of all authors of this manuscript to meet, discuss and strive to reach an expert consensus at the D20 Meeting of the Digital Dental Society (DDS) in Milan, Italy, 16th – 17th September 2016.

Funding
The authors declare that they have not received any funding to write this manuscript.

Authors' contributions

RJ wrote the overall manuscript, while MC, BS, BH and MB provided specific section information which was integrated in this manuscript. Articles were reviewed and manuscript content discussed amongst authors present during the D20 Consensus Meeting of the Digital Dentistry Society (September 2016, Milan, Italy). This allowed further optimizing the paper. Finally, all authors read and approved the final manuscript as such that the present work reflects an expert consensus with recommendations for clinical use.

Authors' information

Not applicable

Competing interests

Michael Bornstein is an associate editor for BMC Oral Health. Other authors declare that they have no competing interests.

Author details

[1]OMFS IMPATH Research Group, Department of Imaging and Pathology, Faculty of Medicine, University of Leuven, Kapucijnenvoer 33, 3000 Leuven, Belgium. [2]Department of Oral and Maxillofacial Surgery, University Hospitals Leuven, Leuven, Belgium. [3]Department of Dental Medicine (DENTMED), Karolinska Institutet, Stockholm, Sweden. [4]EA2496, Orofacial Pathologies, Imaging and Biotherapies Lab, Dental School Paris Descartes University, Sorbonne Paris Cité, Paris, France. [5]Department of Odontology, AP-HP, Nord Val de Seine Hospital (Bretonneau), Paris, France. [6]Unit of Radiology, IRCCS Policlinico San Donato, San Donato Milanese, Italy. [7]Department of Oral Function and Restorative Dentistry, Academic Centre for Dentistry Amsterdam (ACTA), Research Institute MOVE, 1081 LA Amsterdam, The Netherlands. [8]Applied Oral Sciences, Faculty of Dentistry, The University of Hong Kong, Hong Kong SAR, China.

References

1. Jacobs R. Dental cone beam CT and its justified use in oral health care. JBR-BTR. 2011;94:254–65.

2. Van Assche N, van Steenberghe D, Quirynen M, Jacobs R. Accuracy assessment of computer-assisted flapless implant placement in partial edentulism. J Clin Periodontol. 2010;37:398–403.

3. Van Assche N, Vercruyssen M, Coucke W, Teughels W, Jacobs R, Quirynen M. Accuracy of computer-aided implant placement. Clin Oral Implants Res. 2012;23:112–23.

4. Vercruyssen M, Laleman I, Jacobs R, Quirynen M. Computer-supported implant planning and guided surgery: a narrative review. Clin Oral Implants Res. 2015;26(Suppl):69–76.

5. Jacobs R, Quirynen M. Dental cone beam computed tomography: justification for use in planning oral implant placement. Periodontology 2000. 2014;66:203–13.

6. Mozzo P, Procacci C, Tacconi A, Martini PT, Andreis IA. A new volumetric CT machine for dental imaging based on the cone-beam technique: preliminary results. Eur Radiol. 1998;8:1558–64.

7. European Commission. Cone beam CT for dental and maxillofacial radiology (Evidence-based guidelines). Radiation Protection No 172 ISSN 1681-6803. http://sedentexct.eu/files/radiation_protection_172.pdf. Accessed 9 Oct 2016.

8. Bornstein MM, Scarfe WC, Vaughn VM, Jacobs R. Cone beam computed tomography in implant dentistry: a systematic review focusing on guidelines, indications, and radiation dose risks. Int J Oral Maxillofac Implants. 2014;29(Suppl):55–77.

9. Oenning AC, Jacobs R, Pauwels R, Stratis A, Hedesiu M, Salmon B, Dimitra Research Group. Cone-beam CT in paediatric dentistry: DIMITRA project position statement. Pediatr Radiol. 2018;48(3):308–16.

10. Widmann G, Bischel A, Stratis A, Kakar A, Bosmans H, Jacobs R, Gassner EM, Puelacher W, Pauwels R. Ultralow dose dentomaxillofacial CT imaging and iterative reconstruction techniques: variability of Hounsfield units and contrast-to-noise ratio. Br J Radiol. 2016;89:20151055.

11. Pauwels R, Jacobs R, Singer SR, Mupparapu M. CBCT-based bone quality assessment: are Hounsfield units applicable? Dentomaxillofac Radiol. 2015; 44:20140238.

12. Van Dessel J, Huang Y, Depypere M, Rubira-Bullen I, Maes F, Jacobs R. A comparative evaluation of cone beam CT and micro-CT on trabecular bone structures in the human mandible. Dentomaxillofac Radiol. 2013;42:20130145.

13. Pauwels R, Araki K, Siewerdsen JH, Thongvigitmanee SS. Technical aspects of dental CBCT: state of the art. Dentomaxillofac Radiol. 2015;44:20140224.

14. Pauwels R, Stamatakis H, Bosmans H, Bogaerts R, Jacobs R, Horner K, Tsiklakis K, SEDENTEXCT Project Consortium. Quantification of metal artefacts on cone beam computed tomography images. Clin Oral Implants Res. 2013;100(Suppl):94–9.

15. Pauwels R, Stamatakis H, Manousaridis G, Walker A, Michielsen K, Bosmans H, Bogaerts R, Jacobs R, Horner K, Tsiklakis K, SEDENTEXCT Project Consortium. Development and applicability of a quality control phantom for dental cone-beam CT. Appl Clin Med Phys. 2011;12:3478.

16. Horner K, Islam M, Flygare L, Tsiklakis K, Whaites E. Basic principles for use of dental cone beam computed tomography: consensus guidelines of the European academy of dental and maxillofacial radiology. Dentomaxillofac Radiol. 2009;38:187–95.

17. Harris D, Horner K, Gröndahl K, Jacobs R, Helmrot E, Benic GI, Bornstein MM, Dawood A, Quirynen M. Guidelines for the use of diagnostic imaging in implant dentistry 2011: update of the E.A.O. A consensus workshop organized by the European Association for Osseointegration in the Medical University of Warsaw, Poland. Clin Oral Implants Res. 2012;23:1243–53.

18. Harris D, Buser D, Dula K, Gröndahl K, Jacobs R, Lekholm U, Nakielny R, van Steenberghe D, van der Stelt P. E.A.O. Guidelines for the use of diagnostic imaging in implant dentistry. Clin Oral Impl Res. 2002;13:566–70.

19. Tyndall DA, Price JB, Tetradis S, Ganz SD, Hildebolt C, Scarfe WC, American Academy of Oral and Maxillofacial Radiology. Position statement of the American Academy of oral and maxillofacial radiology on selection criteria for the use of radiology in dental implantology with emphasis on cone beam computed tomography. Oral Surg Oral Med Oral Pathol Oral Radiol. 2012;113:817–26.

20. Tyndall DA, Brooks SL. Selection criteria for dental implant site imaging: a position paper of the American Academy of oral and maxillofacial radiology. Oral Surg Oral Med Oral Pathol Oral Radiol Endod. 2000;89:630–7.

21. Brown J, Jacobs R, Levring Jäghagen E, Lindh C, Baksi G, Schulze D, Schulze R, European Academy of DentoMaxilloFacial Radiology. Basic training requirements for the use of dental CBCT by dentists: a position paper prepared by the European Academy of DentoMaxilloFacial Radiology. Dentomaxillofac Radiol. 2014;43:20130291.

22. van Steenberghe D, Malevez C, Van Cleynenbreugel J, Bou Serhal C, Dhoore E, Schutyser F, Suetens P, Jacobs R. Accuracy of drilling guides for transfer from three-dimensional CT-based planning to placement of zygoma implants in human cadavers. Clin Oral Implants Res. 2003;14:131–6.

23. Joda T, Brägger U, Gallucci G. Systematic literature review of digital three-dimensional superimposition techniques to create virtual dental patients. Int J Oral Maxillofac Implants. 2015;30:330–7.

24. Ganz SD. Three-dimensional imaging and guided surgery for dental implants. Dent Clin N Am. 2015;59:265–90.

25. Hämmerle CH, Cordaro L, van Assche N, Benic GI, Bornstein M, Gamper F, Gotfredsen K, Harris D, Hürzeler M, Jacobs R, Kapos T, Kohal RJ, Patzelt SB, Sailer I, Tahmaseb A, Vercruyssen M, Wismeijer D. Digital technologies to support planning, treatment, and fabrication processes and outcome assessments in implant dentistry. Summary and consensus statements. The 4th EAO consensus conference 2015. Clin Oral Implants Res. 2015; 26(Suppl 11):97–101.

26. Flügge TV, Att W, Metzger MC, Nelson K. Precision of dental implant digitization using intraoral scanners. Int J Prosthodont. 2016;29:277–83.

27. Al-Rawi B, Hassan B, Vandenberge B, Jacobs R. Accuracy assessment of three-dimensional surface reconstructions of teeth from cone beam computed tomography scans. J Oral Rehabil. 2010;37:352–8.

28. Hassan B, Giménez Gonzalez B, Tahmaseb A, Jacobs R, Bornstein MM. Three-dimensional facial scanning technology: applications and future trends. Forum Implantol. 2014;10:78–86.

29. Flügge TV, Nelson K, Schmelzeisen R, Metzger MC. Three-dimensional plotting and printing of an implant drilling guide: simplifying guided implant surgery. J Oral Maxillofac Surg. 2013;71:1340–6.

30. Rangel FA, Maal TJJ, Bronkhorst EM, Breuning KH, Schols JGJH, Bergé SJ, Kuijpers-Jagtman AM. Accuracy and reliability of a novel method for fusion of digital dental casts and cone beam computed tomography scans. PLoS One. 2013;8:e59130.

31. Joda T, Zarone F, Ferrari M. The complete digital workflow in fixed prosthodontics: a systematic review. BMC Oral Health. 2017;17(1):124.

32. Ritter L, Reiz SD, Rothamel D, Dreiseidler T, Karapetian V, Scheer M, Zöller JE. Registration accuracy of three-dimensional surface and cone beam computed tomography data for virtual implant planning. Clin Oral Implants Res. 2012;23:447–52.

33. Scherer MD. Presurgical implant-site assessment and restoratively driven digital planning. Dent Clin N Am. 2014;58:561–95.

34. Mora MA, Chenin DL, Arce RM. Software tools and surgical guides in dental-implant-guided surgery. Dent Clin N Am. 2014;58:597–626.

35. Rosati R, De Menezes M, Rossetti A, Sforza C, Ferrario VF. Digital dental cast placement in 3-dimensional, full-face reconstruction: a technical evaluation. Am J Orthod Dentofac Orthop. 2010;138:84–8.

36. Naudi KB, Benramadan R, Brocklebank L, Ju X, Khambay B, Ayoub A. The virtual human face: superimposing the simultaneously captured 3D photorealistic skin surface of the face on the untextured skin image of the CBCT scan. Int J Oral Maxillofac Surg. 2013;42:393–400.

37. Raico Gallardo YN, da Silva-Olivio IR, Mukai E, Morimoto S, Sesma N, Cordaro L. Accuracy comparison of guided surgery for dental implants according to the tissue of support: a systematic review and meta- analysis. Clin Oral Implants Res. 2017;28:602–12.

38. Joda T, Gallucci GO. The virtual patient in dental medicine. Clin Oral Implants Res. 2015;26:725–6.

39. Hassan B, Gimenez Gonzalez B, Tahmaseb A, Greven M, Wismeijer D. A digital approach integrating facial scanning in a CAD/CAM workflow for full mouth implants supported rehabilitation of the edentulous patient: a pilot clinical study. J Prosthet Dent. 2017;117:486–92.

40. Tahmaseb A, Wismeijer D, Coucke W, Derksen W. Computer technology applications in surgical implant dentistry: a systematic review. Int J Oral Maxillofac Implants. 2014;29:25–42.

41. Schulze R, Heil U, Gross D, Bruellmann DD, Dranischnikow E, Schwanecke U, Schoemer E. Artefacts in CBCT: a review. Dentomaxillofac Radiol. 2011;40:265–73.

42. Flügge T, Derksen W, Te Poel J, Hassan B, Nelson K, Wismeijer D. Registration of cone beam computed tomography data and intraoral surface scans – a prerequisite for guided implant surgery with CAD/CAM drilling guides. Clin Oral Implants Res. 2017;28:1113–8.

43. Swennen GR, Barth EL, Eulzer C, Schutyser F. The use of a new 3D splint and double CT scan procedure to obtain an accurate anatomic virtual augmented model of the skull. Int J Oral Maxillofac Surg. 2007;36:146–52.

44. Pascual D, Vaysse J. Guided and computer-assisted implant surgery and prosthetics: the continuous digital workflow. Rev Stomatol Chir Maxillofac Chir Orale. 2016;117:28–35.

45. Ochi M, Kanazawa M, Sato D, Kasugai S, Hirano S, Minakuchi S. Factors affecting accuracy of implant placement with mucosa-supported stereolithographic surgical guides in edentulous mandibles. Comput Biol Med. 2013;43:1653–60.

46. Tahmaseb A, De Clerck R, Aartman I, Wismeijer D. Digital protocol for reference-based guided surgery and immediate loading: a prospective clinical study. Int J Oral Maxillofac Implants. 2012;27:1258–70.

47. Solaberrieta E, Mínguez R, Barrenetxea L, Ramon Otegi J, Szentpétery A. Comparison of the accuracy of a 3-dimensional virtual method and the conventional method for transferring the maxillary cast to a virtual articulator. J Prosthet Dent. 2015;113:191–7.

48. Lam WY, Hsung RT, Choi WW, Luk HW, Pow EH. A 2-part facebow for CAD-CAM dentistry. J Prosthet Dent. 2016;116:843–7.

49. Varga E, Hammer B, Hardy BM, Kamer L. The accuracy of three-dimensional model generation. What makes it accurate to be used for surgical planning? Int J Oral Maxillofac Surg. 2013;42:1159–66.

50. Hassan B, Souza PC, Jacobs R, de Azambuja BS, van der Stelt P. Influence of scanning and reconstruction parameters on quality of three-dimensional

51. Katsumata A, Hirukawa A, Okumura S, Naitoh M, Fujishita M, Ariji E, et al. Relationship between density variability and imaging volume size in cone-beam computerized tomographic scanning of the maxillofacial region: an in vitro study. Oral Surgery, Oral Med Oral Pathol Oral Radiol Endod. 2009;107:420–5.

52. Wang L, Chen KC, Gao Y, Shi F, Liao S, Li G, Yan J, Lee PK, Chow B, Liu NX, Xia JJ, Shen D. Automated bone segmentation from dental CBCT images using patch-based sparse representation and convex optimization. Med Phys. 2014;4:043503.

53. Engelbrecht WP, Fourie Z, Damstra J, Gerrits PO, Ren Y. The influence of the segmentation process on 3D measurements from cone beam computed tomography-derived surface models. Clin Oral Investig. 2013;17:1919–27.

54. Loubele M, Jacobs R, Maes F, Denis K, White S, Coudyzer W, et al. Image quality vs radiation dose of four cone beam computed tomography scanners. Dentomaxillofac Radiol. 2008;37:309–18.

55. Codari M, Caffini M, Tartaglia GM, Sforza C, Baselli G. Computer-aided cephalometric landmark annotation for CBCT data. Int J Comput Assist Radiol Surg. 2017;12:113–21.

56. Kuusisto N, Vallittu PK, Lassila LVJ, Huumonen S. Evaluation of intensity of artefacts in CBCT by radio-opacity of composite simulation models of implants in vitro. Dentomaxillofacial Radiol. 2015;44:20140157.

57. Prell D, Kyriakou Y, Beister M, Kalender WA. A novel forward projection-based metal artefact reduction method for flat-detector computed tomography. Phys Med Biol. 2009;54:6575–91.

58. Wang Q, Li L, Zhang L, Chen Z, Kang K. A novel metal artefact reducing method for cone-beam CT based on three approximately orthogonal projections. Phys Med Biol. 2013;58:1–17.

59. Meilinger M, Schmidgunst C, Schütz O, Lang EW. Metal artefact reduction in cone beam computed tomography using forward projected reconstruction information. Z Med Phys. 2011;21:174–82.

60. Kim J, Nam H, Lee R. Development of a new metal artefact reduction algorithm by using an edge preserving method for CBCT imaging. J Korean Phys Soc. 2015;67:180–8.

61. Tohnak S, Mehnert AJH, Mahoney M, Crozier S. Dental CT metal artefact reduction based on sequential substitution. Dentomaxillofacial Radiol. 2011;40:184–90.

62. Bechara B, McMahan CA, Geha H, Noujeim M. Evaluation of a cone beam CT artefact reduction algorithm. Dentomaxillofacial Radiol. 2012;41:422–8.

63. Bechara BB, Moore WS, McMahan C a, Noujeim M. Metal artefact reduction with cone beam CT: an in vitro study. Dentomaxillofac Radiol. 2012;41:248–53.

64. de-Azevedo-Vaz SL, Peyneau PD, Ramirez-Sotelo LR, Vasconcelos Kde F, PS C, Haiter-Neto F. Efficacy of a cone beam computed tomography metal artefact reduction algorithm for the detection of peri-implant fenestrations and dehiscences. Oral Surg Oral Med Oral Pathol Oral Radiol. 2016;121:550–6.

65. Burgess J. Digital DICOM in dentistry. Open Dent J. 2015;9:330–6.

66. Gan Y, Xia Z, Xiong J, Zhao Q, Hu Y, Zhang J. Toward accurate tooth segmentation from computed tomography images using a hybrid level set model. Med Phys. 2015;42:14–27.

67. Bornstein MM, Al-Nawas B, Kuchler U, Tahmaseb A. Consensus statements and recommended clinical procedures regarding contemporary surgical and radiographic techniques in implant dentistry. Int J Oral Maxillofac Implants. 2014;29(Suppl):78–82.

68. Graham RNJ, Perriss RW, Scarsbrook AF. DICOM demystified: a review of digital file formats and their use in radiological practice. Clin Radiol. 2005;60:1133–40.

69. Suapang P, Dejhan K. Medical image compression and DICOM-format image archive. In: ICROS-SICE international joint conference; 2009. p. 1945–9.

70. Libersa P, Savignat M, Tonnel A. Neurosensory disturbances of the inferior alveolar nerve: a retrospective study of complaints in a 10-year period. J Oral Maxillofac Surg. 2007;65:1486–9.

71. Jacobs R, Quirynen M, Bornstein MM. Neurovascular disturbances after implant surgery. Periodontol 2000. 2014;66:188–202.

72. Yilmaz Y, Ucer C, Scher E, Suzuki J, Renton T. A survey of the opinion and experience of UK dentists: part 1: the incidence and cause of iatrogenic trigeminal nerve injuries related to dental implant surgery. Implant Dent. 2016;25:638–45.

73. Jacobs R, van Steenberghe D. Radiographic planning and assessment of Endosseous oral implants. Heidelberg: Springer-Verlag; 1998.

74. Loubele M, Van Assche N, Carpentier K, Maes F, Jacobs R, van Steenberghe D, Suetens P. Comparative localized linear accuracy of small-field cone-beam CT and multislice CT for alveolar bone measurements. Oral Surg Oral Med Oral Pathol Oral Radiol Endod. 2008;105:512–8.
75. Kühl S, Zürcher S, Zitzmann NU, Filippi A, Payer M, Dagassan-Berndt D. Detection of peri-implant bone defects with different radiographic techniques - a human cadaver study. Clin Oral Implants Res. 2016;27:529–34.
76. Codari M, de Faria VK, Ferreira Pinheiro Nicolielo L, Haiter Neto F, Jacobs R. Quantitative evaluation of metal artifacts using different CBCT devices, high-density materials and field of views. Clin Oral Implants Res. 2017;28:1509–14.

2

Applying the theory of planned behavior to self-report dental attendance in Norwegian adults through structural equation modelling approach

Anne N. Åstrøm[1,2*], Stein Atle Lie[2] and Ferda Gülcan[2]

Abstract

Background: Understanding factors that affect dental attendance behavior helps in constructing effective oral health campaigns. A socio-cognitive model that adequately explains variance in regular dental attendance has yet to be validated among younger adults in Norway. Focusing a representative sample of younger Norwegian adults, this cross-sectional study provided an empirical test of the Theory of Planned Behavior (TPB) augmented with descriptive norm and action planning and estimated direct and indirect effects of attitudes, subjective norms, descriptive norms, perceived behavioral control and action planning on intended and self-reported regular dental attendance.

Method: Self-administered questionnaires provided by 2551, 25–35 year olds, randomly selected from the Norwegian national population registry were used to assess socio-demographic factors, dental attendance as well as the constructs of the augmented TPB model (attitudes, subjective norms, descriptive norms, intention, action planning). A two-stage process of structural equation modelling (SEM) was used to test the augmented TPB model.

Results: Confirmatory factor analysis, CFA, confirmed the proposed correlated 6-factor measurement model after re-specification. SEM revealed that attitudes, perceived behavioral control, subjective norms and descriptive norms explained intention. The corresponding standardized regression coefficients were respectively ($\beta = 0.70$), ($\beta = 0.18$), ($\beta = -0.17$) and ($\beta = 0.11$) ($p < 0.001$). Intention ($\beta = 0.46$) predicted action planning and action planning ($\beta = 0.19$) predicted dental attendance behavior ($p < 0.001$). The model revealed indirect effects of intention and perceived behavioral control on behavior through action planning and through intention and action planning, respectively. The final model explained 64 and 41% of the total variance in intention and dental attendance behavior.

Conclusion: The findings support the utility of the TPB, the expanded normative component and action planning in predicting younger adults' intended- and self-reported dental attendance. Interventions targeting young adults' dental attendance might usefully focus on positive consequences following this behavior accompanied with modeling and group performance.

Keywords: Dental attendance, Young adults, Theory of planned behavior, Structural equation modelling, AMOS

---

* Correspondence: Anne.Aastrom@uib.no
[1]Oral health Centre of Expertise in Western Norway, Bergen, Hordaland, Norway
[2]Department of Clinical Dentistry, Faculty of Medicine, University of Bergen, PO Box 7804, N-5020 Bergen, Norway

Background

The importance of dental attendance is a key measure in health education as regular attendance is associated with good health and well-being. In Norway, the Public Dental Service (PDS) is financed by taxes and provides free dental care to children and adolescents until 20 years of age [1, 2]. The private dental services provides dental care to the general adult population and is organized according to market mechanisms, with dental fees determined by supply and demand and with very limited private or public insurance arrangements [3]. Regardless of the disparities in dental coverage between Norway and other Scandinavian countries, dental attendance rates have been high among Norwegian adults. About 80 and 77% of Norwegian adults above 20 years of age reported having visited a dentist during the last 12 months in 2008 and 2013, respectively [4–6].

Nevertheless, as in other Scandinavian countries, the prevalence of regular dental care utilization among Norwegian adults varies according to age, period and socio-economic status, being smallest in the younger age- and the lower income groups [4–7]. Støle et al. [8] found that 87% of 23–24 year old Norwegian adults visited a dentist every second year in 1983, whereas the corresponding figures in 1994 was 85%. Among 25 year old Norwegian adults, 62 and 44% reported dental attendance once a year in 1997 and 2007, respectively [9]. According to the Official Statistics of Norway, the prevalence of having visited public dental health care services during last year was highest among 45–66 year olds and lowest among 21–24 year olds in 2016 [10]. Previous studies have identified enabling factors, such as cost of treatment and dental anxiety, as important barriers towards regular use of dental care [11, 12]. In a recent population-based study of Swedish adults, financial problems and lack of social support were associated with refraining from seeking dental care [11]. Whereas socio-demographic- and need related factors are important covariates of dental care utilization, relatively few studies have considered modifiable socio-cognitive determinants in the younger adult populations. Influencing younger adults' adherence to continued dental attendance requires understanding of the socio-cognitive factors underlying their decision to comply with advices for regular dental care. A socio-cognitive model that adequately explains variance in regular dental attendance has yet to be validated among younger adults in Norway.

Theoretical approach

The theory of planned behavior, TPB, is a widely applied socio-cognitive model of the attitude–behavior relationship, assuming that most conscious behaviors is rational and goal directed [13, 14]. TPB proposes a causal link between attitudes and behavior mediated by behavioral intentions. Intention directly influences behavior and is shaped by attitudes, subjective norms and perceived behavioral control regarding the behavior. Empirical validations of the TPB have revealed that the model reliably explains 40–50% of the variance in intention and that intention explains between 20 and 40% of the variance in actual behavior [14–16].

In spite of its predictive success, TPB has been criticized for its validity and it has been shown that other variables explain considerable proportions of the variance in intention and behavior [17]. Moreover, descriptive norms and action planning have shown residual effects on intention and behaviour after consideration of the original TPB variables [17, 18]. Evidence suggests that adding action planning would improve the prediction of behavior from the TPB [18, 19]. Thus, formation of action plans can be used to promote the realization of desired outcomes [18, 19]. The role of subjective norms within the TPB has also been considered [20, 21]. Subjective norms have been criticized for its narrow conceptualization, focusing what significant people thinks others ought to do, neglecting descriptive norms referring to what significant others themselves actually do [20–22]. Descriptive norms correlate with behavioral intentions and have shown to be among the strongest correlates of physical activity [23]. The TPB has received considerable empirical support across health- and social behaviors, including oral hygiene behaviors and health screening [15]. However, to our knowledge, only one previous study has examined use of public dental services in the context of TPB [16].

Focusing a representative sample of young Norwegian adults 25–35 years old, this study provides an empirical test of the TPB augmented with descriptive norm and action planning and estimates direct and indirect effects of attitudes, subjective norms, descriptive norms, perceived control, and action planning on intended and self-reported regular dental attendance. Based on the conceptualization of the TPB and previous empirical support it was hypothesized that the responses to 16 observed indicator variables could be explained by 6 latent factors in terms of attitudes, subjective norms, descriptive norms, perceived control, intention and action planning. Further, it was hypothesized that each indicator would have a stronger relation with their corresponding factor than with the competing factors. Finally, it was hypothesized that attitudes, subjective norm, descriptive norm and perceived behavioral control would predict behavioral intention and that intention, action planning and perceived behavioral control, would predict self-reported dental attendance.

Methods

Study design, participants and ethical issues

The present study used data from an electronic, cross-sectional public dental health survey conducted in Norway. A representative sample of 9000 adults (using individuals as the primary sampling unit) aged 25–35 years was randomly selected from the Norwegian national population registry in September 2016. Participation was voluntary and anonymous and the return of a completed questionnaire recognized as the informed consent. Ethical permission to carry out the survey was granted by the Ombudsman, Norwegian Center for Research Data (NO.*49241*). NORSTAT (www.norstat.no) was responsible for the electronically distributed questionnaires and for the data collection. An eligible sample of 9052 adults aged 25–35 years of age received an electronic version of the questionnaire with an introductory letter explaining the purpose of the study. Total response rate was 29% (2635/9052). Eighty-four respondents were removed due to incomplete questionnaires. All participants who provided complete questionnaires were included in the present study ($n = 2551$).

Measures

Dental attendance behavior was measured using one question; "How often do you usually visit a dentist?" the response categories ranged from (1) twice a year or more to (4) more seldom than every second year. Components of an augmented version of Ajzen's TPB [13] was measured in terms of attitudes, subjective norms, perceived behavioral control, descriptive norm and action planning in relation to regular dental attendance. In accordance with recommendations from Ajzen [13], each construct was measured considering the four elements of action (attending), target (dentist), context (on a regular basis), and time (future) (13) (. Intention to attend a dentist regularly was measured by two items, e.g. "I intend to attend a dentist regularly in the future." Responses were indicated on a four-point scale: (1) Strongly disagree, (2) Disagree, (3) Neither agree nor disagree (4) Agree and (4) Strongly agree. Attitude towards regular dental attendance was assessed by four items, e.g. "to attend a dentist regularly in the future do not make sense to me". Responses were indicated on a five-point scale ranging from 1 (strongly disagree) to 5 strongly disagree). Subjective norm was measured by three items, e.g. "My parents (partner/friend, dentist) want me to attend a dentist regularly in the future". Responses were indicated on a five-point scale ranging from 1 (strongly disagree) to 5 (strongly agree). Perceived behavioral control was measured by two items, e.g. "Its totally up to me whether I attend a dentist regularly in the future". Responses were indicated on a five-point scale ranging from 1 (strongly disagree) to 5 (strongly agree). Descriptive norm was measured by two items, e.g. "My friends attend dentist regularly" – with response categories ranging from 1 (strongly disagree) to 5 (strongly agree). Action planning was assessed using the action planning scale adopted from Sniehotta et al. [17], including three items, e.g. "I have made a detailed plan when to attend, where to attend and how to attend a dentist regularly in the future". Response categories ranged from 1 (strongly disagree) to 5 (strongly agree). Parts of the questionnaire used in the present study is available in English in the Additional file 1.

Statistical analyses

Data were analyzed using SPSS version 22.0 (IBM Corp. Released 2013, IBM SPSS Statistics for Windows, Armonk NY: IBM Corp). IBM SPSS AMOS 16.0 [24] was used to test the hypothesized augmented TPB model using a two-step modelling approach whereby the measurement model (step1) and the structural model (step 2) were constructed separately [25]. First, a confirmatory factor analysis, CFA, using maximum likelihood estimation (ML) was conducted to test the adequacy of the measurement model [25]. Modification indices (MI) were used to identify sources of misfit in the model. A prerequisite for testing of invariance across structural paths in the full structural model (step 2) is that the measurement model has configural and metric invariance. Configural invariance was examined by testing the fit of the modified correlated measurement model separately for males and females and by testing the fit of an un-constrained multi-group model. Metric invariance was examined by comparing a multi-group model with all factor loadings constrained equal to the baseline configural model in which the factor loadings were free to vary. The models were assumed non-invariant if the change in chi square was significant and the decrease in comparative fit index, CFI, was less than 0.001 [26].

A full structural equation modelling, SEM, (step 2) examined whether the hypothesized TPB model was acceptable fit to the present data, testing simultaneously the interrelationships specified within the a priori augmented TPB model. To assess how adequately the hypothesized model described the sample data, chi-square test was used together with the following goodness of fit indices; CFI (Comparative fit index), RMSEA (root mean square error of approximation) and AIC (Akaike's information criteria). In line with the conventional recommendations of Hu and Bentler [27], a good model fit was indicated by a RMSEA less or equal to 0.06, a CFI greater or equal to 0.90 and with a model having lower AIC being the more plausible together with a non-significant Chi square. Statistical significance of parameter estimates are the Critical Ration (CR) representing the parameter estimate divided by its standard error. Based on a level of 0.05, the test statistics (CR) needed to be 1.96 before rejection of the null hypothesis.

Results

Sample profile

In spite of the relatively low response rate (29%) obtained, the age distribution of the final sample corresponded with that of the Norwegian population 20–44 years old by December 2016. The age distribution of younger (25–29 years) and older (30–35 years) participants were 43.7 and 56.3%, respectively. Corresponding figures in the population were respectively 46.3 and 53%. Whereas the gender distribution in the sample was 43% men and 56.7% women, the corresponding population distribution was 51.3 and 49.0%. Among the participants, 27.3, 38.6 and 34.1% reported respectively, primary-, bachelor- and college/university level of education. Corresponding figures in the adult population 16 years and above were 26.5, 37.8 and 32.9%. Among the respondents ($n = 2551$), 91.5% were of native Norwegian origin. Eight percent confirmed dental attendance at least twice a year, 47.2% once a year, 21.2% every second year and 21.2% more seldom than every second year (Table 1).

Descriptive statistics of TPB variables

Table 2 depicts mean, standard deviation, minimum and maximum scores and theoretical range for each indicator measuring the latent constructs of attitudes, subjective norms, perceived control, descriptive norms, intention and action planning. On average the study group demonstrated strong intentions with mean values in the range 4.2–4.3, both positive and negative attitudes (mean values 2.4–4.7), moderate to strong subjective norms (mean values 3.9–4.4), moderate descriptive norms (mean values 3.4–3.9), strong perceived behavioral control (mean values 4.4–4.5), and weak action planning (mean values 2.0–2.2).

Evaluation of the measurement model

The default ML estimation with AMOS requires continuous multivariate normality of the observed indicator variables. As multivariate kurtosis represented by Mardia's coefficient was below the recommended value of 3.0, it was not deemed necessary to bias correct estimates through bootstrapping [24]. According to the fit indices (CFI, RMSEA, AIC) employed, CFA indicated that an initially proposed correlated 6-factor model (attitudes, subjective norms, descriptive norms, perceived control, intention, action planning) was not an acceptable fit on any of the fit indices employed (CMIN (df) = 1457.6 (89), CFI = .925, RMSEA =0.058, AIC = 757.666). Inspection of modification indices indicated covariation between

Table 1 Frequency distribution of participants' socio-demographic characteristics and dental attendance behavior, ($n = 2551$) and corresponding percentage figures in the total population

	Category	Participants % (n)	Total population %
Gender	Male	43.3 (1105)	51.3
	Female	56.7 (1446)	49.0[a]
Age	25-29 years	43.7 (1116)	46.3
	30–35 years	56.3 (1435)	53.0[a]
Country of birth	Norway	91.5 (2333)	
	Other Nordic	2.6 (66)	
	Outside Nordic	6.0 (152)	
Civil status	Single	36.6 (935)	
	Married	63.4 (1616)	
Highest level of education	Primary/secondary	27.3 (679)	26.5
	Bachelor degree	38.6 (962)	37.8
	College/university	34.1 (850)	32.9[b]
Income (NOK)	At least 400.000	19.5 (413)	
	400,001–800,000	41.2 (876)	
	> 800,000	39.3 (835)	
Dental attendance	At least twice a year	8.0 (203)	
	Once a year	47.2 (1205)	
	Every second year	21.2 (540)	
	More seldom	21.2 (540)	

[a]Norwegian population 20–44 years by December 2016
[b]Norwegian population above 20 years by December 2016

pairs of error terms, resulting from item overlap, or reflecting biases in responding such as "yea" saying or "no" saying. Attitude had a non-significant loading to one indicator (attend a dentist regularly is intolerable) which was removed from the model. Re-estimation of the 6-factor model gave acceptable fit (CMIN = (df) 655.666 (69), CFI = .96, RMSEA = .058, AIC = 757.666). As shown in Table 3, all factor loadings were in the expected direction and had significant regression weights with their related latent variables (C.R. > 1.96), indicating convergent validity. Most statistically significant items' standardized regression weights were above 0.3, and thus in accordance with the threshold proposed [28]. Higher values of the indicators were associated with stronger (positive) attitudes, stronger subjective norms, descriptive norms, perceived behavioral control, intentions and action planning. The inter-factor correlations (correlations between the 6 latent variables) were below 0.85 indicating acceptable discriminant validity (< 0.85). Figure 1 depicts the modified 6- factor measurement model based on CFA.

Gender specific modified correlated factor models indicated acceptable fit for males (CMIN 306, df 69, $p < 0.000$, CFI = 0.968, RMSEA = 0.056) as well as for

Table 2 Descriptive statistics of all variables related to the augmented model of planned behavior

	Mean	SD	Min	Max	Theoretical range
Intention					
I intend to attend dentist regularly (Q31_1)	4.3	1.0	1	5	Low-high
I have made a decision to attend (Q31_2)	4.2	1.1	1	5	Low-high
Attitudes					
To attend dentist regularly is:					
—reasonable (Q31_4)	4.7	0.7	1	5	Negative-positive
–necessary (Q31_6)	4.3	1.0	1	5	Negative-positive
-economic burden (Q31_5)	2.4	1.3	1	5	Negative-positive
Intolerable Q31_3	4.2	1.1	1	5	Negative-positive
Subjective norm					
My parents want me to attend regularly (Q31_7)	4.0	1.1	1	5	Low-high
My partner want me to attend regularly (Q31_8)	3.9	1.1	1	5	Low-high
My dentist want me to attend regularly (Q31_9)	4.4	0.9	1	5	Low-high
Descriptive norm					
My friends attend regularly (Q31_12)	3.4	1.0	1	5	Low-high
My parents attend regularly (Q31_13)	3.9	1.1	1	5	Low-high
Perceived control					
It's up to me to attend regularly (Q31_10)	4.5	0.8	1	5	Low-high
I am capable to attend regularly (Q31_11)	4.4	1.0	1	5	Low-high
Action planning					
I have made a detailed plan regarding————————					
When attending (Q31_14)	2.0	1.2	1	5	Low-high
Where attending (Q31_15)	2.2	1.4	1	5	Low -high
How attending (Q31_16)	2.0	1.3	1	5	Low-high

Table 3 Standardized regression weights for the different components of the modified correlated 6-factor measure model including intention(INT), attitudes (ATT), subjective norms (SN), descriptive norms (DN), perceived behavioral control (PBC), action planning (AP)

Parameters	Observed variable (figure label)	Parameter estimate (factor loading)
INT	I intend to attend (Q31_1)	0.927 ***
	I have decided to attend (Q3_2)	0.890***
ATT	To attend is reasonable (Q31_4)	0.695***
	To attend is necessary (Q31_6)	0.715***
	To attend is an economic burden (Q31_5)	0.117***
SN	My parents want me to attend (Q31_7)	0.789***
	My friends want me to attend (Q31_8)	0.627***
	My dentist want me to attend (Q31_9)	0.792***
DN	My friends attend (Q31_12)	0.680***
	My parents attend (Q31_13)	0.642***
PBC	Its up to me whether to attend (Q31_10)	0.358***
	I am capable to attend (Q31_11)	0.916***
AP	I have made a detailed plan when (Q31_14)	0.901***
	I have made a detailed plan where (Q31_14)	0.895***
	I have made a detailed plan how (Q31_15)	0.832***

***p < 0.001

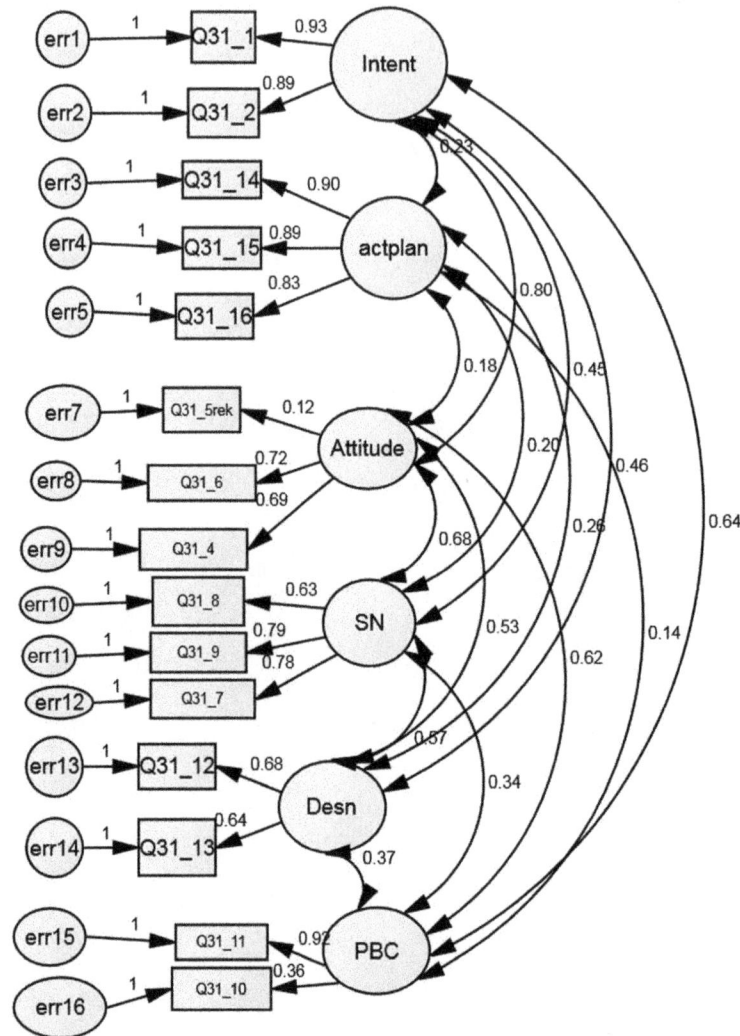

Fig. 1 Modified 6-factor measurement model based on CFA

females (CMIN 402,846, df = 69, $p < 0.000$, CFI = 0.964, RMSEA = 0.058). Multi-group analyses, testing for invariance across males and females simultaneously, revealed acceptable fit for the unconstrained model (CMIN = 709.689, df 138, $p < 0.000$, CFI = 0.966, RMSEA = 0.040) indicating configural invariance (equivalent factor structure). Compared to the unconstrained baseline model, a model with constrained measurement weights were statistically significant (CMIN 738.00 df147, $p < 0.001$, CFI = 0.964, RMSEA = 0.040). As indicated by the slightly increase in CMIN and decline in CFI values as compared to those in the unconstrained configural model, some variance in factor loadings could be expected across males and females. The difference Δ CMIN =28.319, DF 9 was statistically significant at $p < 0.001$ indicating lack of metric invariance or at best partial invariance for the factor loadings.

Structural equation model

Structural equation modelling, SEM, was conducted to estimate the fit of the augmented TPB model and the relationships among the latent constructs. The model with intention (INT), action planning (AP), and dental attendance predicted by attitudes (ATT), subjective norms (SN), descriptive norms (DN) and perceived behavioral control (PBC) was an acceptable fit to the data; CMIN 821.234 (85), $p < 0.001$, CFI = 0.959, RMSEA = 0.058 and AIC = 923,234). Direct paths from attitudes, subjective norms and descriptive norms on dental attendance behavior did not improve the fit of the model and none of those paths was statistically significant. Figure 2 depicts the direct effects for the augmented TPB model.

As hypothesized by the augmented TPB, stronger attitudes $\beta = .70$, $p < 0.001$, perceived behavioral control

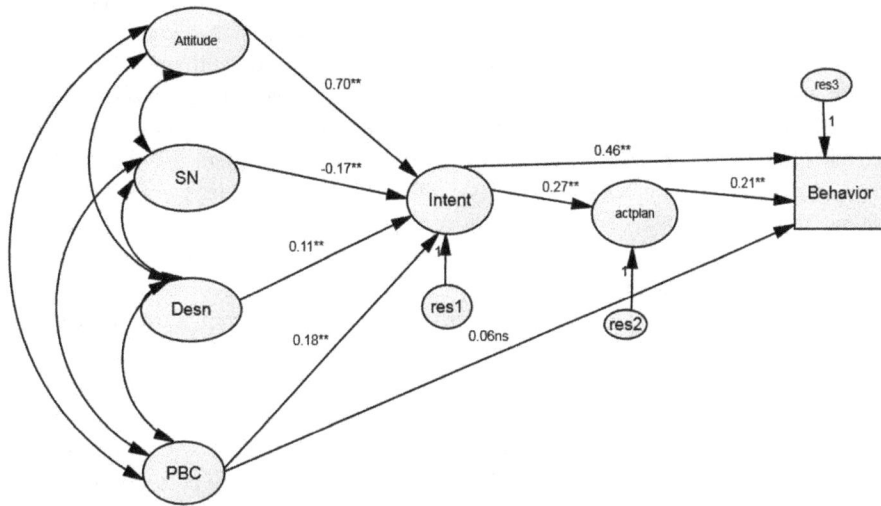

Fig. 2 The augmented Theory of Planned Behavior structural equation model. For ease of interpretation only direct pathways are shown

$\beta = 0.18$, $p < 0.001$ and descriptive norm $\beta = .11$, $p < 0.001$ were all linked to stronger intentions (Table 4). Subjective norm was negatively related to intention $\beta = --17$, $p < 0.001$. Stronger intention was linked to stronger action planning $\beta = .27$, $p < 0.001$ and to more frequent dental attendance $\beta = 0.46$, $p < 0.001$. Stronger PBC was also linked to more frequent dental attendance, however this path was not statistically significantly $\beta = 0.06$, 0.03n.s. Stronger action planning was linked to more frequent dental attendance $\beta = .19$, $p < 0.001$. Attitudes, subjective norms, descriptive norms and perceived behavioral control accounted for 64% of the variance in intention, intention accounted for 7.6% of the variance in action planning and intention, action planning and perceived behavioral control accounted for 32% variance in dental attendance. Specific indirect effects were estimated by multiplying the direct effects of the variables involved in the total pathway. An indirect path from perceived behavioral control to behavior ($\beta = 0.01$) was as follows; Perceived behavioral control-intention ($\beta = .18$), intention-action planning ($\beta = .27$), action planning-behavior ($\beta = .19$). This indicates that the effect of perceived behavioral control on dental attendance was primarily through intention and action planning. An indirect path from intention to behavior ($\beta = 0.05$) was as follows; intention-action planning ($\beta = 0.27$), action planning-behavior ($\beta = 0.19$). The effect of intention on behavior was primarily a direct one.

Discussion

The present study examined, for the first time, the effect of motivational (intention) and volitional (action planning) factors upon regular dental attendance using a

Table 4 Significant direct standardized regression weights for the extended theory of planned behavior- Modified SEM model

	Standardized regression weight	% total effect
Direct standardized effects		
Intention-attitudes	.76 (.70)***	Intention: 64
Intention-subjective norms	.-19 (-.17)***	Action plan: 7.6
Intention-descriptive norm	.11 (.11)***	Behavior: 32
Intention-perceived control	.16 (.18)***	
Intention-Action plan	.27 (.27)***	
Action plan-behavior	.21 (.19)***	
Intention -Behavior	.51(.46)***	
Perceived control-behavior	.06 (.03)ns	
Indirect standardized effects		
Perceived control-intention-action plan - behavior	.01	
Intention-action plan -behavior	.05	

***$p < 0.001$

cross-sectional design, a structural equation modelling approach (SEM) and a representative sample of Norwegian adults 25–35 years of age. The benefit of SEM over other statistical procedures is its ability to test the hypothesized relationships among observed and latent variables in the TPB model completely and simultaneously. Structural equation modelling has gained considerable popularity and whilst modelling the TPB constructs as latent variables shows the ability to account for measurement errors, which may influence the relationships in the model [25, 26].

This study revealed that the proportion of dental attendance at least once a year amounted to 47.2% among 25–35 year old Norwegian adults. This prevalence rate is marginally lower and higher than those reported among 25-year-old Norwegians in 1997 (62%) and 2007 (44.6%), respectively, and deviates with figures from 2013 indicating that 63% of 20–39 year olds had visited a dentist within the previous year [6, 9]. Nevertheless, dental attendance rate is not satisfactory as long as 21% reported dental attendance frequency less than every second year.

In a first step, a modified correlated factor analytical model provided support for the factorial validity of a questionnaire supposed to measure intention, action planning, attitudes, subjective norms, perceived control and descriptive norms thus confirming construct validity of a modified 6-factor model (Fig. 1). Although a small and statistically significant p-value for the chi-square statistics indicated poor fit of the measurement model, by taking sample size into consideration, the comparative fit indices fulfilled the criteria for good fit [24, 26]. In the final model, all inter-factor correlations were below the threshold set to indicate poor discriminative validity [25–27]. Structural equation modelling in a second step showed that the augmented TPB model applied was a good fit to the data explaining large amounts of variation in intention and attendance behavior. In addition, multi-group analysis revealed that the structural part (configural invariance) of the model operated equivalently across males and females, although the factor loadings did not achieve invariance.

The present finings add to previous findings considering the ability of the augmented TPB to account for greater variance in intention and behavior than the TPB alone [28, 29]. The explained variance in intention (64%) and behavior (32%) was higher than that commonly reported in meta-analyses of the TPB, being in the range of 40–49% for intention and 26–36% regarding actual behavior [14, 15]. Thus, the results revealed direct statistically significant pathways to intention from attitude ($\beta = .70$), subjective norm ($\beta = .-.17$), PBC ($\beta = .18$), and descriptive norm ($\beta = .11$). These findings support the hypothesis that TPB augmented with descriptive norm would predict behavior indirectly through behavioral

intention. A direct path from descriptive norm to intention suggests that young adults are guided by what others do regarding their dental visiting behavior. Meta analytical reviews of health related behaviors have also revealed that descriptive norm adds to the prediction of intention independent of the TPB constructs [30, 31]. Nevertheless, attitudes were the strongest motivational determinant implying that younger adults' decision to attend a dentist on a regular basis was almost entirely based on anticipated benefits of that behavior but also on social norms (subjective norm and descriptive norm) and considerations of potential obstacles (perceived behavioral control), in that order. The finding that attitudes and perceived behavioral control are predictive of intended dental attendance is in line with other studies predicting decisions to utilize health care services [1, 16]. These findings imply that reduced perceived control due to barriers, such as for instance dental anxiety and fear, would reduce intention and actual use of dental health care services among younger Norwegian adults. Unexpectedly, the direction of the path from subjective norms to intention was negative implying that higher perceived social approval for dental attendance result in lower motivation for that behavior. Although speculative, the construct of psychological reactance may offer an explanation to this uncommon finding as psychological reactance effects in health related behavior have been observed previously in various domains [20]. In practical terms, however, interventions targeting young adults' dental attendance behavior might usefully focus on informed awareness of the positive oral health consequences following this behavior accompanied with strategies such as modeling and group performance. Educational messages aimed at increasing young adults' regular dental attendance could highlight the prevalence of dental attendance among the youth in the community. If young adults get a sense that everybody at their own age is attending on a regular basis, they might be encourage to abandon their non-attendance.

Intention was by far the strongest predictor of dental attendance ($\beta = .46$), whereas action planning came second ($\beta = .21$). This supports the hypothesis that action planning contributes to the prediction of dental attendance over and above the effect of intention whereas the association between intention and behavior was partly mediated through action planning. Forming action plans considering when, where and how to act facilitates behavioral action by setting situational cues that activate cognitive processes needed to execute the behavior and highlights that intenders may benefit from formulating plans to engage in regular dental attendance [28, 29]. Previous studies have revealed that action planning contributes to the prediction of health service utilization, such as cervical cancer screening [18, 20]. Schutz et al. [28] and Åstrøm [19] examined subsequent flossing in the context of social cognition theory and found that action planning was a significant predictor of actual flossing alongside intentions and previous flossing. Consistent with those studies, but at odds with others [18, 19, 28], the present one found action planning to be a significant predictor of dental attendance. Inconsistent with TPB, perceived behavioral control did not emerge as a significant predictor of dental attendance. This accords, however, with a meta-analysis by Cooke and French [31], where perceived control was an unimportant predictor of screening behavior. Thus, attending a dentist on regular basis seem to be under complete volitional control by younger adults in Norway, who do not require particular resources, opportunities and technical skills for performance [13].

This study should be interpreted within the context of its strengths and limitations. The evidence provided from a large population based study that dental attendance is strongly associated with action planning and intention, which in turn is associated with attitudes, subjective norms, descriptive norms and perceived behavioral control identifies targets for informing dental health care interventions among young adults in Norway. A limitation of the present study was the use of self-reported dental attendance that might be biased by social desirability bias resulting in over reporting as compared with medical records. Evidence suggests that the validity of self-reported use of dental services ranges from poor to excellent, depending on service type [32]. Moreover, the dental attendance question was adopted from previously tested measures and it is reasonable to assume that it was sufficiently simple and unambiguous to achieve a satisfactory degree of reliability. Another weakness associated with the present cross-sectional study, as with most population based electronically administered surveys, is the relatively low response rate. Comparison of sex, age and educational level distributions among participants with the corresponding figures in the population provided by official statistics showed a similar age- and educational level distribution but a moderately different gender distribution that most probably did not affect the generalizability of the findings presented. A further weakness is the use of a cross –sectional design, thus violating Ajzen's recommended longitudinal design for the original TPB model [13]. Measuring intention to attend dentists and self-reported dental attendance in one point in time might have resulted in an unrealistic high explained variance of behavior since the intention behavior gap widens the longer the time interval between intention and behavior [13]. Further studies should incorporate subsequent measures of behavior or use information from dental records to validate the self-report measure utilized in the present study.

Conclusions

The presents study is the first large nationally representative population based study analyzing younger adults' dental attendance behavior within the context of an augmented TPB model and using a structural equation modeling approach. The present findings support the utility of the TPB, the expanded normative component and the construct of action planning in predicting younger adults' intended and self-reported dental attendance. Interventions targeting young adults' dental attendance behavior might usefully focus on positive consequences following this behavior accompanied with modeling and group performance.

Abbreviations
AIC: Aikaikes; AP: Action planning; ATT: Attitudes; CFA: Confirmatory factor analysis; CFI: Comparative fit index; CMIN: minimum discrepancy; CR: Critical ratio; DN: Descriptive norms; INT: Intention; MI: Modification indices; ML: Maximum likelihood; PBC: Perceived behavioral control; RMSEA: root mean square error of approximation; SEM: Structural Equation Modeling; SN: subjective norms; SPSS: Statistical Packages for Social Sciences; TPB: Theory of planned behavior

Acknowledgements
The authors are grateful to the Public Dental Health care Services, Hordaland county for financial support to conduct this study.

Funding
This study did receive funding form the Public Dental Health Care Services in Hordaland County, Norway. The funding body did not have any role in the design of the study, nor in the data collection analysis and interpretation of the data when writing the manuscript.

Authors' contributions
ANÅ planned the study, designed the questionnaire and co0nducted all statistical analyses. She was the main contributor in completing the writing of the manuscript. SAL: Contributed to the conduction of the statistical analyses and provided valuable statistical guidance. FG: Contributed to the study design and completion of the manuscript. Provided valuable technical guidance. All authors read and approved the final manuscript

Competing interests
The authors declare that they have no competing interests.

References
1. Holst D. Varieties of oral health care systems. Public Dental services: Organization and Financing of Oral health Care services in the Nordic countries. In: Pine C, Harris R, editors. Community Oral health. 2nd ed. London: Quintesse Publishing CO. Ltd; 2007.
2. Nihtila A. A Nordic project of quality indicators for oral health care. Finland: Helsinki; 2010.
3. Grytten J. Payment systems and incentives in dentistry. Community Dent Oral Epidemiol. 2017;45:1–11.

4. Vikum E, Krokstad S, Holst D, Westin S. Socio-economic inequalities in dental service utilization in a Norwegian county: the third Nord-Trondelag health survey. Scand J Public Health. 2012;40:648–55.

5. Grytten J, Holst D, Skau I. Demand for and utilization of dental services according to household income in the adults population in Norway. Community Dent Oral Epidemiol. 2012;40:297–305.

6. Grytten J, Holst D, Skau I. Demand for dental services and dental treatment patterns among Norwegian adults. Nor Tannlegeforen Tid. 2014;124:276–83.

7. Suominen AL, Helminen S, Lahti S, Vehkalahati MM, Knuuttila M, Varsio S, Lindblad A. Use of oral health care services in Finnish adults-results from cross-sectional health 2000 and 2011 surveys. BMC Oral Health. 2017;17:78.

8. Støle AC, Holst D, Schuller AA. Decreasing numbers of young adults seeking dental care on yearly basis. A reason for concern? Nor Tannlegeforen Tid. 1999;109:392–5. (in Norwegian)

9. Åstrøm AN, Skaret E, Haugejorden O. Dental anxiety and dental attendance among 25 –year-olds in Norway: time trends from 1997-2007. BMC Oral Health. 2011;11:10.

10. Official Statistics of Norway, 2016 https://www.ssb.no/statistikkbanken.

11. Berglund E, Westerling R, Lytsy P. Social and health related factors associated with refraining from seeking dental care<: a cross-sectional population study. Community Dent Oral Epidemiol. 2017;45:258–65.

12. Åstrøm AN, Ekback G, Ordell S, Nasir E. Long-term routine dental attendance : influrnce on tooth loss and oral health related quality of life in Swedish older adults. Community Dent Oral Epidemiol. 2014:460–9.

13. Ajzen I. The theory of planned behavior. Organ Behav Hum Decis Process. 1991;50:179–211.

14. Armitage CJ, Conner M. Efficacy of the theory of planned behavior. A meta analytic review. Br J Soc Psychol. 2001;40:471–99.

15. McEachan BA, Taylor N, Harrison R, Lawton R, Gardner P, Conner M. Meta-analysis of the reasoned action approach to understanding health beaviors. Ann Behav Med. 2016:50–592.

16. Luzzi L, Spencer AJ. Factors influencing the use of public dental services: an application of the theory of planned behavior. BMC Health Serv Res. 2008;8: 93.

17. Sniehotta F, Scholz U, Schwarzer R. Action plans and coping plans for physical exercise: a longitudinal intervention study in cardiac rehabilitation. Bristish J Health Psychol. 2006;11:23–37.

18. Sheeran P, Orbell S. Using implementation intention to increase attendance for cervical cancer. Health Psychol. 2000;19:283–9.

19. Astrom AN. Applicability of action planning and coping planning to dental flossing among Norwegian adults: a confirmatory factor analysis approach. Eur J Oral Sci. 2008;116:250–9.

20. Sieverding M, Ciccarello L, Matterne U. What role do social norms play in the context of men's cancer screening intention and behavior? Application of an extended theory of planned behavior. Health Psychol. 2010;29:72–81.

21. Lee H. The role of descriptive norm within the theory of planned behavior in predicting Korean American's exercise behavior. Psychol Rep. 2011;109:208–18.

22. Cialdini RB, Reno RR, Kallgren CA. A focus theory of normative conduct: recycling the concept of norms to reduce littering in public places. J Pers and Soc Osychol. 1990;58:1015–26.

23. Rivis A, Sheeran P. Descriptive norms as an additional predictor in the theory of planned behavior: a meta-analysis. Curr Psychol: Dev, Learn Pers, Soc. 2003;22:218–33.

24. Schumacker RE, Lomax RG. A Beginner's guide to structural equation modelling. second ed. London: Lawrence Erlbaum Associates Publishers; 2004.

25. Byrne B. Structural equation modelling with AMOS. Basic concepts, applications and programming. London: Lawrence Erlbaum Associates, Publishers; 2001.

26. Brown T. Confirmatory factor analysis for applied research. London: Guilford; 2006.

27. Hu L, Bentler PM. Cut off criteria for fit indices in co-variance structures analysis: conventional criteria versus new alternatives. Str Eq Mod. 1999;6:1–55.

28. Schutz B, Sniehotta FF, Wiedemann A, Seemann R. Adherence to a daily flossing regimen in university students:effects of planning when, where , how and what to do in face of barriers. J Clin Periodontol. 2006;33:612–9.

29. Gollwitzer PM, Sheeran P. Implementation intention and goal achievement: a meta- analysis of effects and processes. Adv Exp Soc Psychol. 2006;38:69–119.

30. Rivis A, Sheeran P. Descriptive norm as an additional predictor in the theory of planned behavior: a meta-analysis. Curr Psychol. 2003;22:218–33.

31. Cooke R, French DP. How well do the theory of reasoned action and theory of planned behavior predict intentions and attendance at screening programs? A meta- analysis. Psychol Health. 2008;23:745–65.

32. Gilbert GH, Rose JS, Shelton BJ. A prospective study of the validity of self – reported use of specific types of dental services. Public health Rep. 2003; 118:18–26.

3

Relationship between the burden of major periodontal bacteria and serum lipid profile

Youn-Hee Choi[1], Takayuki Kosaka[2], Miki Ojima[3], Shinichi Sekine[3], Yoshihiro Kokubo[4], Makoto Watanabe[4], Yoshihiro Miyamoto[4], Takahiro Ono[2,5] and Atsuo Amano[3*]

Abstract

Background: The association of periodontal bacteria with lipid profile alteration remains largely unknown, although it has been suggested that chronic periodontitis increases the atherosclerotic risk. This cross-sectional study investigated the relationship between the prevalence and total burden of periodontal bacteria and serum lipid profile.

Methods: Saliva from enrolled participants was collected to detect 4 major periodontal bacteria (*Porphyromonas gingivalis*, *Treponema denticola*, *Tannerella forsythia*, and *Prevotella intermedia*) using Polymerase Chain Reaction method. High-density lipoprotein (HDL) cholesterol, triglycerides (TG), and low-density lipoprotein cholesterol were assessed using blood samples. We compared the averages of each lipid in association with the prevalence of each bacterial species, their burden (low, moderate, and high), and the combination of bacterial burden and periodontal status, defined as periodontitis, using the Community Periodontal Index, after adjustment for other potential confounding factors, by employing general linear models with least square means.

Results: A total of 385 Japanese individuals (176 men, 209 women; mean age 69.2 years) were enrolled. The number of bacterial species and their co-existence with periodontitis were significantly related to a decrease in HDL (*p* for trend < 0.01) and increase in TG (*p* for trend = 0.04). The adjusted mean HDL levels (mg/dL) in individuals with low, moderate, and high levels of bacterial species were 66.1, 63.0, and 58.9, respectively, and those in the 6 groups defined by combination of the two factors were 67.9, 64.6, 64.3, 65.4, 61.5, and 54.7, respectively.

Conclusion: Periodontal bacterial burden is suggested to be independently involved in lowering serum HDL level. Our findings suggest that bacterial tests in a clinical setting could be a useful approach for predicting the risk of HDL metabolism dysregulation.

Keywords: Microbiology, Obesity, Periodontal-systemic disease interaction

Background

Recent studies have revealed that chronic marginal periodontitis is associated with atherosclerosis (as an intermediate endpoint) and cardiovascular diseases [1–3]. Periodontitis and its severity have been operationally defined by two types of clinical measurements, i.e., pocket depth and/or clinical attachment loss, in population studies [4, 5]. The clinical definition of periodontitis is

dependent on the patient's condition or the characteristics of the target study population, without any established gold standard. Thus, more valid, more reliable, and various measures for the chronic periodontitis associated with cardiovascular diseases seems to be required. Previous studies have suggested that the serum antibody levels against specific periodontal bacteria, such as *Porphyromonas gingivalis* and *Aggregatibacter actinomycetemcomitans*, or periodontitis-related microorganism groups [6] are useful to predict the risk of atherosclerotic diseases [7–9]. Furthermore, periodontal bacteria harbored in gingival pockets, in regard to the burden of total bacterial species possessed by an individual, has been

* Correspondence: amanoa@dent.osaka-u.ac.jp
[3]Department of Preventive Dentistry, Osaka University Graduate School of Dentistry, 1-8 Yamadaoka, Suita-Osaka 565-0871, Japan
Full list of author information is available at the end of the article

suggested to be a risk factor for atherosclerosis [10] and myocardial infarction [1].

As for major periodontal pathogenic bacteria, *P. gingivalis*, *Prevotella intermedia*, and *Treponema denticola*, as well as several other species, have been suggested to be possible causative agents in an in vivo study of atherosclerosis [11]. Another recent study [12] showed that specific bacterial groups, including the Orange-Red complex of *P. intermedia*, *P. gingivalis*, *T. denticola*, and *Tannerella forsythia*, were associated with elevated plasma glucose levels in adults. However, it did not show that those bacterial groups were related to other metabolic syndrome components. In contrast, another recent study [13] suggested that periodontitis, as determined by pocket depth, clinical insertion level, and bleeding on probing, was associated with distorted serum lipid levels, and also noted that the serum levels of *P. gingivalis* and *A. actinomycetemcomitans* antibodies may be a risk factor for decrease high-density lipoprotein (HDL) cholesterol levels. In light of metabolic pathways, *P. gingivalis* and its vesicles, for example, promote multiple cytokines as chronic infection and inflammation status resulting in elevation of triglyceride rich lipoprotein affecting on other lipoproteins. In turn, increase of triglyceride raises low-density lipoprotein (LDL) binding to macrophages and induce macrophages to modify native LDL, which plays an important role in foam cell formation [14, 15]. Notwithstanding, the association of periodontal pathogenic bacteria with serum lipid profile alteration as an atherosclerotic risk factor has not been well investigated, even though periodontitis is thought to be tightly related to the development of atherosclerosis. In addition, the effects of periodontal destruction, as a clinical parameter of the relationship between exposure to periodontal bacteria and lipid profiles in humans, are not well known. Therefore, in the present study, we hypothesized that exposure to periodontal bacteria could alter serum lipid metabolic pathways. We aimed to investigate the relationship between the prevalence of periodontal bacterial species with the total periodontal bacterial burden and the serum lipid profile, and to assess the combined effects of bacterial factors and the presence of periodontitis on the level of serum lipids.

Methods

Study participants

We recruited 1067 Japanese individuals aged 30–79 years who underwent a medical check-up and oral examination between June 2008 and March 2010 as part of the Suita Study, which comprised a random sample of 8360 Japanese urban residents. The Suita Study was originally constructed as a cohort between September 1989 and March 1994, and a regular health examination was performed every 2 years between June 2008 and March

2012. In the beginning of the Suita Study, 6485 of the 12,200 registered residents of Suita City underwent general health checkups at the National Center for Cerebral and Cardiovascular diseases [16]. In 1996, a second recruitment commenced, and 1875 additional individuals underwent basic health examinations, as shown in Fig. 1.

Oral health examination especially for periodontal pathogenic bacterial assessment was underwent as a cross-sectional design for the follow-up period of time. Prior to enrollment, the study protocol was approved by the Ethics Committee of the National Cerebral and Cardiovascular Center (M25–032), and only individuals who provided informed consent after receiving a full explanation of the study purpose and methods, both in writing and orally, were included as study participants.

Inclusion criteria for every participant was the presence of 10 teeth and more in mouth. From a total of 1067, 454 persons were excluded in this study because they had under 10 teeth in their mouth. Among the rest of the people ($n = 613$), individuals were excluded if they had low stimulated salivary flow rate (< 0.5 ml min^{-1}) ($n = 228$). Thus, final sample size was 385.

Assay for bacterial analysis in saliva

The volunteers were asked to chew a piece of paraffin gum for 2 min to stimulate salivary flow, and then spit

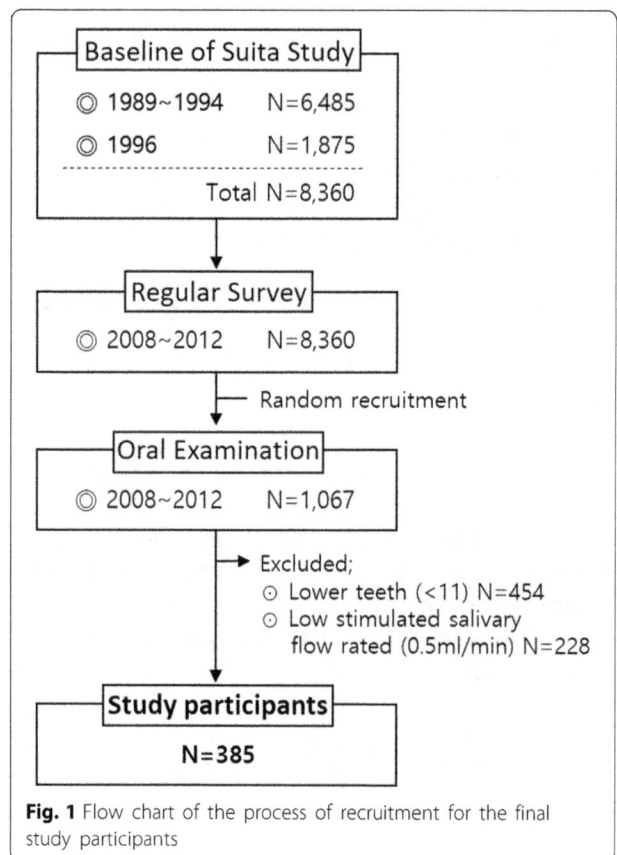

Fig. 1 Flow chart of the process of recruitment for the final study participants

the saliva into a 50 ml Falcon test tube (Corning Inc., Corning, NY, USA), as described previously [17]. After collection, the volume of each saliva sample was determined gravimetrically, and the stimulated salivary flow rates were expressed as ml min^{-1}. Samples were stored at -80 °C until required for analysis. Saliva samples were collected prior to periodontal tissue examination in order to avoid possible side effects.

Bacterial genomic DNA was isolated from the specimens using a Wizard® Genomic DNA Purification Kit (Promega Corporation, Madison, WI, USA), according to the manufacturer's instructions. A 16S RNA-based polymerase chain reaction (PCR) detection method was used to determine the prevalence of four periodontal bacteria (*P. gingivalis, T. denticola, T. forsythia, P. intermedia*), as previously described [18–21]. Table 1 lists the PCR primers used in the study. PCR amplification was performed in a total volume of 25 µL consisting of DNA polymerase (Speed-STAR® HS DNA Polymerase, Takara Bio Inc., Shiga, Japan), 0.5 µM each primer, 10× PCR buffer, dNTP mixture, and 1 µL of the template DNA solution in sterile distilled water. PCR was performed in a thermal cycler (2720 Thermal Cycler, Applied Biosystems, Foster City, CA, USA) with the following cycling parameters: initial denaturation at 95 °C for 2 min, followed by 30 cycles consisting of 95 °C for 10 s and 62 °C for 30 s. Positive and negative controls were included in each PCR set, and when processing all samples. PCR products were analyzed by 2.0% agarose gel (Agarose S, Nippon Gene, Tokyo, Japan) electrophoresis. The gel was stained with 0.5 µg/mL ethidium bromide (Nippon Gene, Tokyo, Japan) and photographed under UV illumination. A 100-bp DNA ladder (EZ Load™, BioRad, CA, USA) was used as a molecular size standard. The detection limit was determined for the simultaneous PCR using known numbers of bacterial cells diluted in distilled water.

Periodontal tissue examination and oral health behavior

Periodontal tissue examinations were performed by 5 dentists (Y. Y., K. T., M. K., T. K., and M. K.) who were appropriately trained and calibrated according to standardized procedures as recommended in the manual

published by the World Health Organization [22]. For each individual, a total of 10 teeth were examined, the maxillary and mandibular left and right first and second molars, maxillary right central incisor, and mandibular left central incisor. When an examination could not be performed because one or both the central incisors was missing, the same tooth on the opposite side was examined. No evaluation was performed when all relevant teeth were missing. Periodontal status was examined at 6 sites of each tooth using a Community Periodontal Index (CPI) probe (YDM, Tokyo, Japan) according to the following criteria, with the highest-value code recorded. The CPI codes were as follows: Code 0, no sign of gingival inflammation; Code 1, bleeding evident after probing; Code 2, dental calculus deposits detected (including those detected by probing up to 4 mm beneath the gingival margin); Code 3, periodontal pocket depth ranging from ≥ 4 mm to < 6 mm; Code 4, periodontal pocket depth ≥ 6 mm. Cohen's κ value for consistency between the periodontal tissue examinations performed by the 5 dentists was 0.78. Clinical periodontitis was defined as a CPI code greater than 2. Information about frequency of tooth brushing (once, twice, more than twice per day) and dental flossing (none, once or more per week, once or more per day) was also used.

Laboratory testing of serum for lipid profile and other general health information

Routine blood tests were used to measure levels of HDL, triglycerides (TG), and LDL cholesterol in serum, with total cholesterol (TC) levels calculated using the following formula: $HDL + LDL + TG/5$. These 4 variables (HDL, TG, LDL, and TC) were used as outcomes. Fasting glucose level was also assessed to define diabetes (fasting glucose ≥ 126 mg/L, or use of diabetic medication). Body mass index (BMI) was calculated by measurement of height and body weight [23]. Well-trained physicians measured systolic (SBP) and diastolic (DBP) blood pressure. Hypertension was defined as $SBP \geq 140$ mmHg and/or $DBP \geq 90$ mmHg or use of antihypertensive treatment [24]. In addition, lifestyle

Table 1 List of Species-specific primers

Primer set	Sequence (5' to 3')	Size (bp)	Detection Limit (No. of cells)	Reference
P. gingivalis	TGT AGA TGA CTG ATG CTG AAA ACC	197	5	(17)
	ACG TCA TCC CCA CCT TCC TC			
T. denticola	AAG GCG GTA GAG CCG CTC A	311	10	(18)
	AGC CGC TGT CGA AAA GCC CA			
T. forsythia	GCG TAT GTA ACC TGC CCG CA	641	25	(15)
	TGC TTC AGT GTC AGT TAT ACC T			
P. intermedia	TTTGTTGGGGAGTAAAGCGGG	575	25	(15)
	TCAACATCTCTGTATCCTGCGT			

details, such as smoking, drinking, and regular exercise, were obtained using a standardized questionnaire by trained physicians or nurses in face-to-face interviews, as previously described [24]. Smoking and drinking were further classified into current, former, and never. The number of times of exercising per week was categorized as none, once or twice, and more than twice.

Statistical methods

Exposure was considered as the total number of periodontal bacteria and the presence of bacteria themselves, and the outcome was considered as each type of serum lipid. Primary exposure and outcome were the number of periodontal pathogens found in saliva, defined as the bacterial burden and the level of HDL, respectively. To understand the demographic, behavioral, and oral health-related factors in study participants according to bacterial type, we performed bivariate analyses of covariates, including age, sex, smoking, drinking, exercise, tooth brushing, dental flossing, periodontitis, number of existing teeth, and the DMFT (decayed, missing, and filled) index according to the 4 bacteria and burden level. For this, chi-square tests or t-tests were performed with SAS version 9.4 (SAS Institute Inc. Cary, NC, USA). The threshold for statistical significance was set at 0.05.

In terms of the operational definition of bacterial burden, the total bacterial burden of periodontal pathogenicity in this study was defined in cases in which the 4 types of periodontal bacteria were found in the saliva. A person was classified as having a high bacterial burden when all 4 bacteria were found in his/her saliva, which indicates a relatively higher exposure to periodontal pathogens. Therefore, the presence of a bacterial species scored 1 point for any of the 4 periodontal bacteria; exposure was considered as low (none of the 4 bacterial species present), moderate (presence of 1–3 bacterial species), or high (all bacterial species present) for statistical analyses.

In second step, to evaluate the crude association between the presence of periodontal bacteria and bacterial burden with periodontitis, and 4 types of serum lipid profiles, bivariate analyses were tested using t-test or one-way Analysis of Variance (ANOVA) with post hoc analysis. Bacterial pathogenicity was measured from not gingival crevicular fluid but stimulated saliva that is easier to quickly collect from many people. In addition, the saliva could include all bacteria originated from the whole periodontal sites of total teeth in mouth.

In order to measure the statistically independent strengths of the association of bacterial burden on lipids, general linear models (GLM) were constructed after adjustment for potential confounding variables, including age, sex, periodontitis, BMI, diabetes, hypertension, smoking,

drinking, exercise, tooth brushing, and dental flossing. To observe the change in effect size, confounders were added step by step into the models and the least square mean (LSM) values for lipid levels were also employed. Their p for trend values were tested as well. Lastly, LSMs were calculated again for the 6 groups categorized by bacterial strains and periodontitis after adjustment for age, sex, BMI, diabetes, hypertension, smoking, drinking, exercise, tooth brushing, and dental flossing for the combined effect on lipid level. The p for trend values were also determined.

Regarding of GLM analysis, the distribution of lipids variables was initially checked whether or not they were normal. The lipids were not normally distributed as a matter of fact so that they were transformed by square root, inverse square root, and natural log. The transformed results were compared to those of GLM. For preference of robust model, GLM analysis was finally selected. Normality test for outcomes, Shapiro-Wilk, Kolmogorov-Smirnov, Cramer-von Mises and Anderson-Darling tests were used for each 4 lipid type. And then the outcomes were transformed by square root, inverse square root, and natural log. The findings of GLM analysis in transformed data were compared to those in unconverted data (not shown).

Results

As shown in Table 2, we examined 385 Japanese study participants (176 men and 209 women, average age 69.2 years). Those with greater numbers of different species of periodontal bacteria were more likely to be a current or ex-smoker ($p = 0.05$) and had periodontitis ($p < 0.01$). Periodontitis group showed a tendency to possess all of the periodontal bacteria, while $P.$ $intermedia$ was more likely to be harbored by ex-smokers and a higher percentage of older people possessed $P.$ $gingivalis$.

Table 3 shows the crude associations between the periodontal bacteria and lipid levels. There were significant relationships between the average HDL level and the presence of each bacterium, except for $P.$ $gingivalis$, the presence of 4 bacteria, and the co-existence of bacteria and clinical periodontitis. Furthermore, the concentration of TG was shown to be significantly elevated along with the increase in the bacterial burden.

In multivariable analysis, the presence of all 4 bacterial species was negatively associated with HDL, after adjustment for clinically defined periodontitis and other potential confounding factors, as shown in Table 4 and Fig. 2. Adjusted mean HDL levels according to the bacterial burn group (low, moderate, and high) were significantly reduced (p for trend = 0.05) (Table 4). Co-existing periodontal bacteria and clinical periodontitis (periodontitis [−] and periodontitis [+]) was significantly related to decreased HDL (Fig. 2). The adjusted mean HDL levels in patients with a combination of periodontitis (−) and

Table 2 Characteristics of demographic, behavioral, and oral health-related factors according to bacterial type

Variable name	Total	Prevalence of periodontal bacteria								Periodontal pathogenic burden		
		P. gingivalis		T. denticola		T. forsythia		P. intermedia		Low	Moderate	High
		Yes	No	Yes	No	Yes	No	Yes	No			
	No. (%)											
Total	385 (100.0)	224(58.2)	161(41.8)	230(59.7)	155(40.3)	285(74.0)	100(26.0)	203(52.7)	182(47.3)	46(11.9)	230(59.7)	109(28.3)
Age (y)												
50–59	**51 (13.2)**	**20(8.9)**	**31 (19.3)**	30 (13.0)	21 (13.5)	37 (13.0)	14 (14.0)	27 (13.3)	24 (13.2)	5 (10.9)	39 (17.0)	7 (6.4)
60 –69	**108 (28.1)**	**64 (28.6)**	**44 (27.3)**	68 (29.6)	40 (25.8)	86 (30.2)	22 (22.0)	57 (28.1)	51 (28.0)	10 (21.7)	64 (27.8)	34 (31.2)
70–82	**226 (58.7)**	**140 (62.5)**	**86 (53.4)**	132 (57.4)	94 (60.6)	162 (56.8)	64 (64.0)	119 (58.6)	107 (58.8)	31 (67.4)	127 (55.2)	68 (62.4)
p-value		**0.01**		0.72		0.29		1.00		0.07		
Gender												
Male	176 (45.7)	108 (48.2)	68 (42.2)	106 (46.1)	70 (45.2)	136 (47.7)	40 (40.0)	98 (48.3)	78 (42.9)	16 (34.8)	107 (46.5)	53 (48.6)
Female	209 (54.3)	116 (51.8)	93 (57.8)	124 (53.9)	75 (54.8)	149 (52.3)	60 (60.0)	105 (51.7)	104 (57.1)	30 (65.2)	123 (53.5)	56 (51.4)
p-value		0.25		0.86		0.18		0.30		0.27		
Smoking												
Current	31 (8.1)	18 (9.2)	13 (9.1)	16 (7.7)	15 (11.5)	22 (8.6)	9 (10.8)	**15 (8.2)**	**16 (10.3)**	**2 (5.1)**	**23 (11.5)**	**6 (6.0)**
Former	100 (26.0)	64 (32.7)	36 (25.2)	67 (32.1)	33 (25.4)	82 (32.0)	18 (21.7)	**65 (35.5)**	**35 (22.4)**	**7 (17.9)**	**55 (27.5)**	**38 (38.0)**
Never	208 (54.0)	114 (58.2)	94 (65.7)	126 (60.3)	82 (63.1)	152 (59.4)	56 (67.5)	**103 (56.3)**	**105 (67.3)**	**30 (76.9)**	**122 (61.0)**	**56 (56.0)**
p-value		0.31		0.27		0.19		**0.03**		**0.05**		
Drinking												
Current	144 (37.4)	90 (45.9)	54 (37.8)	88 (42.1)	56 (43.1)	115 (44.9)	29 (34.9)	77 (42.1)	67 (42.9)	13 (33.3)	87 (43.5)	44 (44.0)
Former	19 (4.9)	11 (5.6)	8 (5.6)	13 (6.2)	6 (4.6)	14 (5.5)	5 (6.0)	9 (4.9)	10 (6.4)	2 (5.1)	12 (6.0)	5 (5.0)
Never	176 (54.0)	95 (48.5)	81 (56.6)	108 (51.7)	68 (52.3)	127 (49.6)	49 (59.0)	97 (53.0)	79 (50.6)	24 (61.5)	101 (50.5)	51 (51.0)
p-value		0.31		0.82		0.28		0.80		0.77		
Exercise (times/week)												
None	110 (28.6)	57 (29.2)	53 (37.1)	68 (32.7)	42 (32.3)	84 (32.9)	26 (31.3)	65 (35.7)	45 (28.8)	16 (41.0)	59 (29.5)	35 (35.4)
≤Twice	228 (59.2)	138 (70.8)	90 (62.9)	140 (67.3)	88 (67.7)	171 (67.1)	57 (68.7)	117 (64.3)	111 (71.2)	23 (59.0)	141 (70.5)	64 (64.6)
p-value		0.13		0.94		0.79		0.18		0.29		
Brushing frequency (times/day)												
Once	75 (19.5)	40 (21.1)	35 (26.7)	46 (22.5)	29 (24.8)	58 (23.4)	17 (23.3)	43 (23.9)	32 (22.7)	9 (28.1)	41 (21.6)	25 (25.3)
Twice	163 (42.3)	96 (50.5)	67 (51.1)	102 (50.0)	61 (52.1)	127 (51.2)	36 (49.3)	93 (51.7)	70 (49.6)	15 (46.9)	101 (53.2)	47 (47.5)
≥ 3 times	83 (21.6)	54 (28.4)	29 (22.1)	56 (27.5)	27 (23.1)	63 (25.4)	20 (27.4)	44 (24.4)	39 (27.7)	8 (25.0)	48 (25.3)	27 (27.3)
p-value		0.32		0.68		0.94		0.81		0.58		
Flossing frequency												

Table 2 Characteristics of demographic, behavioral, and oral health-related factors according to bacterial type *(Continued)*

Variable name	Total	Prevalence of periodontal bacteria								Periodontal pathogenic burden		
		P. gingivalis		T. denticola		T. forsythia		P. intermedia		Low	Moderate	High
		Yes	No	Yes	No	Yes	No	Yes	No			
None	142 (36.9)	80 (41.7)	62 (45.9)	93 (45.4)	49 (40.2)	109 (43.6)	33 (42.9)	81 (45.0)	61 (41.5)	16 (47.1)	78 (40.0)	48 (49.0)
≥ Once/week	55 (14.3)	35 (18.2)	20 (14.8)	29 (14.1)	26 (21.3)	43 (17.2)	12 (15.6)	28 (15.6)	27 (18.4)	5 (14.7)	37 (19.0)	13 (13.3)
≥ Once/day	130 (33.8)	77 (40.1)	53 (39.3)	83 (40.5)	47 (38.5)	98 (39.2)	32 (41.6)	71 (39.4)	59 (40.1)	13 (38.2)	80 (41.0)	37 (37.8)
p-value		0.64		0.24		0.91		0.73		0.85		
Periodontitis by CPI*												
Periodontitis(−)	**195 (54.2)**	**105 (48.8)**	**90 (62.1)**	**100 (44.4)**	**95 (70.4)**	**133 (48.5)**	**62 (72.1)**	**89 (45.2)**	**106 (65.0)**	**27 (75.0)**	**127 (58.5)**	**41 (38.3)**
Periodontitis(+)	**165 (45.8)**	**110 (51.2)**	**55 (37.9)**	**125 (55.6)**	**40 (29.6)**	**141 (51.5)**	**24 (27.9)**	**108 (54.8)**	**57 (35.0)**	**9 (25.0)**	**90 (41.5)**	**66 (61.7)**
p-value		**0.01**		**<.01**		**<.01**		**<.01**		**<.01**		
	mean ± sd											
Age (y)	69.2 ± 7.8	69.8 ± 7.2	68.4 ± 8.4	69.1 ± 7.9	69.3 ± 7.7	68.9 ± 7.8	70.1 ± 7.6	69.3 ± 7.8	69.1 ± 7.83	**71.0 ± 8.0[a]**	**68.3 ± 7.9[b]**	**70.3 ± 7.2[b]**
p-value		0.08		0.78		0.18		0.72		**0.05**		
CPI	1.7 ± 1.6	1.8 ± 1.6	1.5 ± 1.5	**2.1 ± 1.5**	**1.1 ± 1.5**	**1.9 ± 1.5**	**1.1 ± 1.5**	**2.0 ± 1.5**	**1.3 ± 1.5**	**1.0 ± 1.5[a]**	**1.6 ± 1.5[a]**	**2.2 ± 1.5[b]**
p-value		0.08		**<.01**		**<.01**		**<.01**		**<.01**		
No. of present teeth	20.9 ± 7.8	20.8 ± 7.1	21.1 ± 8.7	**21.7 ± 6.4**	**19.8 ± 9.4**	21.2 ± 7.1	20.1 ± 9.5	21.6 ± 6.8	20.1 ± 8.8	18.8 ± 11.0	21.2 ± 7.6	21.2 ± 6.5
p-value		0.70		**0.03**		0.32		0.06		0.22		
DFMT index	18.0 ± 7.1	18.1 ± 7.0	17.8 ± 7.2	18.2 ± 6.8	17.6 ± 7.4	18.1 ± 7.0	17.5 ± 7.1	17.7 ± 6.8	18.3 ± 7.4	18.1 ± 8.1	18.0 ± 6.8	17.9 ± 7.1
p-value		0.75		0.38		0.43		0.38		0.43		

Bold indicates statistical significance shown by chi-square test or t- test (*P-value* < 0.05). Total results for each variable may be different due to missing values
Means with the same letter (a and b) are not significantly different by Tukey test. *Community Periodontal Index

Table 3 Serum lipid profile due to presence of periodontal bacteria, total pathogenic burden, and periodontitis

Exposures	No. (%)	High-density lipoprotein mean ± SD	Triglycerides mean ± SD	Low-density lipoprotein mean ± SD	Total cholesterol mean ± SD
P. gingivalis					
Yes	196 (57.8)	60.7 ± 14.6	108.9 ± 64.9	123.3 ± 28.1	205.8 ± 30.4
No	143 (42.2)	63.0 ± 17.3	101.6 ± 50.7	120.0 ± 29.2	203.3 ± 32.8
p-value		0.21	0.26	0.30	0.47
T. denticola					
Yes	209 (61.7)	**59.8 ± 15.0**	110.1 ± 65.0	121.9 ± 27.0	203.7 ± 30.2
No	130 (38.3)	**64.8 ± 16.8**	98.9 ± 48.4	121.8 ± 31.1	206.4 ± 33.4
p-value		**0.00**	0.07	0.96	0.45
T. forsythia					
Yes	**256 (75.5)**	**60.7 ± 15.7**	**108.7 ± 64.3**	121.8 ± 28.5	204.3 ± 30.6
No	**83 (24.5)**	**64.7 ± 15.9**	**97.0 ± 39.5**	122.0 ± 28.9	206.0 ± 34.1
p-value		**0.05**	**0.05**	1.00	0.66
P. intermedia					
Yes	183 (54.0)	**59.9 ± 15.6**	110.6 ± 67.2	122.4 ± 27.5	204.4 ± 29.9
No	156 (46.0)	**63.9 ± 15.8**	100.3 ± 48.2	121.2 ± 29.8	205.1 ± 33.3
p-value		**0.02**	0.11	0.68	0.84
Periodontal pathogenic burden					
Low	39 (11.5)	**66.2 ± 16.1a**	97.1 ± 44.3	124.1 ± 27.7	209.7 ± 30.2
Moderate	200 (59.0)	**63.3 ± 16.2a**	102.1 ± 51.9	119.7 ± 29.5	203.4 ± 32.8
High	100 (29.5)	**56.7 ± 13.8b**	116.8 ± 75.4	125.3 ± 26.9	204.7 ± 31.4
p-value		**<.01**	0.08	0.19	0.51
Groups based on combination of bacterial burden and periodontitis					
Periodontitis(−) and low	27 (7.0)	**69.5 ± 15.4[a]**	**89.6 ± 43.8 [a]**	128.8 ± 31.2	216.1 ± 30.5
Periodontitis(−) and moderate	127 (33.0)	**64.9 ± 16.0[a]**	**91.9 ± 41.0 [a]**	119.4 ± 28.7	202.7 ± 30.7
Periodontitis(−) and high	41 (10.6)	**64.1 ± 13.1[a]**	**92.5 ± 39.7[a]**	123.8 ± 19.3	206.4 ± 22.3
Periodontitis(+) and low	9 (2.3)	**63.4 ± 13.1[a]**	**107.0 ± 49.1[a]**	112.7 ± 16.4	197.5 ± 28.4
Periodontitis(+) and moderate	90 (23.4)	**61.9 ± 16.6[ab]**	**113.8 ± 63.2[ab]**	118.4 ± 31.0	203.0 ± 35.6
Periodontitis(+) and high	66 (17.1)	**52.8 ± 12.7[b]**	**131.5 ± 87.1[b]**	125.8 ± 30.7	204.8 ± 32.95
p-value		**<.01**	**<.01**	0.38	0.52

P-values by ANOVA test or t- test. Means with the same letter (a and b) are not significantly different by Tukey test

bacterial burden (low, moderate, and high) and periodontitis (+) with the presence of bacterial species (low, moderate, and high) were decreased (*p* for trend < 0.5), while TG levels in those groups showed a trend to increase (*p* for trend < 0.5) as shown in Fig. 3. In reference to transformed lipids analysis, the final results were similar to those shown in Figs. 2 and 3, even though the estimated mean values were slightly different (not shown).

When HDL, as a main outcome, was used for calculation with the group means of bacterial burden, the power of this study exceeded 0.80 as the sample size ranged from 212 to 556 in two-sided tests (not shown).

Discussion

Periodontal health and disease status have not been viewed in the context of a single periodontal pathogen, such as *P. gingivalis*, but rather in terms of the total pathogenicity of a biofilm [25]. The accumulated total burden of the harbored bacterial species has been suggested to complicate the bacterial community and is involved in the microbial shift from symbiosis to dysbiosis [26]. In the present study, persons who harbored all of the 4 different species showed poor HDL values after adjustment for clinically defined periodontitis and other potential behavioral factors. Additionally, the combination of harboring periodontal bacteria and periodontitis

Table 4 Means of serum lipids by periodontal pathogenic burden using multivariable GLM models

| | Means of serum lipids | | | | | |
| | Model 1 | | Model 2 | | Model 3 | |
	MEAN ± SD	LSM	MEAN ± SD	LSM	MEAN ± SD	LSM
High-density lipoprotein (mg/dL)						
Periodontal pathogenic burden						
Low	**66.2 ± 16.1**	65.4	**68.1 ± 14.9**	66.4	**68.1 ± 14.9**	66.1
Moderate	**63.3 ± 16.2**	63.4	**63.6 ± 16.3**	63.1	**63.5 ± 16.3**	63.0
High	**56.7 ± 13.8**	56.9	**56.8 ± 13.9**	58.2	**57.3 ± 13.8**	58.9
	P for trend > 0.05		P for trend = 0.07		P for trend = 0.05	
	Adjusted $R^2 = 0.10$		Adjusted $R^2 = 0.18$		Adjusted $R^2 = 0.19$	
Triglycerides (mg/dL)						
Periodontal pathogenic burden						
Low	97.1 ± 44.3	100.6	93.6 ± 44.8	100.0	93.6 ± 44.8	101.0
Moderate	102.1 ± 51.9	101.4	101.5 ± 52.7	102.9	101.8 ± 53.1	103.7
High	116.8 ± 75.4	116.8	117.6 ± 75.8	112.9	115.9 ± 76.1	109.6
	P for trend > 0.05		P for trend > 0.05		P for trend > 0.05	
	Adjusted $R^2 = 0.05$		Adjusted $R^2 = 0.12$		Adjusted $R^2 = 0.14$	
Low-density lipoprotein (mg/dL)						
Periodontal pathogenic burden						
Low	124.1 ± 27.7	123.4	125.1 ± 29.1	123.5	125.1 ± 29.1	122.9
Moderate	119.7 ± 29.5	119.6	119.0 ± 29.7	118.9	119.5 ± 29.8	119.3
High	125.3 ± 26.9	125.8	125.1 ± 27.1	125.7	124.9 ± 27.6	126.0
	P for trend > 0.05		P for trend > 0.05		P for trend > 0.05	
	Adjusted $R^2 = 0.14$		Adjusted $R^2 = 0.03$		Adjusted $R^2 = 0.03$	
Total Cholesterol (mg/dL)						
Periodontal pathogenic burden						
Low	209.7 ± 30.2	208.9	211.9 ± 30.6	209.9	211.9 ± 30.6	209.2
Moderate	203.4 ± 32.8	203.2	202.8 ± 32.9	202.6	203.3 ± 32.8	203.1
High	205.4 ± 29.2	206.1	205.5 ± 29.5	206.5	205.4 ± 30.1	206.8
	P for trend > 0.05		P for trend > 0.05		P for trend > 0.05	
	Adjusted $R^2 = 0.04$		Adjusted $R^2 = 0.03$		Adjusted $R^2 = 0.02$	

Model 1: Adjusted for age and gender, Model 2: Additionally adjusted for periodontitis, BMI, diabetes, and hypertension, Model 3: Additionally adjusted for smoking, drinking, exercise, tooth brushing, and dental flossing
Bold indicates statistical significance ($p < 0.05$)

on decreased HDL and increased TG showed significant trends. Our results provide important epidemiological evidence that the accumulated burden of periodontal bacteria from saliva can independently affect regulation of HDL and TG levels, which are critical risk factors for atherosclerotic diseases, regardless of periodontitis. Such findings have not been reported previously, even though it has been shown that the presence of periodontitis, as defined by typical clinical measures, can contribute to a decrease in serum HDL and increase in TG [14, 27, 28], as well as to the development of atherosclerosis-related cardiovascular disease [29].

Interest in the role of the total periodontal bacterial burden, rather than that of a specific pathogen, in development of cardiovascular disease has emerged from studies reporting only one or two periodontal bacteria in relation to the occurrence of atherogenesis [30] and coronary heart disease [31]. Several recent case–control studies [32–35] and a cohort study [1] have investigated the role of co-existing major periodontal bacteria in a cardiovascular disease event, and their findings have suggested that a higher inflammatory burden of periodontal bacteria could elevate the risk of stroke, myocardial infarction, and coronary artery disease.

In addition to the importance of the impact of bacterial exposure on the development of cardiovascular diseases as an end-point health outcome, it is vital to highlight biomarkers associated with atherosclerosis medication, such

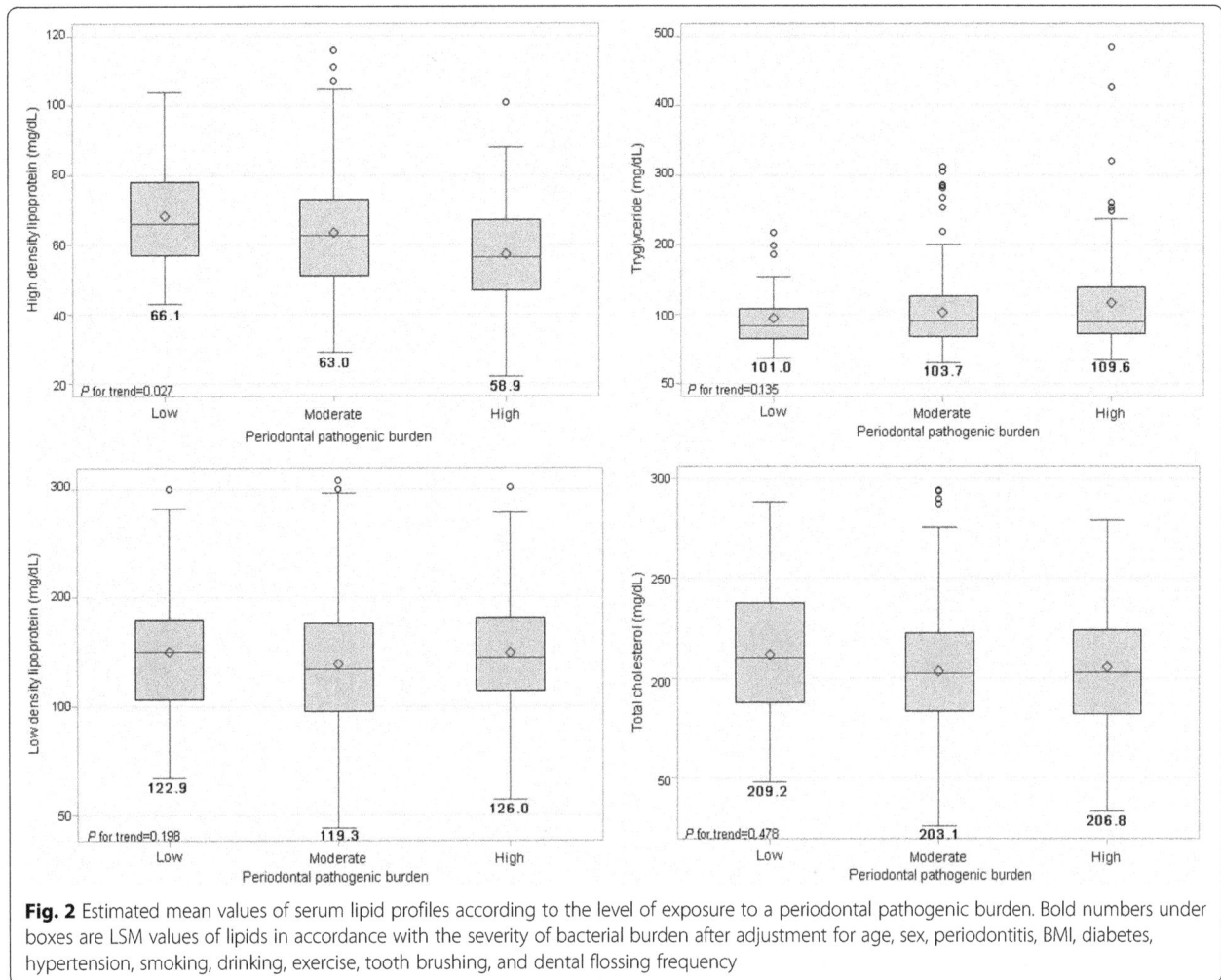

Fig. 2 Estimated mean values of serum lipid profiles according to the level of exposure to a periodontal pathogenic burden. Bold numbers under boxes are LSM values of lipids in accordance with the severity of bacterial burden after adjustment for age, sex, periodontitis, BMI, diabetes, hypertension, smoking, drinking, exercise, tooth brushing, and dental flossing frequency

as serum lipid profiles, to gain a better understanding on how infection and/or inflammation induced by periodontal bacteria play a role in altering lipid metabolism. Previous reports have noted that patients with periodontitis diagnosed based on clinical parameters have a risk of dyslipidemia, such as decreased HDL, increased TG, and increased LDL [27, 29, 36]. In addition, control of periodontal inflammation by standard treatment was shown to improve HDL and LDL levels [37], and findings of a recent meta-analysis [38] indicated that periodontal treatment enhanced the levels of atherosclerotic biomarkers, including HDL, TG, and TC.

The present findings provide evidence suggesting that the total inflammation burden induced by exposure to major periodontal bacteria could induce dyslipidemia by lowering HDL and possibly increasing TG, after adjustment for periodontitis as a clinical parameter. The mean differences in HDL lowered by bacterial burden seem to be clinically small; thus, the effect of the oral pathogenic burden on low HDL or hyper-triglycerides beyond the normal range is unclear. However, we could not ignore

this independent, albeit small effect from exposure to oral infection or inflammation, which may trigger the development of dyslipidemia and even atherosclerosis in individuals harboring several risk factors [14, 29]. A recent cross-sectional study [13] reported that the presence of *A. actinomycetemcomitans* and *P. gingivalis* reduced the plasma level of HDL, while another study [39], which used a scoring method for 3 pathogen antibodies, combined with herpes simplex virus, showed association with decreased HDL. In a Japanese prospective study [40], increased tooth brushing frequency caused improvement in hypertriglyceridemia. Consistent with the findings from previous studies, our findings established that inflammation related to oral bacteria contributes to deterioration of the lipid metabolic pathway, although some evidence regarding this association remains lacking. Nevertheless, an important strength of this study is empirical evidence showing a connection between the total burden of exposure to *P. intermedia*, *P. gingivalis*, *T. denticola*, and *T. forsythia*, detected from stimulated saliva, with decreased HDL and a trend for

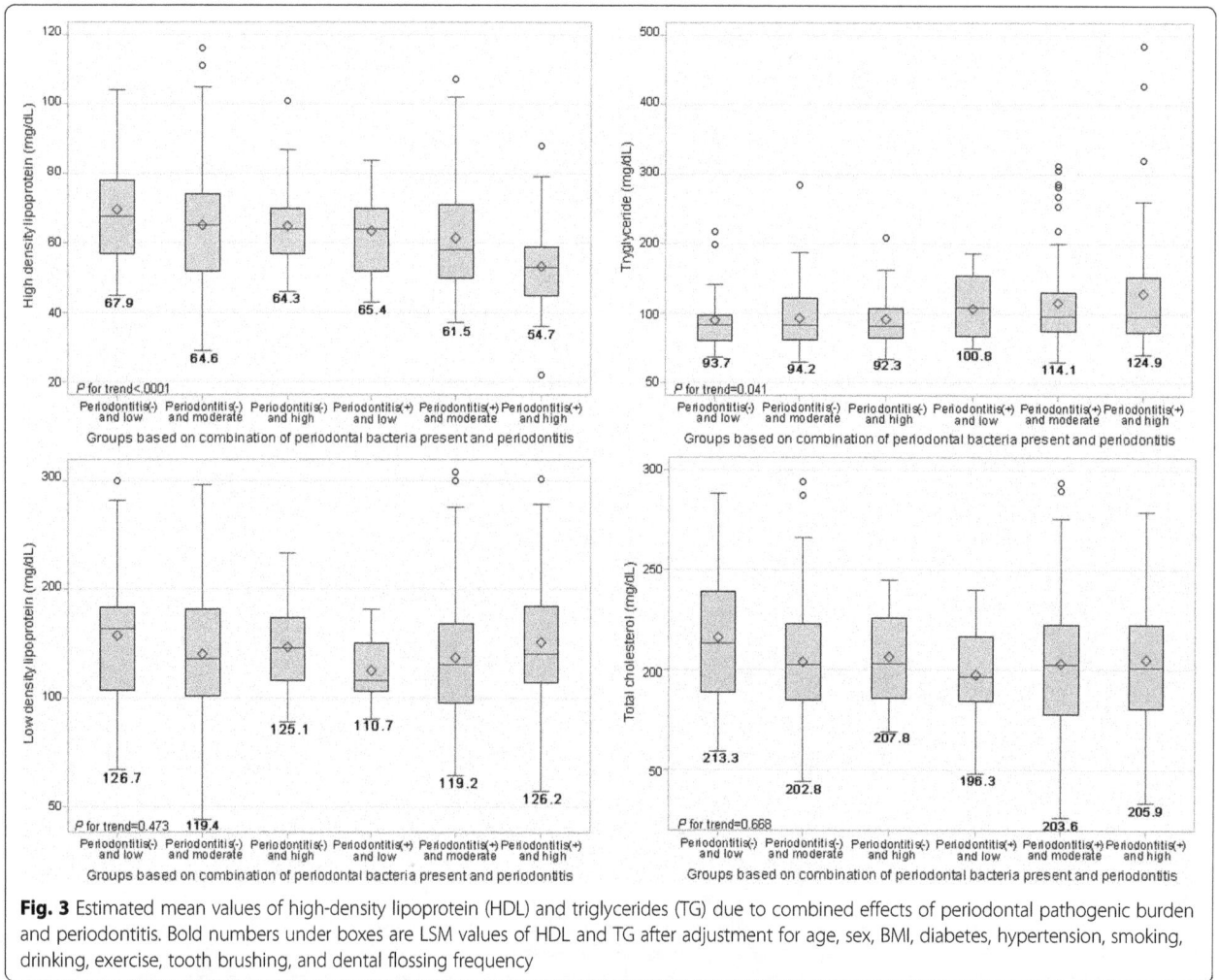

Fig. 3 Estimated mean values of high-density lipoprotein (HDL) and triglycerides (TG) due to combined effects of periodontal pathogenic burden and periodontitis. Bold numbers under boxes are LSM values of HDL and TG after adjustment for age, sex, BMI, diabetes, hypertension, smoking, drinking, exercise, tooth brushing, and dental flossing frequency

increasing TG in serum. Saliva seems to be the sample most readily obtainable from a number of subjects, and the bacterial burden, which can deflect the metabolic pathway, must be sufficient for bacterial detection in saliva (even though plaque specimens are a better medium for sensitive bacterial detection) [18, 24].

In this study, we exploited GLM models, with calculation of LSMs, although the level of lipids was not normally distributed, as we were concerned about the major limitation of transformed data (lack of a real value, which makes it difficult to interpret). We assume that the 4 lipid values were normally distributed, because the distribution of the lipids in the general population is normal and, furthermore, the implication of such a robust model is easier to understand.

This study had some limitations. Since it was cross-sectional in nature, we were not able to examine the causal relationship between exposure and outcome, and the interplay between periodontal inflammation and lipid dysregulation via host response reaction is complex. To improve our understanding of the role of the oral

bacterial burden in lipid metabolism, well-designed studies, such as prospective or randomized controlled trials, are needed to verify these results. On the other hand, the sample size of this study was small, as the sample size calculation was implemented after the study had been finished, rather than prior to commencement, as this was an exploratory study. Based on the results of this study, statistical power was confirmed using final sample size whether the power was at least 0.80 or not. In addition, this study focused on only 4 primary bacterial species related to periodontitis, originating from gingival pockets. Nevertheless, other bacterial species have been found to be associated with the risk of systemic disease [12]; for this reason, pathogenic burden levels were classified as low, moderate, or high, instead of 0, 1–3, and 4. Despite this disadvantage, the present results suggest that a clinical bacterial test for the 4 well-known periodontal bacteria could be useful for screening patients with a greater risk of serum lipid profile deterioration and development of atherosclerotic disease. It is possible that oral microorganisms interact with each other; thus, each organism should be quantified to assess the individual contribution to the total pathogenic burden and modification of lipid metabolism. Moreover, no information was obtained about changed host responses, such as inflammatory serum cytokines, induced by periodontal infection and that resulted in lipid metabolic modification. Other variables may also not have been assessed, even though some crucial potential confounders were adjusted for in our statistical models. For instance, reduced chewing ability related to low number of remain teeth affects proper mastication, which also influences lipids metabolism negatively considering inclusion criteria (10 teeth and more in mouth). Finally, generalization of the study results may be limited, as only a small number of elderly Japanese persons living a metropolitan area were examined in this study. Further studies that consider host metabolic dysfunction after exposure to major periodontal pathogens, and that also include various populations, as well as the general population of Japan, with larger sample sizes, are necessary.

Conclusions

The results of this research suggest that a higher burden of bacteria was independently associated with lower HDL in serum after adjustment for periodontitis and other potential risk factors. This could show a possible link between exposure to major periodontal bacteria, in terms of the total burden, and increased risk of dysregulation of serum lipid metabolism. Furthermore, screening for the presence of periodontal bacteria could be beneficial to detect lipid changes earlier than atherogenesis, thus reducing the risk for development of atherosclerotic disease. Future studies that provide additional evidence about these issues are needed.

Abbreviations

A. actionomycetemconitans: Aggregatibacter actinomycetemcomitans; ANOVA: Oneway Analysis of Variance; BMI: Body mass index; CPI: Community Periodontal Index; DBP: Diastolic blood pressure; DMFT: Decayed, Missing, and Filled Teeth; GLM: General linear models; HDL: High-density lipoprotein; LDL: Low-density lipoprotein; LSM: Least square mean; *P. gingivalis: Porphyromonas gingivalis; P. intermedia: Prevotella intermedia*; PCR: Polymerase Chain Reaction; SBP: Systolic blood pressure; *T. denticola: Treponema denticola; T. forsythia: Tannerella forsythia*; TC: Total cholesterol; TG: Triglycerides

Acknowledgements

The authors thank 5 dentists (Yoko Yoshimuta, Kayoko Takemura, Momoyo Kida, Takayuki Kosaka, and Miki Kikui) who had conducted oral examination for this study in Department of Prosthodontics, Gerontology and Oral rehabilitation, Osaka University Graduate School of Dentistry.

Funding

This work was supported by a Grant-in-Aid (A) (262530940) from the Japan Society for the Promotion of Science, Tokyo, Japan, and a grant from the "Challenge to Intractable Oral Diseases" Project of Osaka University Graduate School of Dentistry, Suita-Osaka, Japan.

Authors' contributions

YHC and AA contributed to statistical analysis, data interpretation, and manuscript drafting and revision. TK, MO, and SS had been involved in acquisition of data. YK, MW, and YM constructed study design and preliminary statistical analysis. TO contributed to drafting and advice for revisions of manuscript. All authors read and approved the final manuscript.

Competing interest

The authors declare that they have no competing interests.

Author details

[1]Department of Preventive Dentistry, School of Dentistry, Kyungpook National University, Daegu, Republic of Korea. [2]Department of Prosthodontics, Gerontology and Oral Rehabilitation, Osaka University Graduate School of Dentistry, Suita-Osaka, Japan. [3]Department of Preventive Dentistry, Osaka University Graduate School of Dentistry, 1-8 Yamadaoka, Suita-Osaka 565-0871, Japan. [4]Department of Preventive Cardiology, National Cerebral and Cardiovascular Center, Suita-Osaka, Japan. [5]Division of Comprehensive Prosthodontics, Niigata University Graduate School of Medical and Dental Sciences, Niigata, Japan.

References

1. Andriankaja O, Trevisan M, Falkner K, Dorn J, Hovey K, Sarikonda S, Mendoza T, Genco R. Association between periodontal pathogens and risk of nonfatal myocardial infarction. Community Dent Oral Epidemiol. 2011;39(2):177–85.
2. Desvarieux M, Demmer RT, Jacobs DR, Papapanou PN, Sacco RL, Rundek T. Changes in clinical and microbiological periodontal profiles relate to progression of carotid intima-media thickness: the oral infections and vascular disease epidemiology study. J Am Heart Assoc. 2013;2(6):e000254.
3. Seymour GJ, Ford PJ, Cullinan MP, Leishman S, West MJ, Yamazaki K. Infection or inflammation: the link between periodontal and cardiovascular diseases. Futur Cardiol. 2009;5(1):5–9.
4. Choi YH, McKeown RE, Mayer-Davis EJ, Liese AD, Song KB, Merchant AT. Association between periodontitis and impaired fasting glucose and diabetes. Diabetes Care. 2011;34(2):381–6.
5. Humphrey LL, Fu R, Buckley DI, Freeman M, Helfand M. Periodontal disease and coronary heart disease incidence: a systematic review and meta-analysis. J Gen Intern Med. 2008;23(12):2079–86.
6. Socransky SS, Haffajee AD. Periodontal microbial ecology. Periodontol. 2005; 2000(38):135–87.
7. Furuichi Y, Shimotsu A, Ito H, Namariyama Y, Yotsumoto Y, Hino Y, Mishige Y, Inoue M, Izumi Y. Associations of periodontal status with general health conditions and serum antibody titers for Porphyromonas gingivalis and Actinobacillus actinomycetemcomitans. J Periodontol. 2003;74(10):1491–7.
8. Hanaoka Y, Soejima H, Yasuda O, Nakayama H, Nagata M, Matsuo K, Shinohara M, Izumi Y, Ogawa H. Level of serum antibody against a periodontal pathogen is associated with atherosclerosis and hypertension. Hypertens Res. 2013;36(9):829–33.
9. Pussinen PJ, Alfthan G, Rissanen H, Reunanen A, Asikainen S, Knekt P. Antibodies to periodontal pathogens and stroke risk. Stroke. 2004;35(9):2020–3.
10. Spahr A, Klein E, Khuseyinova N, Boeckh C, Muche R, Kunze M, Rothenbacher D, Pezeshki G, Hoffmeister A, Koenig W. Periodontal infections and coronary heart disease: role of periodontal bacteria and importance of total pathogen burden in the coronary event and periodontal disease (CORODONT) study. Arch Intern Med. 2006;166(5):554–9.
11. Kebschull M, Demmer RT, Papapanou PN. "gum bug, leave my heart alone!"–epidemiologic and mechanistic evidence linking periodontal infections and atherosclerosis. J Dent Res. 2010;89(9):879–902.

12. Shrestha D, Choi YH, Zhang J, Hazlett LJ, Merchant AT. Relationship between serologic markers of periodontal bacteria and metabolic syndrome and its components. J Periodontol. 2015;86(3):418–30.

13. Jaramillo A, Lafaurie GI, Millan LV, Ardila CM, Duque A, Novoa C, Lopez D, Contreras A. Association between periodontal disease and plasma levels of cholesterol and triglycerides. Colomb Med (Cali). 2013;44(2):80–6.

14. Feingold KR, Grunfeld C. The effect of inflammation and infection on lipids and lipoproteins. In: De Groot LJ, Beck-Peccoz P, Chrousos G, Dungan K, Grossman A, Hershman JM, Koch C, McLachlan R, New M, Rebar R, et al., editors. Endotext. South Dartmouth: MDText.com, Inc; 2000. https://www.ncbi.nlm.nih.gov/books/NBK326741.

15. Morimoto Y, Nakatani T, Yokoe C, Kudo C, Hanamoto H, Niwa H. Haemostatic management for oral surgery in patients supported with left ventricular assist device–a preliminary retrospective study. Br J Oral Maxillofac Surg. 2015;53(10):991–5.

16. Kokubo Y, Kamide K, Okamura T, Watanabe M, Higashiyama A, Kawanishi K, Okayama A, Kawano Y. Impact of high-normal blood pressure on the risk of cardiovascular disease in a Japanese urban cohort: the Suita study. Hypertension. 2008;52(4):652–9.

17. Jensen JL, Karatsaidis A, Brodin P. Salivary secretion: stimulatory effects of chewing-gum versus paraffin tablets. Eur J Oral Sci. 1998;106(4):892–6.

18. Ashimoto A, Chen C, Bakker I, Slots J. Polymerase chain reaction detection of 8 putative periodontal pathogens in subgingival plaque of gingivitis and advanced periodontitis lesions. Oral Microbiol Immunol. 1996;11(4):266–73.

19. Kuboniwa M, Amano A, Kimura KR, Sekine S, Kato S, Yamamoto Y, Okahashi N, Iida T, Shizukuishi S. Quantitative detection of periodontal pathogens using real-time polymerase chain reaction with TaqMan probes. Oral Microbiol Immunol. 2004;19(3):168–76.

20. Tran SD, Rudney JD. Multiplex PCR using conserved and species-specific 16S rRNA gene primers for simultaneous detection of Actinobacillus actinomycetemcomitans and Porphyromonas gingivalis. J Clin Microbiol. 1996;34(11):2674–8.

21. Watanabe K, Frommel TO. Porphyromonas gingivalis, Actinobacillus actinomycetemcomitans and Treponema denticola detection in oral plaque samples using the polymerase chain reaction. J Clin Periodontol. 1996;23(3 Pt 1):212–9.

22. World Health Organization. Oral health surveys: basic methods. 4th ed. Switzerland: Geneva; 1997.

23. Iwashima Y, Kokubo Y, Ono T, Yoshimuta Y, Kida M, Kosaka T, Maeda Y, Kawano Y, Miyamoto Y. Additive interaction of oral health disorders on risk of hypertension in a Japanese urban population: the Suita study. Am J Hypertens. 2014;27(5):710–9.

24. Kosaka T, Kokubo Y, Ono T, Sekine S, Kida M, Kikui M, Yamamoto M, Watanabe M, Amano A, Maeda Y, et al. Salivary inflammatory cytokines may be novel markers of carotid atherosclerosis in a Japanese general population: the Suita study. Atherosclerosis. 2014;237(1):123–8.

25. Hajishengallis G, Lamont RJ. Beyond the red complex and into more complexity: the polymicrobial synergy and dysbiosis (PSD) model of periodontal disease etiology. Mol Oral Microbiol. 2012;27(6):409–19.

26. Berezow AB, Darveau RP. Microbial shift and periodontitis. Periodontol. 2011;55(1):36–47.

27. Penumarthy S, Penmetsa GS, Mannem S. Assessment of serum levels of triglycerides, total cholesterol, high-density lipoprotein cholesterol, and low-density lipoprotein cholesterol in periodontitis patients. J Indian Soc Periodontol. 2013;17(1):30–5.

28. Pussinen PJ, Jauhiainen M, Vilkuna-Rautiainen T, Sundvall J, Vesanen M, Mattila K, Palosuo T, Alfthan G, Asikainen S. Periodontitis decreases the antiatherogenic potency of high density lipoprotein. J Lipid Res. 2004;45(1):139–47.

29. Schenkein HA, Loos BG. Inflammatory mechanisms linking periodontal diseases to cardiovascular diseases. J Periodontol. 2013;84(4 Suppl):S51–69.

30. Honda T, Oda T, Yoshie H, Yamazaki K. Effects of Porphyromonas gingivalis antigens and proinflammatory cytokines on human coronary artery endothelial cells. Oral Microbiol Immunol. 2005;20(2):82–8.

31. Matthews D. Possible link between periodontal disease and coronary heart disease. Evid Based Dent. 2008;9(1):8.

32. Hyvarinen K, Laitinen S, Paju S, Hakala A, Suominen-Taipale L, Skurnik M, Kononen E, Pussinen PJ. Detection and quantification of five major periodontal pathogens by single copy gene-based real-time PCR. Innate Immun. 2009;15(4):195–204.

33. Hyvarinen K, Mantyla P, Buhlin K, Paju S, Nieminen MS, Sinisalo J, Pussinen PJ. A common periodontal pathogen has an adverse association with both acute and stable coronary artery disease. Atherosclerosis. 2012;223(2):478–84.

34. Leishman SJ, Ford PJ, Do HL, Palmer JE, Heng NC, West MJ, Seymour GJ, Cullinan MP. Periodontal pathogen load and increased antibody response to heat shock protein 60 in patients with cardiovascular disease. J Clin Periodontol. 2012;39(10):923–30.

35. Palm F, Lahdentausta L, Sorsa T, Tervahartiala T, Gokel P, Buggle F, Safer A, Becher H, Grau AJ, Pussinen P. Biomarkers of periodontitis and inflammation in ischemic stroke: a case-control study. Innate Immun. 2014;20(5):511–8.

36. Rufail ML, Schenkein HA, Koertge TE, Best AM, Barbour SE, Tew JG, van Antwerpen R. Atherogenic lipoprotein parameters in patients with aggressive periodontitis. J Periodontal Res. 2007;42(6):495–502.

37. Buhlin K, Hultin M, Norderyd O, Persson L, Pockley AG, Pussinen PJ, Rabe P, Klinge B, Gustafsson A. Periodontal treatment influences risk markers for atherosclerosis in patients with severe periodontitis. Atherosclerosis. 2009;206(2):518–22.

38. Teeuw WJ, Slot DE, Susanto H, Gerdes VE, Abbas F, D'Aiuto F, Kastelein JJ, Loos BG. Treatment of periodontitis improves the atherosclerotic profile: a systematic review and meta-analysis. J Clin Periodontol. 2014;41(1):70–9.

39. Vilkuna-Rautiainen T, Pussinen PJ, Roivainen M, Petays T, Jousilahti P, Hovi T, Vartiainen E, Asikainen S. Serum antibody response to periodontal pathogens and herpes simplex virus in relation to classic risk factors of cardiovascular disease. Int J Epidemiol. 2006;35(6):1486–94.

40. Kobayashi Y, Niu K, Guan L, Momma H, Guo H, Cui Y, Nagatomi R. Oral health behavior and metabolic syndrome and its components in adults. J Dent Res. 2012;91(5):479–84.

4

A retrospective study on molar furcation assessment via clinical detection, intraoral radiography and cone beam computed tomography

Wenjian Zhang[1]* (iD), Keagan Foss[2] and Bing-Yan Wang[3]

Abstract

Background: Accurate determination of bone loss at the molar furcation region by clinical detection and intraoral radiograph is challenging in many instances. Cone beam computed tomography (CBCT) is expected to open a new horizon in periodontal assessment. The purpose of this study was to compare and correlate accuracy of molar furcation assessment via clinical detection, intraoral radiography and CBCT images.

Methods: Eighty-three patients with chronic periodontitis who had existing CBCT scans were included. Furcation involvement was assessed on maxillary and mandibular first molars. Periodontal charts (modified Glickman's classification), intraoral (periapical and/or bitewing) radiographs (recorded as presence or absence) and axial CBCT reconstructions were used to evaluate furcation involvement on buccal and palatal/lingual sites. The correlation of furcation assessment by the three methods was evaluated by Pearson analysis.

Results: There were significant correlations ($p < 0.05$) between clinical detection and intraoral radiography, clinical detection and CBCT, as well as intraoral radiography and CBCT at all the measured sites (r values range between 0.230 to 0.644). CBCT generally exhibited higher correlation with clinical detection relative to intraoral radiography, especially at distal palatal side of maxillary first molar ($p < 0.05$). In addition, CBCT provided more accurate assessment, with bone loss measurement up to 2 decimals in millimeters, whereas clinical detection had 3 classes and the intraoral radiographs usually only detected the presence of furcation involvement in Glickman Class 2 and 3.

Conclusions: This study validates that CBCT is a valuable tool in molar furcation assessment in addition to clinical detection and intraoral radiography.

Keywords: Furcation involvement, Clinical detection, Intraoral radiography, CBCT

Background

Furcation involvement (FI) refers to the condition when periodontal disease has caused bone resorption into the bifurcation or trifurcation of a multi-rooted tooth [1]. Dentists commonly encounter the difficulty of accurately assessing molars with FI, due to limited physical access, morphological variations and measurement errors [2–4]. Any discrepancies between pre-and intra-surgical findings of FI may lead to alterations of surgical treatment

plan [5] and unanticipated treatment costs (financially and temporally) [6]. Therefore, management of FI has presented as one of the greatest challenges to the success of periodontal therapy [7].

Traditionally, FI is assessed with a combination of clinical detection and intraoral radiographs [8]. Clinically, FI is evaluated with a Nabers probe, and categorized according to Glickman's or Hamp's classification system based on horizontal bone loss at the furcation area [9, 10]. However, the accuracy of clinical detection largely depends on operator technique, and many times, the measurement is reflective of penetration depth into the inflamed connective tissue, instead of the actual depth of the inter-radicular

* Correspondence: Wenjian.Zhang@uth.tmc.edu
[1]Department of Diagnostic & Biomedical Sciences, University of Texas School of Dentistry at Houston, 7500 Cambridge Street, Houston, TX 77054, USA
Full list of author information is available at the end of the article

bony defect [11]. In addition, factors such as tooth position, inclination, root morphology, length of root trunk, degree of root separation and configuration of residual inter-radicular bone, all affect accuracy of clinical furcation assessment [12, 13]. Periapical (PA) or bitewing (BW) radiographs are commonly used intraoral projections to supplement clinical detection for furcation assessment [8, 14]. These 2D imaging are generally considered to have low sensitivity but high specificity for furcation detection, mainly due to inherent shortcomings of 2D projections, such as superimposition and angulation problems [15]. Detectability of early FI by intraoral radiographs is especially limited and inconsistent [16].

Cone beam computed tomography (CBCT) is capable of generating accurate and reliable submillimeter-resolution images in all spatial dimensions, with cost and absorbed doses much lower than conventional CT [17, 18]. The applications of CBCT in dentistry are increasing rapidly, including in periodontology [19, 20]. CBCT is expected to reveal marginal bone contours as well as infrabony and furcation defects [21], therefore plays a role in the assessment and treatment planning of molars with FI. Currently, there are limited studies comparing diagnostic accuracy of FI by clinical detection, intraoral radiography and CBCT [12, 22, 23]. The aim of the present study was to compare and correlate assessment of molar FI via these three methods, to help further develop evidence on the applicability of CBCT in molar FI assessment.

Methods

Subjects

An Institutional Review Board (IRB) approval was granted prior to the start of the study (HSC-DB-17-0370). The patients who visited the University of Texas School of Dentistry at Houston dental clinic from 2012 to 2016 were retrospectively screened according to the selection criteria. The inclusion criteria were: 1) subject was diagnosed as having generalized moderate or severe chronic periodontitis; 2) subject had comprehensive periodontal examination and information had been stored in the school's Electronic Health Record (EHR); 3) subject had diagnostic quality periapical and/or bitewing radiographs covering posterior dentition; 4) subject had diagnostic quality CBCT scan with coverage of entire maxilla and mandible. Majority of the patients had CBCT scans for implant treatment planning purpose, and the time interval between periodontal clinical exam and CBCT scan was less than 3 months. All of the patients who met the inclusion criteria were included in the study, and their first molars of maxilla and mandible bilaterally were assessed according to the following methods.

Intraoral radiographic acquisition

All the intraoral radiographs were acquired with Focus wall-mounted unit (Instrumentarium Dental, Charlotte,

NC, USA). The unit was operated at 70 peak kilovolt (kVp), 7 mA (mA), and an exposure time corresponding to the exposed area. All the radiographs were taken with XCP receptor-holding devices (Dentsply Rinn, Elgin, IL, USA) and the paralleling technique. Photostimulable phosphor (PSP) plates (Air Techniques, Melville, NY, USA) were utilized as the receptor, and were scanned with the Scan-X Intraoral scanner (Air Techniques) after exposure. The images were stored in the EHR of the School of Dentistry, displayed on a 19-in. flat panel screen (HP Development Company, Palo Alto, CA, USA) with a 1920 X 1080 pixel resolution, and observed under a dimly lit environment.

CBCT imaging acquisition

All of the CBCT scans were taken at the Imaging Clinic of University of Texas School of Dentistry at Houston. The included scans covered maxillary and mandibular arches with a field of view (FOV) of 150×90 mm^2. The scans were acquired at 90 kVp, 10 mA, 16 s and a 0.2 mm^3 voxel size with a Kodak 9500 unit (Carestream Health, Inc., Rochester, NY, USA). CBCT images were reconstructed with Anatomage Invivo 5 software (Anatomage Inc., San Jose, CA, USA) at 1 mm thickness. All images were viewed on the same monitor and environment as the intraoral radiographs.

Comprehensive periodontal evaluation

Clinical periodontal assessment

All subjects had comprehensive periodontal examination by the pre-doctoral dental students under the supervision and approval of a periodontal faculty. The evaluation included an assessment of molar furcation involvement according to modified Glickman's classification [10] (Fig. 1). Briefly, this classification was defined as: Class I, incipient or early stage of furcation involvement, bone destruction is less than 2 mm into the furca; Class II, horizontal bone destruction extending deeper than 2 mm but less than 6 mm into the furca; Class III, horizontal bone destructions communicate between furcae of the tooth, and result in a through-and-through tunnel.

Intraoral radiographic assessment

First molar furcation status was evaluated on molar PA and/or BW radiographs. Presence of triangular radiolucency at the furcation area, and/or alveolar bone level was observed below furcation were radiographic signs for FI. FI was recorded as presence or absence based on the intraoral radiographs (Fig. 2).

CBCT imaging measurements

First molar furcation assessment was conducted mainly on reconstructed CBCT sagittal and axial views. Presence of FI was demonstrated as loss of trabecular bone

Fig. 1 Periodontal chart demonstrates classification of molar furcation involvement

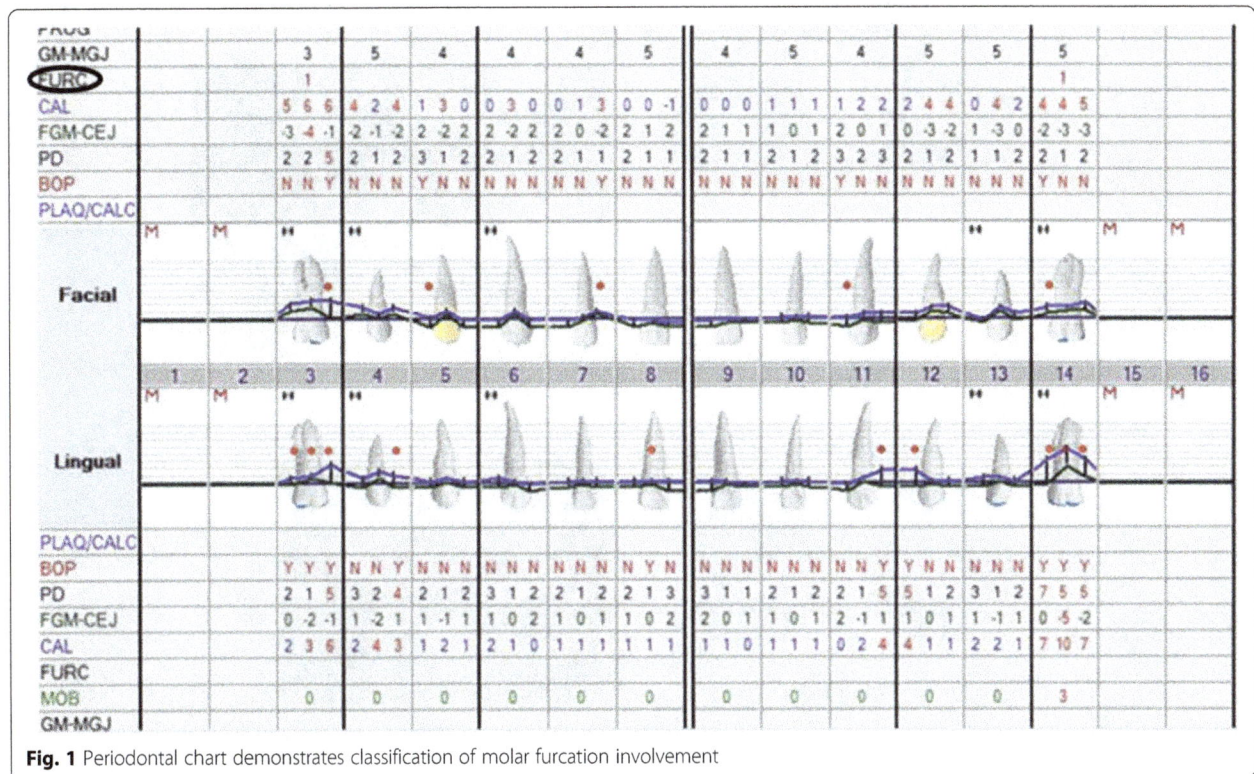

at the furcation region on both axial and sagittal view. The depth of FI was measured on axial view where the slice showed the greatest amount of bone loss. On this slice, a line was drawn tangentially to the adjacent root surfaces. The distance from this line to the deepest point of bone loss was designated as the amount of furcation bone loss. If applicable, buccal and/or lingual furcation bone loss was measured for mandibular first molar, and buccal, mesial palatal, and distal palatal furcation bone loss were measured for maxillary first molars (Fig. 3).

All the data were analyzed by one of the co-authors KF, who was a first-year dental student and received adequate training on molar furcation assessment via intraoral radiographs and CBCT scans. The data were reanalyzed in 7 months to evaluate intra-rater reliability and reproducibility.

Statistical analysis

Spearman's correlation analysis was used to determine the correlations between clinical detection and intraoral radiography, clinical detection and CBCT, as well as intraoral radiography and CBCT at all the measured sites. The difference in the correlation coefficients was analyzed using Steiger's Z-test. Intra-class correlation coefficient (ICC) was calculated to assess intra-rater reliability and reproducibility. The statistical difference was set at $p < 0.05$. The statistical analysis were run with SPSS program (version 24, IBM, Armonk, NY, USA).

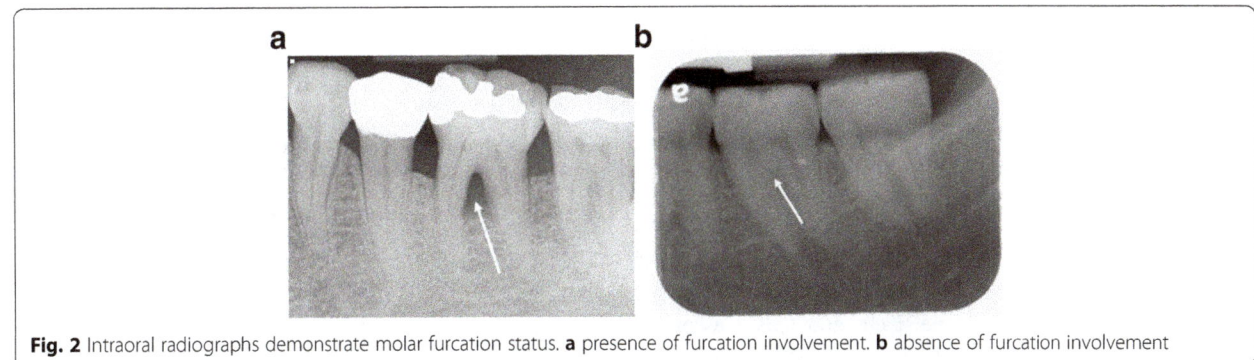

Fig. 2 Intraoral radiographs demonstrate molar furcation status. **a** presence of furcation involvement. **b** absence of furcation involvement

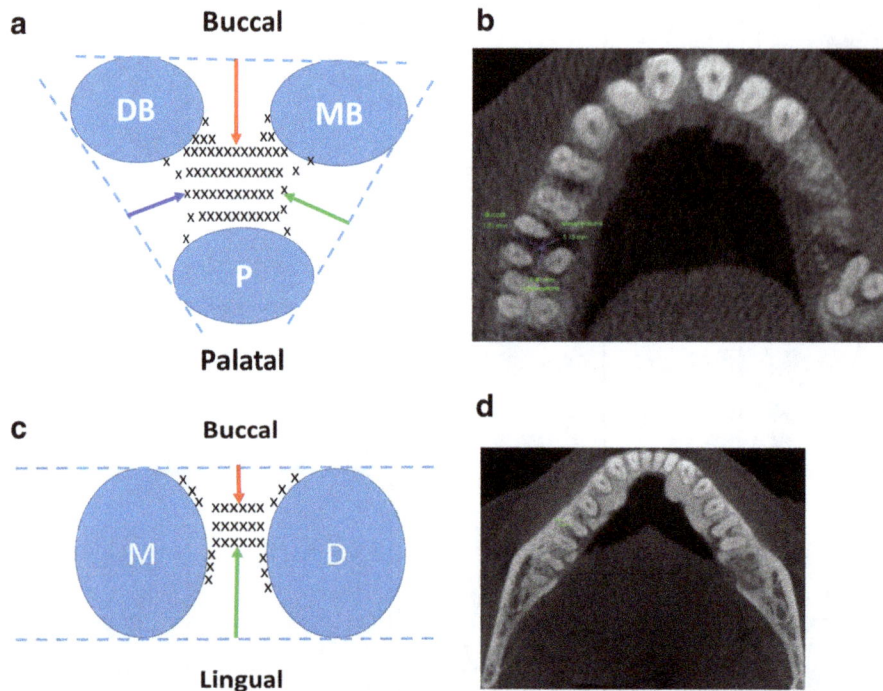

Fig. 3 Measurement of molar furcation involvement on CBCT scans. **a** a schematic diagram illustrates measurement of furcation bone loss of a maxillary first molar. Dotted line represents tangent line connecting two adjacent root surfaces. Arrows represent distances from the middle of tangent line to the deepest point of bone loss at the different surfaces. Red, green, and blue arrows denote furcation bone loss at buccal, mesial palatal, and distal palatal surface of the molar, respectively. MB, mesial buccal root; DB, distal buccal root; and P, palatal root. **b** a representative CBCT axial view demonstrates measurements of furcation bone loss of a maxillary first molar. **c** a schematic diagram illustrates measurement of furcation bone loss of a mandibular first molar. Dotted line represents tangent line connecting buccal or lingual surfaces of the two roots, respectively. Arrows represent distances from the middle of tangent line to the deepest point of bone loss at the different surfaces. Red and green arrows denote furcation bone loss at buccal and lingual surface of the molar, respectively. M, mesial root; and D, distal root. **d** a representative CBCT axial view demonstrates measurements of furcation bone loss of a mandibular first molar

Results

Based on a previous study conducted by Qiao et al. [13] who compared molar furcation assessment between clinical probing and CBCT, a power analysis was performed which demonstrated that a sample size of 51 subjects would achieve 80% power to detect the association between these two evaluation methods on a significance level of 0.05. To ensure adequate sample size, a total of 83 patients were included in the study. Among these patients, 41 were males, 42 were females, and an age range of 31–86 with a mean age of 59.03 ± 13.08 years old.

First molar FI assessed by clinical detection, BW/PA and CBCT were illustrated in Tables 1, 2 and 3, respectively. For maxillary first molar B, MP and DP FI, clinical detection demonstrated a mean modified Glickman's classification of 0.75 ± 0.08, 0.41 ± 0.08, 0.33 ± 0.07, respectively, and CBCT assessment revealed a mean 1.55 ± 0.22, 0.58 ± 0.05, 0.67 ± 0.12 mm bone loss, respectively. For mandibular first molar B and L FI, clinical detection demonstrated a mean modified Glickman's classification of 0.66 ± 0.10 and 0.69 ± 0.09, respectively, and CBCT assessment revealed a mean 1.52 ± 0.19 and 1.15 ± 0.18 mm bone

Table 1 First molar furcation involvement assessed by periodontal probing

Modified Glickman classification[a]	Maxillary first molar				Mandibular first molar		
	B	MP	DP	Average	B	L	Average
Not present[b]	49.1%	78.4%	83.6%	70.4%	60.8%	53.9%	57.4%
Class I	34.5%	7.8%	5.2%	15.8%	18.6%	27.5%	23.1%
Class II	9.5%	6.9%	6.0%	7.5%	13.7%	11.8%	12.8%
Class III	6.9%	6.9%	5.2%	6.3%	6.9%	5.9%	6.4%
Total	100%	100%	100%	100%	100%	100%	100%

Data are presented as percentage of assayed surfaces without or with furcation involvement of corresponding category based on periodontal charting
Abbreviations: B buccal, MP mesial palatal, DP distal palatal, L lingual
[a]Modified Glickman classification: Class I, incipient or early stage of furcation involvement, bone destruction is less than 2 mm into the furca; Class II, horizontal bone destruction extending deeper than 2 mm but less than 6 mm into the furca; Class III, horizontal bone destructions communicate between furcae of the tooth, and result in a through-and-through tunnel
[b]Not present: no furcation involvement

Table 2 First molar furcation involvement assessed by periapical or bitewing radiographs

Radiographic assessment	Maxillary first molar	Mandibular first molar
Absence of furcation involvement	71.8%	66.0%
Presence of furcation involvement	28.2%	34%
Total	100%	100%

Data are presented as percentage of assayed first molars without or with furcation involvement based on radiographic assessment

loss, respectively (data were presented as mean ± SD). All of the three evaluation methods demonstrated more frequent FI of mandibular first molars relative to maxillary counterpart. Of maxillary first molars, both clinical detection and CBCT revealed that buccal surface was more vulnerable for FI compared to palatal side.

Comparison of first molar FI assessment between CBCT and clinical detection showed that, when CBCT demonstrated no furcation involvement, 18.7% of these cases were documented as FI on clinical detection. On the contrary, of the 26.7% cases identified as having 0.1–2.0 mm or 2.1–6.0 mm bone loss on CBCT, clinical detection showed no FI (Table 4). For comparison between intraoral radiographic evaluation and clinical detection, there were situations when no FI was detected on intraoral radiographs, 25.6% of these cases were demonstrated to have Class I-III FI by clinical detection. In addition, for 18.2% cases identified as FI on radiographs, clinical detection failed to detect any bone loss (Table 5).

Spearman's correlation and Steiger's Z-test analysis demonstrated that clinical detection, BW/PA and CBCT were significantly correlated with each other in the assessment of first molar FI, with r values ranged between 0.230 to 0.644 ($P < 0.05$, Table 6). Compared with BW/PA, CBCT appeared to have higher correlation coefficients with clinical detection, especially at distal palatal side of maxillary first molar, which reached statistically significant difference ($p < 0.05$, Table 6). Between the two sets of measurements by the same rater, the ICC was 0. 903, with 95% confidence interval of (0.858, 0.934),

Table 3 First molar furcation involvement measured by CBCT

Depth of furcation involvement (mm)	Maxillary first molar				Mandibular first molar		
	B	MP	DP	Average	B	L	Average
0.0	46.7%	81.5%	73.9%	67.4	45.9%	54.1%	50.0%
0.1–2.0	21.7%	5.4%	16.3%	14.5	15.3%	25.9%	20.6%
2.1–6.0	25.0%	13.0%	6.5%	14.8	36.5%	17.6%	27.1%
> 6.0	6.5%	0.0%	3.3%	3.3	2.4%	2.4%	2.4%
Total	100%	100%	100%	100%	100%	100%	100%

Data are presented as percentage of assayed surfaces without or with furcation involvement of corresponding category based on CBCT assessment
Abbreviations: B buccal, MP mesial palatal, DP distal palatal, L lingual

Table 4 Cross tabulation of CBCT with periodontal probing for evaluation of furcation involvement for maxillary and mandibular first molars

Count		Periodontal probing				Total
		0	1	2	3	
CBCT (mm)	0.0	213	36	10	3	262
	0.1–2.0	40	24	7	0	71
	2.1–6.0	38	22	13	6	79
	> 6.0	1	2	3	5	11
Total		292	84	33	14	423

which demonstrated great reliability and repeatability of the evaluator.

Discussion

Our results demonstrated that all three FI assessment methods had significant correlations among each other. CBCT had stronger correlation to clinical detection than PA/BW, especially on distal palatal side of maxillary first molar. The results validate applicability of CBCT in FI assessment. Although all of the included patients had diagnosis of generalized moderate or severe chronic periodontitis, more than a half of them were not found to have FI based on the three evaluation methods.

When CBCT showed no furcation involvement, clinical detection identified 18.7% of cases with FI, indicating over-detection by clinical measurement. On the contrary, of the 26.7% cases demonstrated bone loss on CBCT, clinical detection showed no FI, suggesting under-detection by clinical detection. This was consistent with what was reported by Darby [12] and Walter [23], who also found over- and under-estimation of FI by clinical probing relative to CBCT analysis. It is speculated that probing angulation and force, soft tissue inflammation, and inter-radicular bone and root morphology, all contribute to variations of clinical detection.

Between intraoral radiographic examination and clinical detection, there were situations when no FI was identified on intraoral radiographs, about one quarter of these cases were demonstrated having FI by clinical detection. In addition, for 18.2% cases identified as FI on radiographs, probing failed to detect any bone loss. This observation confirmed the necessity of supplementing

Table 5 Cross tabulation of intraoral radiograph with periodontal probing for evaluation of furcation involvement for maxillary and mandibular first molars

Count		Periodontal probing				Total
		0	1	2	3	
Intraoral radiograph	0 (absence)	258	75	13	2	352
	1 (presence)	58	17	39	28	142
Total		316	92	52	34	494

Table 6 Correlation coefficients of periodontal probing with CBCT or BW/PA in assessment of furcation involvement for maxillary and mandibular first molars

Periodontal charting (Modified Glickman)	CBCT	BW/PA
Maxillary buccal	0.599[a]	0.579[a]
Maxillary mesial palatal	0.591[a]	0.499[a]
Maxillary distal palatal	0.644[a,c]	0.424[a,c]
Mandibular buccal	0.372[a]	0.362[a]
Mandibular lingual	0.264[b]	0.230[b]

Abbreviations: *CBCT* cone beam computed tomography, *BW/PA* bitewing/periapical radiographs
[a]Correlation is significant at *p* < 0.01, between CBCT and periodontal charting, or between BW/PA and periodontal charting
[b]Correlation is significant at *p* < 0.05, between CBCT and periodontal charting, or between BW/PA and periodontal charting
[c]CBCT demonstrated significantly stronger correlation (*p* < 0.05) with periodontal charting relative to BW/PA at assessment of distal palatal side of maxillary first molars

clinical detection with intraoral radiographs for the diagnosis of FI, which is reflective of the consensus in the literature [8, 14]. The inconsistency between these two methods could be due to measurement errors from either or both detecting techniques. Anatomic complexity, such as superimposition of palatal root at the furcation region may contribute to under-diagnosis of FI for maxillary molars on intraoral radiographs [5, 24], and sinus tract extending into furcation due to intrapulpal infection may lead to over-diagnosis of FI on intraoral radiographs [25], respectively.

The current study identified that mandibular first molars had more FI than maxillary first molars. In a study conducted in a Swede population, Svärdström [26] found that the prevalence of furcation involved molars was higher in the maxilla than in the mandible, based on clinical detection and intraoral radiographs. Hou et al. [27] concluded that the highest prevalence of FI was in the mandibular first molar in a Japanese population based on clinical detection. It appears that geographical locations, racial origins and evaluation modalities are among the factors contributing to variations of prevalence for molars with FI. Current study also found that FI was more frequently associated with and more severe at buccal side of maxillary first molars relative to palatal side, similarly as reported by Porciuncula [28].

Although considered a valuable addition in molar furcation assessment, CBCT is not without its shortcomings. Scatter, partial volume averaging and beam hardening artifacts could compromise its diagnostic quality, especially for patients with heavy metallic restorations, multiple endodontic treatment, orthodontic appliances, or implant prosthesis [29–31]. In addition, detectability of FI by CBCT depends on how sensitive it is to reveal bone loss at furcation area. Generally, demineralization may not be evident radiographically until it reaches approximately 30–40% [32]. This makes it challenge to detect and initiate early intervention for incipient FI of molars. In general,

periodontal probing and intraoral radiographs should be used as routine examinations for detection of FI. For complicated cases when routine exams fail to provide adequate information for diagnosis and/or treatment planning, CBCT may be attempted with the smallest field of view possible and optimal exposure settings.

There were limitations for the study. It was a retrospective investigation, and the clinical detection was performed by different dental students under the supervision of board-certified periodontist, and the results were confirmed by the supervising faculty before being entering in the EHR. Still, inter-operator variations could contribute to inconsistence in the clinical detection. Also, in the present study, a relative old model of CBCT unit, Kodak 9500 was used, since this was the only CBCT unit in the Imaging Clinic of the school. This unit had a smallest voxel size of 200 μm. Compared to newer CBCT units with much smaller voxel size, such as 80 μm for Accuitomo [33], the much larger voxel size of current unit had limited spatial resolution, therefore, could limit the accuracy in the assessment of FI. In addition, current study only measured horizontal bone loss at the furcation area on CBCT scan, in order to correlate with clinical detection. Modified Glickman Classification was utilized in clinical detection, which only recorded horizontal furcation involvement of the molars. Future study could consider incorporating vertical bone loss measurement on CBCT, to gain better appreciation on furcation status. Intra-surgical FI assessment (gold standard) could be implemented, if possible, to further evaluate the accuracy of CBCT in the diagnosis of FI.

Conclusions

CBCT has been validated as a valuable supplemental tool for assessment of molar FI in addition to periodontal probing and intraoral radiographic examinations.

Abbreviations
BW: Bitewing; CBCT: Cone beam computed tomography; EHR: Electronic Health Record; FI: Furcation involvement; FOV: Field of view; IRB: Institutional Review Board; kVp: Kilovolt; mA: Milliampere; PA: Periapical; PSP: Photostimulable phosphor

Funding
This study was partially supported by the Research Office, University of Texas School of Dentistry at Houston.

Authors' contributions
WZ conceived the ideas, designed the experiments, and composed the manuscript. KF did all the measurements and performed initial data analysis. BW refined the ideas, performed in-depth data analysis and interpretations, and critically revised the manuscript. All authors read and approved the final manuscript.

Competing interests

The authors declare that they have no competing interests.

Author details

[1]Department of Diagnostic & Biomedical Sciences, University of Texas School of Dentistry at Houston, 7500 Cambridge Street, Houston, TX 77054, USA. [2]University of Texas School of Dentistry at Houston, 7500 Cambridge Street, Houston, TX 77054, USA. [3]Department of Periodontics & Dental Hygiene, University of Texas School of Dentistry at Houston, 7500 Cambridge Street, Houston, TX 77054, USA.

References

1. Cate T. Glossary of terms. J Periodontol. 1977;48(9):611–2.
2. Al-Shammari KF, Kazor CE, Wang HL. Molar root anatomy and management of furcation defects. J Clin Periodontol. 2001;28(8):730–40.
3. Hempton T, Leone C. A review of root resective therapy as a treatment option for maxillary molars. J Am Dent Assoc. 1997;128(4):449–55.
4. Muller HP, Eger T. Furcation diagnosis. J Clin Periodontol. 1999;26(8):485–98.
5. Walter C, Weiger R, Zitzmann NU. Periodontal surgery in furcation-involved maxillary molars revisited–an introduction of guidelines for comprehensive treatment. Clin Oral Investig. 2011;15(1):9–20.
6. Walter C, Weiger R, Dietrich T, Lang NP, Zitzmann NU. Does three-dimensional imaging offer a financial benefit for treating maxillary molars with furcation involvement? A pilot clinical case series. Clin Oral Implants Res. 2012;23(3):351–8.
7. Ramfjord SP, Caffesse RG, Morrison EC, Hill RW, Kerry GJ, Appleberry EA, Nissle RR, Stults DL. Four modalities of periodontal treatment compared over five years. J Periodontal Res. 1987;22(3):222–3.
8. Mol A. Imaging methods in periodontology. Periodontol. 2004;34:34–48.
9. Hamp SE, Nyman S, Lindhe J. Periodontal treatment of multirooted teeth. Results after 5 years. J Clin Periodontol. 1975;2(3):126–35.
10. Knowles JW, Burgett FG, Nissle RR, Shick RA, Morrison EC, Ramfjord SP. Results of periodontal treatment related to pocket depth and attachment level. Eight years. J Periodontol. 1979;50(5):225–33.
11. Moriarty JD, Hutchens LH Jr, Scheitler LE. Histological evaluation of periodontal probe penetration in untreated facial molar furcations. J Clin Periodontol. 1989;16(1):21–6.
12. Darby I, Sanelli M, Shan S, Silver J, Singh A, Soedjono M, Ngo L. Comparison of clinical and cone beam computed tomography measurements to diagnose furcation involvement. Int J Dent Hyg. 2015;13(4):241–5.
13. Qiao J, Wang S, Duan J, Zhang Y, Qiu Y, Sun C, Liu D. The accuracy of cone-beam computed tomography in assessing maxillary molar furcation involvement. J Clin Periodontol. 2014;41(3):269–74.
14. Laky M, Majdalani S, Kapferer I, Frantal S, Gahleitner A, Moritz A, Ulm C. Periodontal probing of dental furcations compared with diagnosis by low-dose computed tomography: a case series. J Periodontol. 2013;84(12):1740–6.
15. Vandenberghe B, Jacobs R, Yang J. Detection of periodontal bone loss using digital intraoral and cone beam computed tomography images: an in vitro assessment of bony and/or infrabony defects. Dentomaxillofac Radiol. 2008;37(5):252–60.
16. Hishikawa T, Izumi M, Naitoh M, Furukawa M, Yoshinari N, Kawase H, Matsuoka M, Noguchi T, Ariji E. The effect of horizontal X-ray beam angulation on the detection of furcation defects of mandibular first molars in intraoral radiography. Dentomaxillofac Radiol. 2010;39(2):85–90.
17. Ito K, Gomi Y, Sato S, Arai Y, Shinoda K. Clinical application of a new compact CT system to assess 3-D images for the preoperative treatment planning of implants in the posterior mandible a case report. Clin Oral Implants Res. 2001;12(5):539–42.
18. Aljehani YA. Diagnostic applications of cone-beam CT for periodontal diseases. Int J Dentistry. 2014;2014:865079.
19. Acar B, Kamburoglu K. Use of cone beam computed tomography in periodontology. World J Radiol. 2014;6(5):139–47.
20. Mozzo P, Procacci C, Tacconi A, Martini PT, Andreis IA. A new volumetric CT machine for dental imaging based on the cone-beam technique: preliminary results. Eur Radiol. 1998;8(9):1558–64.
21. du Bois AH, Kardachi B, Bartold PM. Is there a role for the use of volumetric cone beam computed tomography in periodontics? Aust Dent J. 2012; 57(Suppl 1):103–8.
22. Cimbaljevic MM, Spin-Neto RR, Miletic VJ, Jankovic SM, Aleksic ZM, Nikolic-Jakoba NS. Clinical and CBCT-based diagnosis of furcation involvement in patients with severe periodontitis. Quintessence Int. 2015;46(10):863–70.
23. Walter C, Kaner D, Berndt DC, Weiger R, Zitzmann NU. Three-dimensional imaging as a pre-operative tool in decision making for furcation surgery. J Clin Periodontol. 2009;36(3):250–7.
24. Bragger U. Radiographic parameters: biological significance and clinical use. Periodontol. 2005;39:73–90.
25. Rotstein I, Simon JH. Diagnosis, prognosis and decision-making in the treatment of combined periodontal-endodontic lesions. Periodontol. 2004;34:165–203.
26. Svardstrom G, Wennstrom JL. Prevalence of furcation involvements in patients referred for periodontal treatment. J Clin Periodontol. 1996;23(12):1093–9.
27. Hou GL, Lin IC, Tsai CC, Shieh TY. The study of molar furcation involvements in adult periodontitis. II. Age, sex, location and prevalence. Kaohsiung J Med Sci. 1996;12(9):514–21.
28. Porciuncula HF, da Porciuncula MM, Zuza EP, de Toledo BE. Biometric analysis of the maxillary permanent molar teeth and its relation to furcation involvement. Braz Oral Res. 2004;18(3):187–91.
29. Draenert FG, Coppenrath E, Herzog P, Muller S, Mueller-Lisse UG. Beam hardening artefacts occur in dental implant scans with the NewTom cone beam CT but not with the dental 4-row multidetector CT. Dentomaxillofac Radiol. 2007;36(4):198–203.
30. Schulze R, Heil U, Gross D, Bruellmann DD, Dranischnikow E, Schwanecke U, Schoemer E. Artefacts in CBCT: a review. Dentomaxillofac Radiol. 2011;40(5):265–73.
31. Brito-Junior M, Santos LA, Faria-e-Silva AL, Pereira RD, Sousa-Neto MD. Ex vivo evaluation of artifacts mimicking fracture lines on cone-beam computed tomography produced by different root canal sealers. Int Endod J. 2014;47(1):26–31.
32. White SC, Pharoah MJ. Oral radiology principle and interpretation. 7th ed. St. Louis: Elsevier Inc.; 2014.
33. Pauwels R, Faruangsaeng T, Charoenkarn T, Ngonphloy N, Panmekiate S. Effect of exposure parameters and voxel size on bone structure analysis in CBCT. Dentomaxillofac Radiol. 2015;44(8):20150078.

5

Effects of dental treatment and systemic disease on oral health-related quality of life in Korean pediatric patients

Ji-Soo Song[1], Hong-Keun Hyun[2], Teo Jeon Shin[2] and Young-Jae Kim[2]* ⓘ

Abstract

Background: The findings that not only dental caries but also systemic disease can exert a negative effect on oral health-related quality of life (OHRQoL), and that dental treatment can improve OHRQoL have been confirmed in multiple studies. The purpose of this study is to investigate the impact of dental treatment on OHRQoL of Korean pediatric patients and the differences in OHRQoL between patients with and without systemic disease.

Methods: All the primary caregivers of pediatric patients who underwent dental treatments under either general anesthesia or intravenous deep sedation at Seoul National University Dental Hospital completed abbreviated versions of the Child Oral Health Impact Profile (COHIP-14) and Family Impact Scale (FIS-12) surveys on OHRQOL pre- and post-treatment (average: 2.4 ± 1.7 months after dental treatment). This is a case control study with patients divided into two groups according to the presence or absence of systemic disease.

Results: Data from 93 pediatric patients (46 male and 47 female, average patient age: 5.0 ± 3.4 years) were analyzed to compare OHRQoL before and after treatment with the Wilcoxon signed-rank test and to calculate the effect size using Cohen's d. All of the patients exhibited an improvement in OHRQoL (COHIP-14: $p < 0.001$, effect size = 1.0; FIS-12: $p < 0.001$, effect size = 0.7). Patients with systemic diseases demonstrated lower OHRQoL in both pre- and post-treatment surveys than patients without systemic diseases (Wilcoxon Rank-sum test, both COHIP-14 and FIS-12: $p < 0.05$). The COHIP-14 appears to have a greater impact on the FIS-12 in patients with systemic disease than those without (explanatory power of 65.3 and 44.6%, respectively).

Conclusions: Based on the primary caregivers' perceptions, dental treatment can improve the OHRQoL in Korean pediatric patients. Systemic disease results in a reduced OHRQoL, and the awareness of patients' oral health appeared to have a greater impact on OHRQoL for family members of patients with a systemic disease.

Keywords: Child, Dental treatment, Systemic disease, Oral health-related quality of life

---

* Correspondence: neokarma@snu.ac.kr
[2]Department of Pediatric Dentistry, Dental Research Institute, School of Dentistry, Seoul National University, Seoul National University Dental Hospital, 101, Daehakno, Jongno-gu, 03080 Seoul, Republic of Korea
Full list of author information is available at the end of the article

Background

Dental caries is the most common chronic oral disease, with a high prevalence in children and adolescents worldwide [1]. The prevalence of active caries in primary teeth was as high as 34.5%, and that of dental caries experience in primary teeth was as high as 62.2% in 2012 Korean study [2]. Oral health-related quality of life (OHRQoL) is a multidimensional concept that includes a subjective evaluation of the individual's oral health status, functional well-being, social and emotional well-being, expectations of and satisfaction with care, and sense of self-image [3]. Its importance is widely emphasized in both research and clinical settings, given the increasing demand for active participation of patients in the treatment process, and the lack of basic treatment for certain chronic diseases (e.g., dental caries, periodontal disease) that require long-term treatment and follow-up. Nevertheless, research about the OHRQoL of pediatric patients in Korea has only recently been initiated despite the high prevalence of dental caries. The only study that has conducted a full-scale reliability and validity test in Korea was reported by Ahn et al., in which a Korean version of the Child Oral Health Impact Profile (COHIP) was used in 2236 children and adolescents aged 8–15 years [4].

The findings that dental caries can exert a negative effect on OHRQoL and that dental treatment can improve OHRQoL have been confirmed in several studies [5–9]. Pain caused by dental caries can interfere with normal masticatory function and sleep, which can inhibit normal body growth [10]. Unpleasant smiles associated with the destruction of tooth structure also can negatively influence the social life of children [11]. In addition, the perceptions and attitudes of primary caregivers on oral health influence the behavioral patterns regarding their child's oral health [12]. Chronic disease such as dental caries in children can affect family life [13, 14], and patients with systemic disease have been shown to have low OHRQoL [15–17]. Their underlying disease may be associated with poor oral health, but they may also have difficulties maintaining their oral health and accessing adequate dental care due to underlying disease [18]. There are no studies that have been conducted to identify the relationship between dental caries and the OHRQoL of pediatric patients and their families, and to compare the OHRQoL between patients with and without systemic diseases in Korea. Therefore, this study examined the impact of dental treatment on OHRQoL of Korean pediatric patients and the differences in the OHRQoL between patient with and without systemic disease.

Methods

Subjects

This study involved all primary caregivers or parents of pediatric dental patients who underwent dental treatment under either general anesthesia or intravenous deep sedation at Seoul National University Dental Hospital pediatric department from February 2013 to February 2014. Five professors who were all experienced in general anesthesia and intravenous sedation in the pediatric dentistry department conducted all the dental treatments, and standardized treatment protocols were followed. Patients who received dental treatment without general anesthesia or intravenous sedation were not included in the study. The use of general anesthesia or intravenous sedation is decided by the anesthesiologist based on the physical condition of the airway and respiratory system, not on the severity of dental caries. Primary caregivers accompanying the patients on the day of treatment were invited to participate in the survey. The study was performed with the approval of the Seoul National University Dental Hospital Research Ethics Board (IRB Number: CRI12006). We fully explained the study to the primary caregivers only if they were the legal guardians of the patients and only included participants with written consent on the day of treatment.

Study design

This study was a case control study to compare OHRQoL between the patients with and without systemic disease in each cohort. Accordingly, patients were categorized into two groups. The patient group without systemic disease did not exhibit conditions that encumbered everyday life, but required either general anesthesia or intravenous deep sedation due to dental phobia and a large number of dental caries. The group with systemic disease included patients with special health care needs, such as intellectual disability (ID), autism, or developmental disorders, as well as conditions that affect everyday life (e.g., cancer, cerebral palsy, convulsive disorders, genetic disorders, and cardiovascular disorders) [19, 20]. Cases with dental treatments that did not involve pulp treatment or restorations—including periodontal treatment, such as scaling, or minor oral surgery, such as removal of supernumerary teeth—were excluded from the study.

Primary caregivers were asked to fill out surveys on OHRQoL, pre-treatment as well as post-treatment when the patients returned for a follow-up visit. As calculated from our pilot study performed in the initial stage of this study with 20 patients (10 patients without systemic disease and 10 patients with systemic disease), the power calculation indicated that 104 cases were required to compensate for a 20% drop-out rate at 5% significance level and 80% statistical power. The pre-treatment survey included responses from 109 cases and follow-up post-treatment surveys were completed for 93 of these cases within 6 months. These cases were selected for analysis. Sixteen cases were excluded, as the patient did not have a follow-up appointment, a different primary caregiver accompanied the patient for the post-treatment visit, or the primary caregiver declined to complete the post-treatment survey. The post-treatment survey was completed in an average of 2.4 ± 1.7 months after dental treatment.

Surveys

In order to assess OHRQoL, the Child Oral Health Impact Profile (COHIP) and Family Impact Scale (FIS) were utilized. An abbreviated version of the COHIP, "COHIP-14", which included 10 items from the Oral Health subscale (OH) and 4 items from the Functional Limitation subscale (FL), was used in this study [21]. Similarly, the "FIS-12" scale used in the study included 5 items from the Parental/Family Activity subscale (PA), 4 items from the Parental Emotion subscale (PE), 2 items from the Family Conflict subscale (FC), and 1 item from the Financial Burden subscale (FB) [21]. Because pediatric patients requiring general anesthesia or intravenous sedation were usually younger than the target age of COHIP and FIS, these subscales and items were selectively chosen from the original questionnaires to be reasonably assessed among the primary caregivers of these patients. Several items that caregivers could not answer correctly or required an active response from

the patient were removed through an active discussion between two experienced dentists [21]. The resultant subscales and items are outlined in Tables 1 and 2. The pre-treatment COHIP-14 survey assessed the frequency of issues arising from dental disorders in pediatric patients from the primary caregiver's perspective, and the FIS-12 assessed the impact on everyday life activities and emotions of the patient and family members in the 3 months prior to the survey. For the post-treatment survey, the primary caregivers were instructed to reflect on changes post-treatment when completing both the COHIP-14 and FIS-12. Both measurements utilized a 5-point Likert scale, where the COHIP-14 and the FIS-12 ranged from 0, being "Never", to 4, being "Almost every day". Because the items of COHIP-14 were negatively worded, the scores in COHIP-14 were reversed [22]. The scores of the items were added to calculate subscale scores, which were then summed to obtain the finalized COHIP-14 and FIS-12 scores. The COHIP-14 score ranged from 0 to 56, while FIS-12 score ranged from 0 to 48. Higher COHIP scores and lower FIS scores corresponded to a better OHRQoL.

In addition to the COHIP and FIS, global ratings of OHRQoL also known as single-item ratings, were used to assess the general oral health of the pediatric patients and their overall QoL. These questions were answered

Table 1 Prevalence and mean values of the 14-item Child Oral Health Impact Profile (COHIP-14) scores before and after dental treatment (average 2.4 ± 1.7 months' follow-up period) (n = 93)

	Before COHIP-14 score	After COHIP-14 score	Difference (after-before)		
	Mean(SD)	Mean(SD)	Mean(SD)	Effect size [a]	p-value
COHIP-14	37.5(7.9)	45.2(7.7)	7.7(8.1)	1.0	< 0.001*
Oral Health subscale (OH)	26.0(5.4)	31.9(5.7)	5.8(6.0)	1.0	< 0.001*
Pain/tooth ache	2.7(1.0)	3.4(0.8)	0.7(1.2)	0.6	
Breathing through mouth	2.0(1.1)	2.5(1.2)	0.5(1.2)	0.4	
Discoloration of teeth	1.9(1.4)	3.4(1.1)	1.5(1.6)	0.9	
Crooked teeth or spaces	2.5(1.5)	3.5(1.0)	1.0(1.6)	0.6	
Sores or sore spots	3.4(0.8)	3.6(0.7)	0.2(0.8)	0.3	
Bad breath	2.1(1.3)	2.8(1.2)	0.6(1.2)	0.5	
Bleeding gums	3.2(1.0)	3.3(0.9)	0.1(0.9)	0.1	
Food sticking	2.1(1.0)	2.5(1.1)	0.4(1.3)	0.3	
Sensitivity to hot/cold	3.1(1.0)	3.6(0.7)	0.5(1.2)	0.4	
Dry mouth	3.1(1.1)	3.3(0.9)	0.2(1.0)	0.2	
Functional Limitations subscale (FL)	11.4(4.0)	13.3(3.0)	1.9(3.6)	0.5	< 0.001*
Trouble chewing firm foods	2.3(1.5)	2.9(1.4)	0.6(1.5)	0.4	
Difficulty eating	2.8(1.3)	3.3(1.0)	0.6(1.3)	0.5	
Trouble sleeping due to teeth/face	3.6(0.8)	3.9(0.4)	0.3(0.8)	0.4	
Difficulty keeping teeth clean	2.8(1.4)	3.2(1.2)	0.4(1.4)	0.3	

Wilcoxon signed-rank test
*Significant at α = 0.05 level
[a]Calculated using Cohen's d (= difference / SD)

Table 2 Prevalence and mean values of the 12-item Family impact scale (FIS-12) scores before and after dental treatment (average 2.4 ± 1.7 months' follow-up period) (n = 93)

	Before FIS-12 score	After FIS-12 score	Difference (after-before)		
	Mean(SD)	Mean(SD)	Mean(SD)	Effect size [a]	p-value
FIS-12	15.7(9.2)	10.3(8.3)	5.4(8.3)	0.7	< 0.001*
Parental/family Activity subscale (PA)	7.4(4.8)	4.7(4.5)	2.7(4.7)	0.6	< 0.001*
Taken time off work	0.6(1.0)	0.3(0.7)	0.3(1.0)	0.3	
Required more attention	2.8(1.3)	1.9(1.5)	0.8(1.5)	0.5	
Had less time for yourself	1.5(1.4)	1.0(1.4)	0.5(1.6)	0.3	
Sleep disrupted	1.5(1.3)	0.8(1.1)	0.7(1.2)	0.6	
Family activity interrupted	1.0(1.3)	0.6(1.0)	0.4(1.3)	0.3	
Parental Emotion subscale (PE)	6.1(3.8)	4.0(3.4)	2.1(3.2)	0.7	< 0.001*
Been upset	1.3(1.2)	0.9(1.0)	0.4(1.1)	0.4	
Felt guilty	1.8(1.3)	1.2(1.1)	0.6(1.1)	0.5	
Worried about less opportunity	2.0(1.2)	1.3(1.2)	0.7(1.1)	0.6	
Felt uncomfortable	1.0(1.3)	0.7(1.0)	0.3(1.3)	0.2	
Family Conflict subscale (FC)	1.4(1.7)	1.0(1.2)	0.4(1.3)	0.3	0.004*
Argued with child	0.8(1.1)	0.7(1.0)	0.1(1.0)	0.1	
Caused conflict in the family	0.6(0.9)	0.3(0.6)	0.3(0.8)	0.4	
Financial Burden subscale (FB)	0.8(1.1)	0.6(0.8)	0.2(1.0)	0.2	0.095
Cause financial difficulties	0.8(1.1)	0.6(0.8)	0.2(1.0)	0.2	

Wilcoxon's signed-rank test
*Significant at α = 0.05 level
[a]Calculated using Cohen's d (= difference / SD)

on a 6-point Likert scale from "Very bad" to "Very good".

Statistical analysis

Statistical analysis of the survey responses was performed using SPSS 21.0 (SPSS Inc., Chicago, IL, USA). The missing data was 4.39% of the total response. Before statistical analysis, the missing values of COHIP and FIS items were replaced by the variables' means to obtain sum scores. Since there were no statistically significant differences in the number of decayed teeth and the results of the OHRQoL questionnaire between general anesthesia and intravenous deep sedation, we have performed statistical analysis with the combined results. First, the Cronbach's alpha coefficient was used to measure internal consistency. As the Kolmogorov–Smirnov test indicated the COHIP-14 and FIS-12 scores did not follow a normal distribution, the Wilcoxon's signed-rank test was utilized to compare OHRQoL pre- and post-treatment. Cohen's d indicated the effect size and was calculated by dividing the average difference in OHRQoL scores between pre- and post-treatment by the standard deviation. An effect size of $0.2 < d \leq 0.5$ was considered small, $0.5 < d \leq 0.8$ was considered intermediate, and $d > 0.8$ was considered large. To assess convergent validity, the partial Spearman correlation was examined between the COHIP and global ratings and

between FIS score and global ratings. The Wilcoxon's rank-sum test was used to compare findings in patients with and without systemic disease and to compare individuals of different ages and genders. This test was also used to investigate effects of treatment variables, including number of decayed teeth, number of treated teeth and pulp treatment.

Finally, to understand the correlation between the utilized scales, a structural equation model was designed using IBM SPSS Amos 23.0.0 to build a Multi-indicator model. The hypotheses for the structural equation model were as follows. First, the subscales of COHIP and FIS could have different explanatory power on COHIP and FIS, and COHIP would have a significant explanatory power on FIS. The rationale for these hypotheses is that a chronic illness such as dental caries in children can affect the quality of life of the family, which is based on the family member's recognition of chronic diseases in children [13]. Second, the magnitude of the explanatory power in the structure equation model would be different depending on the presence or absence of systemic disease. Accordingly, the individual SEMs for patients with and without systemic disease were constructed by confirmatory factor analysis. This study included COHIP and FIS subscales as observed variables and COHIP-14 and FIS-12 per se as latent variables. To assess the fitness of the structural equation model, the chi-square *p*-value, Goodness of Fit Index (GFI), and Normed Fit Index (NFI) were calculated. In general, if the GFI and NFI values are above 0.9, the suggested model is appropriate and seems to have good explanatory power.

Results

Analysis was carried out on data from 93 pediatric patients (46 males and 47 females) and their primary caregivers. Among caregiver participants, 91 (97.8%) were parents (81 mothers and ten fathers) and two (2.2%) were grandmothers. A mean age of the 93 pediatric patients was 5.0 ± 3.4 years. There were 43 patients without systemic diseases (21 male and 22 female) with a mean age of 4.0 ± 2.1 years, while the remaining 50 patients had systemic diseases (25 male and 25 female), and a mean age of 5.9 ± 3.9 years. Patients with systemic disease were significantly older than those without ($p = 0.012$).

The average dmft index and the average number of treated teeth due to dental caries were 10.8 ± 4.8 and 8.8 ± 4.4, respectively. There was no significant difference in dmft index or number of treated teeth between the groups with (10.6 ± 4.5, 8.7 ± 4.7) and without (11.0 ± 5.1, 9.0 ± 4.0) systemic diseases ($p = 0.648, 0.640$). Dental treatment included direct resin restoration, pulp treatment, prefabricated crown restoration and early extraction of carious teeth. The average number of teeth according to type of dental treatment was as follows: 5.6 ± 3.3 for direct resin restoration, 2.6 ± 2.8 for pulp treatment, 2.7 ± 2.9 for prefabricated crown restoration, and 0.5 ± 1.3 for early extraction. There was no statistically significant difference between the two groups according to type of treatment.

In the 16 patients excluded from the analysis, the mean age, the average dmft index and the average number of treated teeth were 5.8 ± 3.5, 11.8 ± 5.8 and 8.8 ± 4.4, respectively. These results were not statistically different from the results of the 93 patients included in the analysis ($p = 0.426, 0.409$ and 0.943, respectively).

Cronbach's alpha coefficient, indicating internal consistency, for COHIP-14, OH, and FL were 0.737, 0.624, and 0.769, respectively. For FIS-12, PA, PE, and FC, the values were 0.866, 0.810, 0.770, and 0.532, respectively.

COHIP scores were higher and FIS scores were lower post-treatment than pre-treatment. Therefore, the absolute value of the difference between pre- and post-treatment scores was used. Each of the item, pre- and post-treatment scores, as well as the difference in scores for COHIP-14 and FIS-12 are outlined in Tables 1 and 2. COHIP-14 and its subscale OH and FL scores were significantly and clinically improved at post-treatment (all $p < 0.001$ and effect size = 1.0, 1.0, 0.5 respectively). Before dental treatment, the most frequent dental problem pointed out in OH was discoloration of the teeth (37.6%), while discomfort during mastication (33.3%) was indicated for FL.

FIS-12 and its subscale PA and PE scores were all significantly and clinically improved post-treatment (all $p < 0.001$ and effect size = 0.7, 0.6, 0.7). Before dental treatment, the most frequently reported concern in PA was "required more attention" (66.7%), while that in PE was "worried about less opportunity in future due to dental problems" (37.6%). In all the subcategories of FC and FB, more than half of the responders reported "never" (57.0, 60.2, 55.9%), or "almost never" (11.8, 20.4, 20.4%).

As shown in Table 3, partial Spearman correlations indicated statistically significant associations between the COHIP-14/FIS-12 scores and the global oral health status and overall QoL both before and after dental treatment. For COHIP-14 before treatment, r(s) = 0.438, $p < 0.001$ and r(s) = 0.241, $p = 0.02$, respectively, and for FIS-12 before treatment, r(s) = − 0.251, $p = 0.015$, r(s) = − 0.391, p < 0.001, respectively. For COHIP-14 after treatment, r(s) = 0.429, $p < 0.001$ and r(s) = 0.287, $p = 0.005$, respectively, and for FIS-12 after treatment, r(s) = − 0.396, p < 0.001, r(s) = − 0.372, p < 0.001, respectively. Correlations with the global oral health status were of moderate magnitude, and correlations with the overall QoL were of low magnitude.

As shown in Table 4, the presence of systemic disease accompanied lower OHRQoL. Gender did not play a significant role in pre- and post-treatment scores of either the COHIP-14 or FIS-12 or in improvement level ($p > 0.05$). Age was not a significant factor for the FIS-12 score, but improvement in the COHIP-14 was significantly greater in patients aged 1–6 years than in those 7 years or older (8.8 ± 7.9, 3.6 ± 7.4, $p = 0.012$). And COHIP-14 and FIS-12 were not associated with number

Table 3 Partial Spearman correlations between COHIP-14 and FIS-12 scores and global oral health status and overall quality of life

	Global oral health status		Overall quality of life	
	r(s)	p-value	r(s)	p-value
COHIP-14 before dental treatment	0.438	< 0.001	0.241	0.02
FIS-12 before dental treatment	−0.251	0.015	−0.391	< 0.001
COHIP-14 after dental treatment	0.429	< 0.001	0.287	0.005
FIS-12 after dental treatment	−0.396	< 0.001	− 0.372	< 0.001

Table 4 COHIP and FIS scores according to gender, age, and medical condition of patients

		Gender		Age		Systemic Disease	
		Male	Female	< 7 years	≥ 7 years	Healthy[a]	Diseased[b]
		Mean(SD)					
COHIP-14	B	38.0(7.7)	37.0(7.1)	36.9(7.8)	39.6(8.3)	40.2(6.1)	34.9(8.6)*
	A	45.6(7.2)	44.7(8.3)	45.7(7.4)	43.3(9.0)	47.2(6.7)	43.3(8.2)*
	D	7.7(7.6)	7.7(8.6)	8.8(7.9)	3.6(7.4)*	7.0(6.9)	8.4(9.1)
FIS-12	B	16.0(9.3)	15.4(9.2)	15.2(9.4)	17.5(8.2)	11.5(6.9)	19.4(9.4)*
	A	10.2(8.6)	10.4(8.1)	9.4(8.0)	13.5(8.9)	6.5(5.5)	13.7(8.9)*
	D	5.7(6.8)	5.0(9.5)	5.8(8.1)	4.0(8.8)	5.0(5.0)	5.7(10.3)

Wilcoxon's rank-sum test
B: Before treatment
A: After treatment
D in COHIP-14: Difference between B and A (A - B)
D in FIS-12: Difference between B and A (B - A)
Healthy[a]: Patients without systemic disease
Diseased[b]: Patients with systemic disease
*: Significantly different between groups ($p < 0.05$)

of decayed teeth, number of treated teeth, and pulp treatment before and after dental treatment, respectively (all $p > 0.05$). But more than five treated teeth and pulp treatment resulted in greater improvement in the COHIP-14 score ($p = 0.016$ and 0.024, respectively).

Figures 1 and 2 shows the structure equation model flow-chart for pediatric patients without and with systemic disease respectively, as affected by COHIP and FIS variables. The coefficients estimated in this model represent the degree of explanatory power of the independent variable on the dependent variable, which indicates the degree to which the increment of one unit in independent variable changes the dependent variable including the error term. If the value is large, it has stronger explanatory power. The COHIP-14 score negatively affected the FIS-12 score, with explanatory power of 44.6 and 65.3% respectively. The reason for the negative direction is that higher COHIP and lower FIS scores indicate better OHRQoL. The magnitude of the explanatory power between COHIP and COHIP subscales and between FIS and FIS subscales was also greater in patients with systemic disease compared to patients without systemic disease. The chi-square test p-value, the GFI score

and the NFI score were 0.807, 0.972, and 0.937 in the former model and were 0.060, 0.917, and 0.904 in the latter model, respectively. These results indicate exceptional fitness and explanatory power of the models.

Discussion

This is the first study to examine the potential association between dental treatment and OHRQoL in pediatric patients in Korea, using a Korean version of the COHIP, which is the only questionnaire that has undergone reliability and validity testing in Korean pediatric patients [4]. OHRQoL is a subjective concept that relies strongly on patient's awareness. Particularly in pediatric patients, teeth and facial development as well as psychological development vary markedly with age. The age of 6 years marks the beginning of abstract thinking and self-concept [23], and the understanding of even basic health concepts may be problematic in younger aged children, like the subjects of this study [24]. And pediatric patients with systemic disease often exhibit negative behavioral patterns during dental treatment due to the previous experiences in the medical hospital. They may also exhibit cognitive impairment,

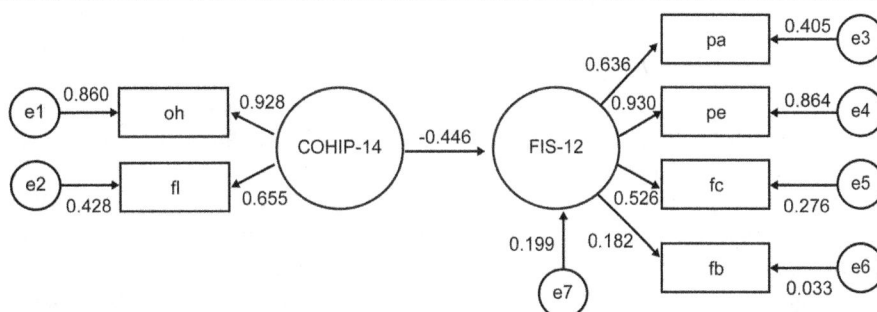

Fig. 1 Structure Equation Model of COHIP and FIS in pediatric patients without systemic disease

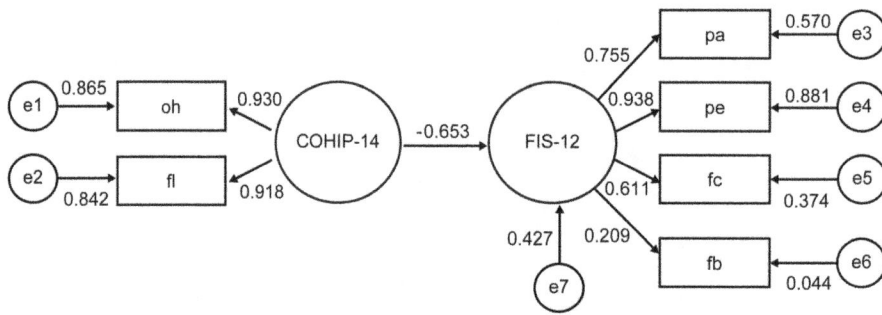

Fig. 2 Structure Equation Model of COHIP and FIS in pediatric patients with systemic disease

which makes it difficult to understand their cognitive processes and consequently results in unreliable measurement of QoL [7]. Therefore, studies on pediatric patients' OHRQoL often rely on the awareness of their primary caregivers [25]. Previous studies have shown that there was greater agreement for observable oral conditions and lesser agreement for non-observable oral conditions between ratings of children's OHRQoL made by parents and the children themselves [25]. In this context, the COHIP-14 and FIS-12 questionnaires used in this study were shortened from the original measurements for the primary caregiver to respond more appropriately. In order to supplement the modifications of the items, internal consistency and convergent validity were confirmed in this study.

The COHIP and FIS scores of pediatric patients were significantly and clinically improved after dental treatments under general anesthesia or intravenous deep sedation (Tables 1 and 2). These results were in agreement with those of previous studies that reported reduced OHRQoL due to a large number of dental caries [5, 6, 26] and assessed the OHRQoL of pediatric patients treated under general anesthesia [7–9, 16, 27–29]. These previous studies showed statistical and clinical improvements in all subscales including oral symptoms and function. And the effect size of FL was lower than that of OH, this is probably because the caregivers might have difficulties to recognize oral function objectively. This tendency is also observed in previous studies in which the caregivers responded to the questionnaire [7–9, 27, 29]. In contrast to these consistent results about dental caries on OHRQoL, the results of dental trauma and malocclusion, which are also common oral disorders in young pediatric patients, exhibited somewhat conflicting results [26, 30–32]. Overall, dental caries seems to have a greater impact on OHRQoL than dental trauma or malocclusion in young pediatric patients. This is likely because the OHRQoL questionnaires for young children are mostly completed by their caregivers, and dental caries in children are strongly influenced by the caregiver's daily oral hygiene care, but the trauma and

malocclusion are not directly related to the caregiver's daily care.

Among the items in the COHIP, the most evident improvements were reported in the items of "discoloration of teeth" and "difficulty chewing firm food" before dental treatment, which are easy-to-notice changes for primary caregivers. This observation was slightly different from what was reported by Ahn et al. [4], where improvement in discoloration was reported at a low frequency, while improvements in food sticking in the teeth, crooked teeth, spaces between teeth, and difficulty in maintaining oral hygiene had high frequency. The age difference in the patient cohorts, as well as the targets of the investigation, patients versus primary caregivers, could account for the differences observed.

According to the study by Abanto et al. [5], dental caries exhibited a negative impact on the total FIS score and PA, PE and FB subscales. These are similar to our results except for the FB subscales. In our study, there was little change observed in the FB subscale, with the most frequent responses being "never" or "almost never" in items of the FB subscale. In cases where treatment is carried out under general anesthesia or intravenous deep sedation at Seoul National University Hospital, there is a possibility that the primary caregivers could either bear the financial burden for the treatment or received financial support from outside organizations. Among the items in the FIS, most evident improvements in this study were reported in the items of "required more attention" and "worried about less opportunity". These results are also similar to those of Abanto et al..

The results of Table 4 indicate that OHRQoL is lower in patients with systemic disease before and after dental treatment. These findings were in accordance with previous reports that found that patients with systemic diseases, such as cerebral palsy [17, 33], autism [34, 35], cancer [10, 36], and craniofacial anomalies [37], suffered from a lower OHRQoL.

Gender was not an important factor in OHRQoL, in agreement with reports by Broder et al. in 2007 and de Paula et al. in 2015 [22, 38]. Greater improvement in the

COHIP score in patients aged 6 years or younger may be related to the significantly higher average number of treated teeth compared to patients aged 7 years or older (9.9 vs. 4.9, $p < 0.001$). And this is consistent with the results that a large number of treated teeth and pulp treatments showed greater improvement in COHIP-14. A previous study reported that age is not an important factor, but that study did not consider the number of treated teeth when considering the effect of age [6].

The COHIP-14 appears to have a greater impact on the FIS-12 in patients with systemic disease (Figs. 1 and 2). Therefore, the diagnosis and understanding of oral health would exert a greater impact on the family's OHRQoL for patients with systemic disease. In other words, dental treatment and improvement in oral health can result in an overall increase in the OHRQoL of families of patients with systemic disease.

General anesthesia or intravenous deep sedation was performed by a single anesthesiologist. However, dental treatment was performed by five professors in pediatric dentistry working at Seoul National University Dental Hospital. Therefore, the follow-up period varied among the dentists, resulting in inconsistent time-lapses between pre- and post-treatment surveys. To minimize the effect of the inconsistencies, only cases in which the duration between surveys was less than 6 months were included for analysis. In addition, we removed several items from original COHIP and FIS questionnaires to compensate the differences of patient age and respondents to the questionnaire. Despite of the validity and reliability tests conducted in this study, the COHIP-14 and FIS-12 were not fully validated. And the magnitude of correlations between the COHIP-14/FIS-12 and the overall QoL were low. This is probably because more than half of the patients had systemic disease, and systemic disease itself, apart from oral health status, could have a negative impact on the overall QoL. Therefore, further research to confirm the overall reliability and validity of COHIP-14 and FIS-12 are required. A difference in the mean age of patients with and without systemic disease and the fact that there was no equivalent cohort of children with similar systemic condition who were treated without general anesthesia or intravenous deep sedation may be other confounders.

Conclusion

Dental treatment under either general anesthesia or intravenous deep sedation can improve the OHRQoL in Korean pediatric patients, which can be recognized by their primary caregivers. Systemic disease results in reduced OHRQoL, and the COHIP-14 appears to have a greater impact on the FIS-12 in patients with systemic disease than on patients without. In other words, the impact on the OHRQoL of the family is more pronounced in patients with systemic diseases, and thus treating dental caries in these patients will greatly improve the OHRQoL of the family members.

Abbreviations
COHIP-14: Child oral health impact profile; FB: Financial burden subscale; FC: Family conflict subscale; FIS-12: Family impact Scale; FL: Functional limitation subscale; GFI: Goodness of fit index; NFI: Normed fit index; OH: Oral Health subscale; OHRQoL: Oral health-related quality of life; PA: Parental/family activity subscale; PE: Parental emotion subscale

Funding
This research was supported by a grant of the Korea Health Technology R&D Project through the Korea Health Industry Development Institute (KHIDI), funded by the Ministry of Health & Welfare, Republic of Korea (grant number: HI15C1503).

Authors' contributions
JS and YK conceived the ideas, TS is the anesthesiologist who performed general anesthesia and intravenous deep sedation in this study, and contributed to collect anesthesia related data. JS and HH contributed to statistical analysis of the collected data and led the writing. All authors have revised the manuscript, and have approved the final manuscript prior to its submission.

Authors' information
Dr. Ji-Soo Song is a specialist of pediatric dentistry and a clinical professor in the department of pediatric dentistry, Seoul National University Dental Hospital.
Dr. Hong-Keun Hyun is a specialist of pediatric dentistry and an associate professor in the department of pediatric Dentistry, dental research institute, school of dentistry, Seoul National University, Seoul National University Dental Hospital.
Dr. Teo Jeon Shin is an anesthesiologist and an associate professor in the department of pediatric Dentistry, dental research institute, school of dentistry, Seoul National University, Seoul National University Dental Hospital.
Dr. Young-Jae Kim is a specialist of pediatric dentistry, a professor and the chairman in the department of pediatric Dentistry, dental research institute, school of dentistry, Seoul National University, Seoul National University Dental Hospital.

Competing interests
The authors declare that they have no competing interests.

Author details
[1]Department of Pediatric Dentistry, Seoul National University Dental Hospital, 101, Daehakno, Jongno-gu, 03080 Seoul, Republic of Korea. [2]Department of Pediatric Dentistry, Dental Research Institute, School of Dentistry, Seoul National University, Seoul National University Dental Hospital, 101, Daehakno, Jongno-gu, 03080 Seoul, Republic of Korea.

References
1. Kassebaum NJ, Smith AGC, Bernabe E, et al. Global, regional, and national prevalence, incidence, and disability-adjusted life years for oral conditions

for 195 countries, 1990-2015: a systematic analysis for the global burden of diseases, injuries, and risk factors. J Dent Res. 2017;96:380–7.

2. Ministry of Health and Welfare. The report of Korean National Oral Health Survey in 2012. Available in Korean at: "http://www.mohw.go.kr/react/jb/sjb030301vw.jsp?PAR_MENU_ID=03&MENU_ID=032901&CONT_SEQ=337111&page=1". Accessed: 2018-05-23. (Archived by WebCite® at "http://www.webcitation.org/6zcipMdG6").

3. Sischo L, Broder HL. Oral health-related quality of life: what, why, how, and future implications. J Dent Res. 2011;90:1264–70.

4. Ahn YS, Kim HY, Hong SM, Patton LL, Kim JH, Noh HJ. Validation of a Korean version of the child oral health impact profile (COHIP) among 8- to 15-year-old school children. Int J Paediatr Dent. 2012;22:292–301.

5. Abanto J, Paiva SM, Raggio DP, Celiberti P, Aldrigui JM, Bonecker M. The impact of dental caries and trauma in children on family quality of life. Community Dent Oral Epidemiol. 2012;40:323–31.

6. Acharya S, Tandon S. The effect of early childhood caries on the quality of life of children and their parents. Contemp Clin Dent. 2011;2:98–101.

7. Jabarifar SE, Eshghi AR, Shabanian M, Ahmad S. Changes in children's oral health related quality of life following dental treatment under general anesthesia. Dent Res J. 2009;6:13–6.

8. Gaynor WN, Thomson WM. Changes in young children's OHRQoL after dental treatment under general anaesthesia. Int J Paediatr Dent. 2012;22:258–64.

9. Yawary R, Anthonappa RP, Ekambaram M, McGrath C, King NM. Changes in the oral health-related quality of life in children following comprehensive oral rehabilitation under general anaesthesia. Int J Paediatr Dent. 2016;26:322–9.

10. Sheiham A. Dental caries affects body weight, growth and quality of life in pre-school children. Br Dent J. 2006;201:625–6.

11. BaniHani A, Deery C, Toumba J, Munyombwe T, Duggal M. The impact of dental caries and its treatment by conventional or biological approaches on the oral health-related quality of life of children and carers. Int J Paediatr Dent. 2018;28:266–76.

12. Amin MS, Harrison RL. Understanding parents' oral health behaviors for their young children. Qual Health Res. 2009;19:116–27.

13. Locker D, Jokovic A, Stephens M, Kenny D, Tompson B, Guyatt G. Family impact of child oral and oro-facial conditions. Community Dent Oral Epidemiol. 2002;30:438–48.

14. Pahel BT, Rozier RG, Slade GD. Parental perceptions of children's oral health: the early childhood oral health impact scale (ECOHIS). Health Qual Life Outcomes. 2007;5:6–10.

15. McMillan AS, Pow EH, Leung WK, Wong MC, Kwong DL. Oral health-related quality of life in southern Chinese following radiotherapy for nasopharyngeal carcinoma. J Oral Rehabil. 2004;31:600–8.

16. Baens-Ferrer C, Roseman MM, Dumas HM, Haley SM. Parental perceptions of oral health-related quality of life for children with special needs: impact of oral rehabilitation under general anesthesia. Pediatr Dent. 2005;27:137–42.

17. Abanto J, Ortega AO, Raggio DP, Bonecker M, Mendes FM, Ciamponi AL. Impact of oral diseases and disorders on oral-health-related quality of life of children with cerebral palsy. Spec Care Dent. 2014;34:56–63.

18. Espinoza KM, Heaton LJ. Communicating with patients with special health care needs. Dent Clin N Am. 2016;60:693–705.

19. American Academy of Pediatric Dentistry. Management of dental patients with special health care needs. Pediatr Dent. 2017;39:229–34.

20. Glassman P. Interventions focusing on children with special health care needs. Dent Clin N Am. 2017;61:565–76.

21. Chang J, Patton LL, Kim HY. Impact of dental treatment under general anesthesia on the oral health-related quality of life of adolescents and adults with special needs. Eur J Oral Sci. 2014;122:363–71.

22. Broder HL, Wilson-Genderson M. Reliability and convergent and discriminant validity of the child oral health impact profile (COHIP Child's version). Community Dent Oral Epidemiol. 2007;35(Suppl 1):20–31.

23. Jokovic A, Locker D, Stephens M, Kenny D, Tompson B, Guyatt G. Validity and reliability of a questionnaire for measuring child oral-health-related quality of life. J Dent Res. 2002;81:459–63.

24. Tsakos G, Blair YI, Yusuf H, Wright W, Watt RG, Macpherson LM. Developing a new self-reported scale of oral health outcomes for 5-year-old children (SOHO-5). Health Qual Life Outcomes. 2012;10:62.

25. Eiser C, Morse R. Can parents rate their child's health-related quality of life? Results of a systematic review. Quality Life Res. 2001;10:347–57.

26. Abanto J, Carvalho TS, Mendes FM, Wanderley MT, Bonecker M, Raggio DP. Impact of oral diseases and disorders on oral health-related quality of life of

preschool children. Community Dent Oral Epidemiol. 2011;39:105–14.

27. Malden PE, Thomson WM, Jokovic A, Locker D. Changes in parent-assessed oral health-related quality of life among young children following dental treatment under general anaesthetic. Community Dent Oral Epidemiol. 2008;36:108–17.

28. Jankauskiene B, Narbutaite J. Changes in oral health-related quality of life among children following dental treatment under general anaesthesia. A systematic review. Stomatologija. 2010;12:60–4.

29. Ridell K, Borgstrom M, Lager E, Magnusson G, Brogardh-Roth S, Matsson L. Oral health-related quality-of-life in Swedish children before and after dental treatment under general anesthesia. Acta Odontol Scand. 2015;73:1–7.

30. Carvalho AC, Paiva SM, Viegas CM, Scarpelli AC, Ferreira FM, Pordeus IA. Impact of malocclusion on oral health-related quality of life among Brazilian preschool children: a population-based study. Braz Dent J. 2013;24:655–61.

31. Gomes MC, Pinto-Sarmento TC, Costa EM, Martins CC, Granville-Garcia AF, Paiva SM. Impact of oral health conditions on the quality of life of preschool children and their families: a cross-sectional study. Health Qual Life Outcomes. 2014;12:55.

32. Kramer PF, Feldens CA, Ferreira SH, Bervian J, Rodrigues PH, Peres MA. Exploring the impact of oral diseases and disorders on quality of life of preschool children. Community Dent Oral Epidemiol. 2013;41:327–35.

33. Abanto J, Carvalho TS, Bonecker M, Ortega AO, Ciamponi AL, Raggio DP. Parental reports of the oral health-related quality of life of children with cerebral palsy. BMC Oral Health. 2012;12:15.

34. Pani SC, Mubaraki SA, Ahmed YT, Alturki RY, Almahfouz SF. Parental perceptions of the oral health-related quality of life of autistic children in Saudi Arabia. Spec Care Dent. 2013;33:8–12.

35. Yashoda R, Puranik MP. Oral health status and parental perception of child oral health related quality-of-life of children with autism in Bangalore, India. J Indian Soc Pedod Prev Dent. 2014;32:135–9.

36. Shavi GR, Thakur B, Bhambal A, Jain S, Singh V, Shukla A. Oral health related quality of life in patients of head and neck cancer attending cancer hospital of Bhopal City, India. J Int Oral Health. 2015;7:21–7.

37. Pope AW, Speltz ML. Research of psychosocial issues of children with craniofacial anomalies: progress and challenges. Cleft palate Craniofac J. 1997;34:371–3.

38. de Paula JS, Sarracini KL, Meneghim MC, et al. Longitudinal evaluation of the impact of dental caries treatment on oral health-related quality of life among schoolchildren. Eur J Oral Sci. 2015;123:173–8.

6

General anxiety, dental anxiety, digit sucking, caries and oral hygiene status of children resident in a semi-urban population in Nigeria

Morenike O. Folayan[1,2,3*], Kikelomo A. Kolawole[1,2,3], Nneka K. Onyejaka[2,3], Hakeem O. Agbaje[2,3], Nneka M. Chukwumah[2,3] and Titus A. Oyedele[2,3]

Abstract

Background: Digit sucking can represent untreated anxiety or other emotional problems. The aim of this study was to determine if digit sucking is a predictor of general anxiety and dental anxiety; and if general and dental anxiety are associated with caries and oral hygiene status of children resident in sub-urban Nigeria.

Methods: This was a secondary data analysis of a household survey conducted in Ile-Ife, Nigeria. The level of general anxiety and dental anxiety of 450 6 to12 year old children were measured using the Revised Child Manifest Anxiety Scale and Dental Subscale of the Child Fear Survey Schedule respectively. Presence of digit sucking habit, caries and oral hygiene status were determined. General anxiety and dental anxiety scores were dichotomized into low and high levels respectively. Logistic regression was conducted to determine if digit sucking was a predictor of general anxiety and dental anxiety; and if general anxiety and dental anxiety were predictors caries and good oral hygiene status. Adjustments were made for age and sex.

Results: Digit sucking is not a significant predictor of dental anxiety ($p = 0.99$) and general anxiety ($p = 0.79$). Children with high general anxiety (AOR: 5.02; 95% CI: 2.9–9.74; $p < 0.001$) and high dental anxiety (AOR: 1.74; 95% CI: 1.15–2.65; $p = 0.009$) had higher odds of having caries and good oral hygiene respectively.

Conclusion: Digit sucking was not a significant predictor of general anxiety and dental anxiety. General and dental anxiety however, had effects on the likelihood of having caries and good oral hygiene.

Keywords: Anxiety, General, Dental, Caries, Oral hygiene, Children, Nigeria

Background

Non-nutritive sucking (NNS) habits are common oral habits, observed in children and in some adults. Digit sucking and nail biting are referred to as nervous NNS habits [1]. These habits are prevalent in normally developing preschool children, and they reflect the state of the mood [1]. Some suggested etiological factors for nail biting include anxiety, stress, loneliness, imitation of others, heredity and inactivity [2]. Nail biting is considered a transitional behavior from thumb sucking [2].

Digit sucking is a normal behavior for young children because they are born with a natural sucking instinct [3]. For most infants, this instinct can last up to the sixth month of life, while for some sucking the habit can continue beyond the sixth month of life when it becomes a soothing and comforting behavior for scared, hungry, sleepy, bored or anxious children [3]. When the habit persists beyond 4 years of age, it can represent untreated anxiety or other emotional problems [4].

General anxiety has been well linked to dental anxiety. Winer [5] suggested that dental fear in children might not be a specific form of fear, but instead may reflect general

* Correspondence: toyinukpong@yahoo.co.uk
[1]Department of Child Dental Health, Obafemi Awolowo University, Ile-Ife, Nigeria
[2]Oral Habit Study Group, Ile-Ife, Nigeria
Full list of author information is available at the end of the article

fear, as there is usually a decline in the prevalence of both general and dental fear with age: the same kind of decline observed with thumb sucking. Klingberg [6] therefore, suggested that children predisposed to general fears should be regarded as having a potential risk of developing dental fear. However, Neverlien [7] found no direct associations between general fear and self-reported dental anxiety, though there was a significant correlation between these two factors for girls who showed signs of clinical anxiety. Folayan et al. [8] however, showed a significant but moderate correlation between dental anxiety and general anxiety.

While Tyron [9] concluded there was no relationship between digit sucking and general anxiety [9], Mahalski and Stanton [10] demonstrated such a relationship through a 5 year longitudinal study. The link between digit sucking and dental anxiety has however not been demonstrated. There is a possibility for such link since prior studies had shown an association between general anxiety and dental anxiety [5, 6, 8]; and an association between digit sucking, other NNS habits and general anxiety [10]. This study will therefore determine if digit sucking is a predictor of dental and general anxiety in children.

Digit sucking has deleterious effects on the oral health of children older than 4 years [11, 12]. Shimura et al. [13] had highlighted the role of emotional stress and the associated psychosomatic responses as a predisposing factor for caries. The association between dental anxiety and poor oral hygiene in adults has also been highlighted [14–16]. We authors found no information in the dental literature on general and dental anxiety being predictors of caries and oral hygiene status in children. Though de Carvalho et al. [17] demonstrated a correlation between dental anxiety oral hygiene frequency and caries, their target population were adolescents not children. This study will therefore, also determine if general anxiety and dental anxiety are associated with caries and oral hygiene status of children resident in sub-urban Nigeria.

Method

This study retrieved the data of children 6 to 12 years old from the data of a larger study conducted to explore the relationship between non-nutritive oral habits and caries [18]. The primary study was a cross sectional study utilising a household survey for study participants' recruitment. A household survey was conducted in order to recruit a representative sample of children from the community since 40.0% of primary school aged children and 60.0% of secondary school aged children are out of school [19].

Study setting

The study was conducted in Ife Central Local Government area of Osun State, a semi-urban area. Ife Central

was chosen as the study location due to its proximity to the Obafemi Awolowo University and the Obafemi Awolowo University Teaching Hospitals Complex, the host institutions of the authors.

Participants were recruited from the National Population Enumeration sites in the Local Government Area. The Enumeration sites were the same used for the 2010 National Antenatal Sero-sentinel Survey [20] and the 2012 National Adolescent Reproductive Health Survey [21]. These study sites were selected because it was assumed that participants in these geographical sites may have been familiar with the conduct of such surveys and thus, be more open to discussing with the field workers.

Study population

The study population for the primary study included 1–7 year old children whose parents gave consent for study participation, and 8–12 year old children who gave assent for study participation in addition to parental consent. Only children who were living with their biological parents or legal guardians and who were at home at the time of data collection were included in the study. The lower age limit for study participants was fixed at 6 years because some of the study tools were designed to collect data for children 6 years and above. The children included in the study were therefore those with in the age-range of children with mixed dentition.

Sample size

Sample size for the primary study as calculated using Leslie Fischer's formula [22] for study population > 10,000. A previous study [23] reported a prevalence of 34.1% for oral habits in 4–15 year old Nigerian children. Based on a prevalence of 34.1%, it was found that it would be necessary to examine 1011 children to capture 345 children with oral habits, with a fall out rate of 10%.

Sampling technique

The sampling procedure used a multi-stage cluster sampling method to select eligible persons. First, there was the random selection of enumeration areas within the Local Government Area. Next, every third household on each street at the enumeration areas was identified for study participant recruitment. In each household, eligible individuals were listed and one eligible child randomly selected for study participation using balloting.

Study procedure

Experienced trained field workers administered a structured questionnaire developed in English to collect data for the study using an approach had had been used successfully for prior studies conducted in multi-lingual communities in Nigeria [24–29].

The field workers collected information from the respondent and submitted the completed questionnaires to the survey supervisor daily. The supervisor reviewed all filled questionnaires and raised queries where gaps were identified in the filled questionnaire, or the consenting process. The queries were addressed latest by the next day by the field worker where this was feasible. This may involve returning to the household to collect missing data or the need to entire essential documentation details in the filled questionnaires.

The questionnaires assessing dental anxiety and general anxiety were only administered to children 6–12 years old. The questionnaires were filled by the mothers of children 6–7 years and by children 8–12 years. Mothers were requested to fill the questionnaire on behalf of their children because prior studies conducted in the same environment showed that the correlation between child's general and dental anxiety level best correlated with the mother's assessment of these situations when compared to correlation with the father's assessment [8]. Dental and general anxiety levels were classified as high or low using the cut off established for the study population by Folayan et al. [8]. However, where the mother was unavailable, fathers completed the questionnaires.

Data collection tools

The questionnaire asked for details on the child's socio-demographic characteristics (age, sex), if digit sucking habit was present, general anxiety and dental anxiety (Sections 1, 3, 18 and 19 of the Additional file 1 respectively). Details of the child's medical and dental history which explored possible medical and dental health issues that could interfere with oral health were also collected (Section 17 of the Additional file 1). Any child who had any form of cognitive impairment was excluded from the study.

General anxiety

The Revised Child Manifest Anxiety Scale (RCMAS) [30] was used to measure level and nature of self-reported trait anxiety. The instrument had been used on prior studies conducted among children in Nigeria [31, 32] and its reliability for use among school children in Nigeria determined [19]. Cross-cultural validity of the tool had also been determined [33]. It consists of 28 anxiety items and 9 lie (social desirability) yes-or-no items. A response of "Yes" indicates that the item is descriptive of the subject's feelings or actions, whereas a response of "No" indicates that the item is generally not descriptive. Scores are provided for total anxiety and four sub-scales namely the 10 item physiological anxiety scale, the 11 item worry/oversensitivity scale, the 7 item social concerns/concentration scale, and the 9 item lie scale. The possible total score ranged

from 0 to 37. Scores were derived from affirmative responses. A high score indicates a high level of anxiety or lie [23]. A prior study had used a cut-off point of 19 to identify children experiencing clinically significant levels of anxiety [33]. For this study, children with scores 19 and below were categorized as having low general anxiety and those with scores above 19 were categorized as having high trait anxiety.

Dental anxiety

The dental anxiety of each child was assessed using Dental Subscale of the Child Fear Survey Schedule (CFSS-DS) described by Cuthbert and Melamed [34]. The CFSS-DS is a 5-point Likert scale with scores ranging from 1 (not afraid at all) to 5 (very afraid) for each of the 15 items. These covered different aspects of the dental situation. Total scores ranged from 15 to 75. The scale had been used in a prior study conducted in the same population in Nigeria, to measure dental anxiety [23]. Children with scores equal to and less than median score for the group were classified as having low anxiety while those who scored above the median score were classified as having high anxiety. This method of categorization had been used by Folayan et al. [35]. For this study, children with scores below 35 were categorized as having low dental anxiety and those with scores 35 and above were categorized as having high dental anxiety.

Intra-oral examination

All children eligible to participate in the study had an oral examination conducted in their homes on the day of study visits. The children were examined under natural light while sitting down on the chair, using sterile dental mirrors by trained dentists attached to each field worker. The teeth were examined wet. Intraoral examination was conducted to determine presence of caries and its severity and oral hygiene status. Radiographs were not used in the study.

Oral hygiene status

The most commonly used index to assess the oral hygiene status, the oral hygiene index was used for assessment in this study. The Oral Hygiene Index (Simplified) OHI-S described by Greene and Vermillion [36] was used to determine the oral hygiene status. It is composed of the Debris Index and Calculus index, each of which was obtained based on 6 numerical determinations representing the amount of debris or calculus found on the surfaces of the index teeth. 11, 16, 26, 31, 36 and 46 and 51, 55, 65, 71, 75, 85 in the permanent and deciduous dentitions respectively. For each individual, the debris and calculus scores were totaled and divided by the number of surfaces scored. The scores were graded as 0.0–1.2 = Good oral hygiene, 1.3–3.0 = Fair oral hygiene and > 3.1 = Poor oral hygiene.

Caries profile

The teeth were examined for caries after the OHI-S was determined. Debris was removed from the wet teeth using gauze prior to assessment for caries status. The teeth present were charted using the FDI tooth numbering system. Caries diagnosis was based on the recommendation of the World Health Organisation Oral Health Survey methods [37]. The caries status was assessed using the Decayed Missing and Filled/decayed missing and filled teeth (DMFT/dmft) index. For ease of analysis, caries status was further divided into caries present or caries absent. Children were classified as having caries present when a tooth was identified to be decayed.

To arrive at a dmft/DMFT score for an individual child, three values were determined: the number of teeth with carious lesions, the number of extracted teeth due to caries, and the number of teeth with fillings or crowns [38]. Parents of children were asked to explain the loss of any teeth that was not found during the oral examination. Only tooth extracted due to caries were recorded as missing. The number of teeth are summed together to give the dmft score for the primary dentition and the DMFT score for the permanent dentition.

Calibration of examiners

Clinical investigators were postgraduate Paedodontists and Orthodontists residents. They were calibrated on the use of the WHO criteria for caries diagnosis and the OHI-S. The intra-examiner scores ranged from 0.89 to 0.94, while inter-examiner variability ranged from 0.82 to 0.90 for caries detection and OHI-S [18].

Data analysis

Descriptive analysis was conducted using a variety of measures of location and dispersion. This was represented as Tables. A test of association was conducted to determine the association between the general anxiety subscales and the presence of caries, or the oral hygiene status. Multivariate logistic regression was conducted to determine the predictors of presence of caries and good oral hygiene; and if digit sucking was a predictor of general anxiety and dental anxiety. The age of the study participants were grouped into two: 6–8 years and 9–12 years. The effect of age and sex were controlled for. Statistical analysis was conducted with Intercooled STATA (release 12) for windows. Statistical significance was inferred at $p \leq 0.05$.

Results

Four hundred and ninety seven participants were eligible to participate in the study. Only 450 (90.5%) participants had data complete enough for analysis of information on both dental and general (state and trait) anxiety. These included 226 (50.2%) 6-8 year olds and 222 (49.3%) male participants. Very few study participants (4.5%) had poor oral hygiene and very few sucked their digits (6.0%). Table 1 highlights the profile of the study participants.

The general anxiety scores measured using the RCMAS ranged from 0 to 36. The mean score was 11.8 ± (7.6) and the median score was 9. The mean physiological anxiety score was 2.42 ± (2.36). The mean worry/oversensitivity score was 3.03 ± (3.34). The social concerns/concentration score was 1.77 ± (2.01). The mean lie score was 4.52 ± (1.84). Three hundred and ninety two (87.1%) participants had low clinically significant trait anxiety (anxiety scores less than 19) while

Table 1 Frequency distribution of demographic variables, caries status, oral hygiene status and anxiety status (N = 450)

Demographic profile	N = 450 Number (%)
Age	
6 years – 8 years	226 (50.2%)
9 years – 12 years	224 (49.8%)
Gender	
Male	222 (49.3%)
Female	228 (50.7%)
Caries status	
Caries present	76 (16.6%)
Caries free	374 (83.1%)
dmft	
0	386 (85.8%)
1–2	48 (10.7%)
3–6	16 (3.5%)
DMFT	
0	428 (95.1%)
1–2	18 (4.0%)
3–4	4 (0.9%)
Oral hygiene status	
Good	172 (38.4%)
Fair	256 (57.1%)
Poor	20 (4.5%)
Dental anxiety	
Low	226 (50.2%)
High	224 (49.8%)
General anxiety	
Low	392 (87.1%)
High	58 (12.9%)
Digit sucking	
Present	27 (6.0%)
Absent	423 (94.0%)

58 (12.9%) participants had high clinically significant trait anxiety (anxiety scores between 19 and 28).

The dental anxiety scores measured using the CFSS-DS ranged from 15 to 75. The mean score was 38.6± (14.4) and the median score was 35. Two hundred and thirteen (47.3%) participants had low dental anxiety (dental anxiety scores less than 35) while 237 (52.7%) respondents had high dental anxiety (dental anxiety scores 35 and above).

Seventy six (16.6%) participants had caries. The dmft scores ranged from 0 to 6 and the DMFT scores ranged from 0to 4. The mean dmft was $0.29 \pm (0.84)$ and the mean DMFT was $0.08 \pm (0.44)$.

Digit sucking and anxiety

Table 2 highlights the association between digit sucking, dental anxiety and general anxiety having controlled for age and sex. Digit sucking was not significantly associated with dental anxiety ($p = 0.99$) and general anxiety ($p = 0.79$). Neither was it a general anxiety (AOR: 0.83; 95% CI: 0.23–3.07) or dental anxiety (AOR: 1.01; 95% CI: 0.44–2.31) a predictor of digit sucking habit.

Caries and anxiety

Table 3 shows the results of the test of association between the general anxiety subscale and caries status. Children who had caries had significant higher means scores ($p < 0.001$) on the physiological anxiety, worry/oversensitivity and social concerns/concentration scales respectively.

Table 4 highlights the predictors of presence of caries. Children who had high general anxiety (OR: 5.07; 95% CI: 2.79–9.20; $p < 0.001$) had higher odds of having caries when compared with children with low general anxiety. Also children who had high dental anxiety (OR: 1.69; 95% CI: 1.02–2.80; $p = 0.04$) had higher odds of having caries when compared with children with low dental anxiety. After adjusting for age, sex and dental anxiety, general anxiety was still a significant predictor of presence caries: children who had high general anxiety (AOR: 5.02; 95% CI: 2.59–9.74; $p < 0.001$) had higher odds of having caries when compared with children with low general anxiety.

Oral hygiene and anxiety

Table 5 shows the results of the test of association between the general anxiety subscale and oral hygiene status. Children with fair oral hygiene had significant lower mean scores on each of the subscales.

Table 6 highlights the predictors of good oral hygiene. Children who had high dental anxiety (OR: 2.27; 95% CI: 1.52–3.32; p < 0.001) had higher odds of having good oral hygiene when compared with children with low dental anxiety. Also children who had high general anxiety (OR: 2.38; 95% CI: 1.35–4.20; $p = 0.002$) had higher odds of having good oral hygiene when compared with children with low general anxiety. After adjusting for age, sex and general anxiety, dental anxiety was still a significant predictor of presence good oral hygiene: children who had high dental anxiety (AOR: 1.87; 95% CI: 1.23–2.84; $p = 0.003$) had higher odds of having good oral hygiene when compared with children with low dental anxiety. Age was also a significant predictor of good oral hygiene children in the unadjusted and adjusted models: older children had lower odds of having good oral hygiene when compared with younger children (AOR: 0.66; 95% CI:0.44–0.98; $p = 0.04$).

Table 2 Frequency distribution and logistic regression analysis of digit sucking as predictor of general anxiety and dental anxiety ($N = 450$)

Variables	Digit sucking				Simple regression		Multiple regression	
	Absent ($N = 423$)	Percent	Present ($N = 27$)	Percent	OR (95% CI)	p-value	AOR (95% CI)	p-value
Sex								
Male	206	48.7	16	59.3	1	–	1	–
Female	217	51.3	11	40.7	0.65 (0.30–1.44)	0.29	0.66 (0.29–1.46)	0.30
Age group								
6–8 years	212	50.1	14	51.9	1	–	1	–
9–12 years	211	49.9	13	48.1	0.93 (0.43–2.03)	0.86	0.96 (0.43–2.11)	0.91
Dental Anxiety								
Low	212	50.1	14	51.9	1	–	1	–
High	211	49.9	13	48.1	0.93 (0.43–2.03)	0.86	1.01 (0.44–2.31)	0.99
General anxiety								
Low	368	87.0	24	88.9	1	–	1	–
High	55	13.0	3	11.1	0.84 (0.24–2.87)	0.78	0.83 (0.23–3.07)	0.79

Table 3 Association between general anxiety subscales and caries status

Subscales	Caries status	Number	Mean ± sd	t	df	p value
Physiological anxiety	Present	76	3.4 ± 2.9	3.9	448	< 0.001
	Absent	374	2.2 ± 2.2			
Worry/oversensitivity	Present	76	4.6 ± 4.1	4.5	448	< 0.001
	Absent	374	2.7 ± 3.1			
Social concerns/concentration	Present	76	2.5 ± 2.4	3.6	448	< 0.001
	Absent	374	1.6 ± 1.9			
Lie	Present	76	4.6 ± 1.9	0.4	448	0.72
	Absent	374	4.5 ± 1.8			

Discussion

The study highlighted the association between dental anxiety, general anxiety, digit sucking, caries and oral hygiene status of children in the age range for mixed dentition, in the study population. We found that digit sucking was not a significant predictor of dental anxiety or general anxiety. The prevalence of high dental anxiety was high in the study population; children with high dental anxiety and younger children were significantly more likely to have good oral hygiene. About an eight of the population had high general anxiety; children with high general anxiety were significantly more likely to have caries.

First, like Tyron [9] and unlike Mahalski and Stanton [10], we found that digit sucking was not a significant predictor of general anxiety and dental anxiety in this study population. We however were unable to explain these observations though we assume it may be linked with the ways culture influences expression of anxiety: we assume that the African culture promotes internalization of problems and its expressions unlike other cultures where externalizing problems and anxiety are welcome and accepted [8].

Second, unlike many prior studies that had found an association between dental anxiety and the increased risk for caries [39–44], our studies could not establish such association. Some of these studies had conducted bivariate analysis (tests of associations) to establish these associations [39, 40] and others had conducted the studies in older children [34, 35]. Studies that have conducted more robust analysis using logistic regression models reported an association between presence of caries and dental anxiety in older children [43, 44]. The difference in study methodology including differences in the age of the study population and method of data analysis, are factors that can significantly influence study outcome. Our study illustrated this in that with simple logistic regression analysis, dental anxiety was associated with presence of caries. However, when the model was adjusted for age, sex and general anxiety, the observed significance was lost. A few other studies [45–47] had also found no association between presence of caries and dental anxiety.

Table 4 Frequency distribution and logistic regression on predictors of presence of caries (N = 450)

Variables	Caries				Simple regression		Multiple regression	
	Absent (N = 374)	Percent	Present (N = 76)	Percent	OR (95% CI)	p-value	AOR (95% CI)	p-value
Sex								
Male	189	50.5	33	43.4	1	–	1	–
Female	185	49.5	43	56.6	1.33 (0.81–2.19)	0.26	1.35 (0.80–2.27)	0.26
Age group								
6–8 years	185	49.5	41	53.9	1	–	1	–
9–12 years	189	50.5	35	46.1	0.84 (0.51–1.37)	0.48	0.91 (0.54–1.54)	0.73
Dental Anxiety								
Low	196	52.4	30	39.5	1	–	1	–
High	178	47.6	46	60.5	1.69 (1.02–2.80)	0.04	1.00 (0.56–1.79)	0.99
General anxiety								
Low	341	91.2	51	67.1	1	–	1	–
High	33	8.8	25	32.9	5.07 (2.79–9.20)	< 0.001	5.02 (2.59–9.74)	< 0.001

Table 5 Association between general anxiety subscales and oral hygiene status

Subscales	Oral hygiene status	Number	Mean ± sd	F(df)	p value
Physiological anxiety	Good	172	2.9 ± 2.6	5.67 (2, 445, 447)	0.004
	Fair	256	2.1 ± 2.1		
	Poor	20	2.7 ± 2.3		
Worry/ oversensitivity	Good	172	3.7 ± 3.7	7.52 (2, 445, 447)	0.001
	Fair	256	2.5 ± 3.0		
	Poor	20	3.9 ± 3.5		
Social concerns/ concentration	Good	172	2.1 ± 2.3	5.39 (2, 445, 447)	0.005
	Fair	256	1.5 ± 1.7		
	Poor	20	2.4 ± 2.4		
Lie	Good	172	4.8 ± 1.8	3.55 (2, 445, 447)	0.03
	Fair	256	4.3 ± 1.8		
	Poor	20	4.7 ± 1.9		

Third, we also noticed that age and sex were not predictors of caries for children with mixed dentition in this study population. Other studies on dental caries in the mixed dentition had reported similar findings [48, 49] while others had reported observations different from ours [40, 50]. This disparity in study findings may point to residential and cultural differences in risk factors for caries. 'Genderization' of diseases and disease processes are also a reflection of how societies and communities 'genderize' behaviors that increase risk for diseases [51–53]. Ile-Ife is still considered a sub-rural area where the impact of genderized' behaviors is seen much later in life than during the mixed dentition stage. Thus, children and teenagers still, for the most part, have homogenized behaviors [54] with distinct age and sexual behaviors occurring at a later age than observed in urbanized communities. Such differences in behavior like being disorganized, self-consciousness and low esteem, increased independency [55] may increase the risk for caries [56]. The homogenized behavior of children in this study population may be a reason why we did not observe significant sexual and age difference in their caries profile.

Fourth, we observed age differences in the oral hygiene profile. A prior study had highlighted differences in the oral hygiene profile of children with primary dentition (1–5 years) and those with mixed dentition (6–12 years) [57]: younger children had better oral hygiene than older children. This study further highlights that for children with mixed dentition, children (6–8 years) had better oral hygiene than teenagers (9-12 years). We feel tooth brushing of children (6-8 years) are still supervised and so increases the chances of having better oral hygiene profile than teenagers who are free from parental supervision of tooth brushing. Our study may be a reflection of this phenomenon. This however, requires further investigation.

Table 6 Frequency distribution and logistic regression analysis on the predictors of good oral hygiene (N = 448)

Variables	Oral Hygiene				Simple regression		Multiple regression	
	Poor (N = 276)	Percent	Good (N = 172)	Percent	OR (95% CI)	p-value	AOR (95% CI)	p-value
Sex								
Male	142	51.4	78	45.3	1	–	1	–
Female	134	48.6	94	54.7	1.28 (0.87–1.87)	0.21	1.25 (0.84–1.86)	0.27
Age group								
6–8 years	126	45.7	100	58.1	1	–	1	–
9–12 years	150	54.3	72	41.9	0.61 (0.41–0.89)	0.01	0.66 (0.44–0.98)	0.04
Dental Anxiety								
Low	160	58.0	65	37.8	1		1	–
High	116	42.0	105	61.2	2.27 (1.52–3.38)	< 0.001	1.87 (1.23–2.84)	0.003
General anxiety								
Low	251	90.9	139	80.8	1	–	1	–
High	25	9.1	33	19.2	2.38 (1.35–4.20)	0.002	1.71 (0.94–3.11)	0.08

Fifth, the independency of the association between general anxiety, dental anxiety, caries and oral hygiene status when adjusted for age and sex, may suggest the independency of the two phenomena – dental anxiety and general anxiety – contrary to the opinion of Winer [5]. Folayan et al. [8] had also reported a moderate but significant correlation between self report of dental anxiety and general anxiety of 8–13 year old children's in the same study population. This study however, conducted a more robust analysis by adjusting for age and sex as possible confounding variables for dental and general anxiety as highlighted in the literatures. The finding of this regression analysis points to the possibility that the direct relationship observed may be lost in the presence of confounding variables. This postulation needs to be studied further.

This study had a few limitations. First, though the study finding is generalization to the study population, the finding may not be generalizable to a more urban population where culture and behavior of children are more diverse and influenced by multiple variables. Also, this study was based on a secondary data analysis thus the study was not powered to determine differences in digit sucking habit, caries and oral hygiene status based on general anxiety and dental anxiety status. The primary study did not identify caries using radiographs thus it only gave a rough estimate of the prevalence of dental caries in the study population. Examining oral hygiene status in wet conditions without using other aids and without any standardization for the time of examination may also bias the finding. We have however followed standard procedures for assessing oral hygiene status thus making our findings comparable with others that used the OHI-S.Also, when working with children, the lack of attention and poor understanding can generates bias. The finding on the association between general anxiety and caries needs to be taken with caution as the confidence interval is wide. Though we have used a logistic regression analysis to determine digit sucking as a predictor for general and dental anxiety, we recognize that prediction requires a longitudinal design as it involves causality. This study was a cross sectional study thus limited in its ability to truly predict and more powered to determine an association. Despite these limitations, the study has added clarity to our understanding of the association between the variables studied, and suggests that significant associations and effects of general anxiety and dental anxiety on presence of digit sucking, presence of caries and presence of good oral hygiene.

Conclusion

Digit sucking was not a significant predictor of general anxiety and dental anxiety in the study population. General anxiety significantly increases the likelihood of presence of caries while dental anxiety significantly increases the likelihood of good oral hygiene. Further studies are required to understand how dental anxiety and general anxiety play independent roles as the risk factors for dental caries and oral hygiene when past studies had shown direct relationship between dental anxiety and general anxiety [58, 59] and caries and oral hygiene status [52, 53].

Abbreviations
AOR: Adjusted Odds Ratio; CFSS-DS: Dental Subscale of the Child Fear Survey Schedule; dmft/DMFT: Decay, missing, filled teeth; NNS: Non-nutritive sucking; OR: Odds Ratio; RCMAS: The Revised Child Manifest Anxiety Scale; SD: Standard Deviation; WHO: World Health Organisation

Authors' contributions
MOF designed the study. MOF, KAK, NKO, HOA, NMC and TAO were involved with the extraction of datafrom the primary data set and organization of the data for analysis MOF conducted the analysis and developed the framework for the manuscript. MOF, KAK, NKO, HOA, NMC and TAO contributed to the interpretation and discussion of the results. All authors read and approved the final version of the manuscript and agreed to its submission.

Competing interests
The authors declare that they have no competing interests.

Author details
[1]Department of Child Dental Health, Obafemi Awolowo University, Ile-Ife, Nigeria. [2]Oral Habit Study Group, Ile-Ife, Nigeria. [3]Department of Child Dental Health, Obafemi Awolowo University Teaching Hospitals Complex, Ile-Ife, Nigeria.

References
1. Foster LG. Nervous habits and stereotyped behaviors in preschool children. J Am Acad Child Adolesc Psychiatry. 1998;37:711–7.
2. Tanaka OM, Vitral RW, Tanaka GY, Guerrero AP, Camargo ES. Nail biting, or onychophagia: a special habit. Am J Orthod Dentofac Orthop. 2008;134: 305–8.
3. Festila D, Ghergie M, Muntean A, Matiz D, Serbanescu A. Suckling and non-nutritive sucking habit: what should we know? Clujul Med. 2014;87:11–4.
4. Shahraki N, Yassaei S, Moghadam MG. Abnormal oral habits: a review. J Dent Oral Hyg. 2012;4:12–5.
5. Winer GA. A review and analysis of children's fearful behaviour in dental setting. Child Dev. 1982;53:1111–3.
6. Klingberg G. Dental fear and behaviour management problems in children. Swed Dent J. 1995;103:1–78.
7. Neverlien PO. Fear and dental apprehension among school-age children in a rural district. Nor Tannlaegeforen Tid. 1989;99:574–8.
8. Folayan MO, Idehen EE, Ojo OO. Dental anxiety in a subpopulation of African children: parents ability to predict and its relation to general anxiety and behaviour in the dental chair. Eur J Paediatr Dent. 2004;5:19–23.
9. Tyron AF. Thumb-sucking and manifest anxiety: a note. Child Dev. 1968;39:1159–63.
10. Mahalski PA, Stanton WR. The relationship between digit sucking and behaviour problems: a longitudinal study over 10 years. J Child Psychol Psychiatry. 1992;33:913–23.
11. Haryett RD, Hansen FC, Davidson PO, Snadilands ML. Chronic thumb-sucking: the psychologic effects and the relative effectiveness of various methods of treatment. Am J Ortho. 1967;53:569–85.

12. Diwanji A, Jain P, Doshi J, Somani P, Mehta D. Modified bluegrass appliance: a non-punitive therapy for thumb sucking in pediatric patients - a case report with review of the literature. Case Rep Dent. 2013;2013:537120.

13. Shimura N, Nakamura C, Hirayama Y, Yonemitsu M. Anxiety and dental caries. Community Dent Oral Epidemiol. 1983;11:224–7.

14. Nair MA, Shankarapillai R, Rai N, Ragotham K, Charanbabu HS. Dental anxiety and oral hygiene in Udaipur rural women. Inter J Dent Clin. 2010;2:33–5.

15. Kanaffa-Kilijanska U, Kaczmarek U, Kilijanska B, Frydecka D. Oral health condition and hygiene habits among adult. Oral Health Prev Dent. 2014;12: 233–9.

16. DeDonno MA. Dental anxiety, dental visits and oral hygiene practices. Oral Health Prev Dent. 2012;10:129–33.

17. de Carvalho RW, de Carvalho Bezerra Falcão PG, de Luna Campos GJ, de Souza Andrade ES, do Egito Vasconcelos BC, da Silva Pereira MA. Prevalence and predictive factors of dental anxiety in Brazilian adolescents. J Dent Child (Chic). 2013;80(1):41–6.

18. Kolawole KA, Folayan MO, Agbaje HO, Oyedele TA, Oziegbe EO, Onyejaka NK, et al. Digit sucking habit and association with dental caries and oral hygiene status of children aged 6 months to 12 years in semi-urban Nigeria. PLoS One. 2016;11:e0148322.

19. United Nations Children's Fund. National report Nigeria: Global study on child poverty and disparities. Available at: http://www.unicef.org/socialpolicy/files/Nigeria_GLOBAL_STUDY_ON_CHILD_POVERTY_AND_DISPARITIES_smaller.pdf. Accessed 14 Feb 2016.

20. Federal Ministry of Health. Technical report 2010, vol. 2010. Nigeria: National HIV sero-prevalence sentinel survey among pregnant women attending antenatal clinics in Nigeria, Department of Public Health and National AIDS/STI Control Programme.

21. Federal Ministry of Health. National HIV & AIDS and reproductive health survey, Abuja. 2013.

22. Araoye MO. Research methodology with statistics for health and social sciences. Nathadex Publishing, Ilorin. 2003:115–9.

23. Quashie-Williams R, da Costa OO, Isiekwe MC. Oral habits, prevalence and effects on occlusion of 4-15 year old school children in Lagos, Nigeria. Niger Postgrad Med J. 2010;17:113–7.

24. Federal Ministry of Health. National HIV and AIDS reproductive health survey. Abuja: Federal Ministry of Health; 2007.

25. Federal Ministry of Health. National HIV/AIDS and reproductive health survey. Abuja: Federal Ministry of Health; 2005.

26. Federal Ministry of Health. HIV/STI integrated biological and behavioural surveillance survey (IBBSS). Abuja: Federal Ministry of Health; 2008.

27. Federal Ministry of Health. HIV/STI integrated biological and behavioural surveillance survey (IBBSS). Abuja: Federal Ministry of Health; 2010.

28. Folayan MO, Adebajo S, Adeyemo A, Ogungbemi KM. Differences in sexual practices, sexual behavior and HIV risk profile between adolescents and young persons in rural and urban Nigeria. PLoS One. 2015;10:e0129106.

29. Folayan MO, Odetoyingbo M, Brandon B, Harrison A. Differences in sexual behaviour and sexual practices of adolescents in Nigeria based on sex and self-reported HIV status. BMC Reprod Health. 2014;11:83.

30. Reynolds CR, Richmond BO. Factor structure and construct validity of what I think and feel: the revised Children's manifest anxiety scale. J Pers Assess. 1985;43:281–3.

31. Pela OA, Reynolds CR. Cross-cultural application of the revised-children's manifest anxiety scale: normative and reliability data for Nigerian primary school children. Psychol Rep. 1982;51:1135–8.

32. Cuthbert MI, Melamed BG. A screening device for children at risk for dental fear ad management problems. J Dent Child. 1982;49:432–6.

33. Al Jabery MA, Arabiat DH. Psychometric properties of the Arabic translated version of the RCMAS: preliminary indicators from a Jordanian sample. J Int Couns Educ. 2011;3:13–24.

34. Folayan MO, Otuyemi OD. Reliability and validity of a short form of the dental subscale of the child fear survey schedule used in a Nigerian children population. Niger J Med. 2002;11:161–3.

35. Folayan MO, Idehen EE, Ojo OO. Dental anxiety in a subpopulation of African children: parents ability to predict and its relation to general anxiety and behaviour in the dental chair. Eur J Paediatr Dent. 2004;1:19–22.

36. Greene JC, Vermillion JR. The simplified oral hygiene index. J Am Dent Assoc. 1964;68:7–13.

37. World Health Organisation (WHO). Oral health surveys: basic methods. Geneva: World Health Organisation; 1997.

38. Krapp K. Dental indices. Encyclopedia of Nursing & Allied Health. Ed. Vol. 2. Gale Cengage. eNotes.com. http://www.enotes.com/dental-indices-reference/. Accessed 2 Jan 2012.

39. Milsom KM, Tickle M, Humphris GM, Blinkhorn AS. The relationship between anxiety and dental treatment experience in 5-year old children. BDJ. 2003; 194:503–6.

40. Viswanath D, Krishna AV. Correlation between dental anxiety, sense of coherence (SOC) and dental caries in school children from Bangalore north: a cross-sectional study. J Indian Soc Pedod Prev Dent. 2015;33:15–8.

41. Esa R, Ong AL, Humphris G, Freeman R. The relationship of dental caries and dental fear in Malaysian adolescents: a latent variable approach. BMC Oral Health. 2014;14:19.

42. Taani DQ, El-Qaderi SS, Abu Alhaija ES. Dental anxiety in children and its relationship to dental caries and gingival condition. Int J Dent Hyg. 2005;3:83–7.

43. Kruger E, Thomson WM, Poulton R, Davies S, Brown RH, Silva PA. Dental caries and changes in dental anxiety in late adolescence. Community Dent Oral Epidemiol. 1998;26:355–9.

44. Rantavuori K, Lahti S, Hausen H, Seppa L, Karkkainen S. Dental fear and oral healthand family characteristics of Finnish children. Acta Odontol Scand. 2004;62:207–13.

45. Abanto J, Vidigal EA, Carvalho TS, Sá SN, Bönecker M. Factors for determining dental anxiety in preschool children with severe dental caries. Braz Oral Res. 2017;31:e13.

46. Alkarslan ZZ, Erten H, Uzun O, Iseri E, Topun O. Relationship between trait anxiety, dental anxiety and DMFT indexes of Turkish patient attending a dental school clinic. East Mediterr Health J. 2010;16:558–13.

47. Thomson WM, Locker D, Poulton R. Incidence of dental anxiety in young adults in relation to dental treatment experience. Community Dent Oral Epidemiol. 2000;28:289–94.

48. Sudha PA, Bhasin S, Anegundi RT. Prevalence of dental caries among 5-13-year-old children of Mangalore city. J Indian Soc Ped Prev Dent. 2005;23:74–9.

49. Shetty NS, Tandon S. Prevalence of dental caries as related to risk factors in school children of south Kanara. J Indian Soc Ped Prev Dent. 1988;6:30–7.

50. Zander A, Sivaneswaran S, Skinnerr J, Byun R, Jalaludin B. Risk factors for dental caries in rural and urban regional Australian communities. Rural Remote Health. 2013;13:2492.

51. Guerra-Silveira F, Abad-Franch F. Sex bias in infectious disease epidemiology: patterns and processes. PLoS One. 2013;8:e62390.

52. Ferraro M, Vieira AR. Explaining gender differences in caries: a multifactorial approach to a multifactorial disease. Int J Dent. 2010;2010:649643.

53. Klein SL, Roberts CW, editors. Sex and Gender Differences in Infection and Treatments for Infectious Diseases. Springer International Publishing AG; 2015. ISBN 978-3-319-16438-0.

54. Rimmo PA. Aberrant driving behaviour: homogeneity of a four-factor structure in samples differing in age and gender. Ergonomics. 2002;45:569–82.

55. Lewis GJ, Haworth CM, Plomin R. Identical genetic influence underpin behavior problems in adolescence and basictraits of personality. J Child Psychol Psychiatry. 2014;55:865–75.

56. Abreu LG, Elyasi M, Badri P, Paiva SM, Flores-Mir C, Amin M. Factors associated with the development of dental caries in children and adolescents in studies employing the life course approach: a systematic review. Eur J Oral Sci. 2015. https://doi.org/10.1111/eos.12206.

57. Hakeberg M, Hägglin C, Berggren U, Carlsson SG. Structural relationships of dental anxiety, mood, and general anxiety. Acta Odontol Scand. 2001;59:99–103.

58. Sowole A, Sote E, Folayan M. Dental caries, pattern and predisposing oral hygiene related factors in Nigerian preschool children. Eur Arch Paediatr Dent. 2007;8:206–10.

59. Ayele FA, Taye BW, Ayele TA, Gelaye KA. Predictors of dental caries among children 7-14 years in north West Ethiopia: a community based cross-sectional study. BMC Oral Health. 2013;13:7.

7

Oral health promotion practices: a survey of Florida child care center directors

Vinodh Bhoopathi[1*], Ajay Joshi[2], Romer Ocanto[3] and Robin J. Jacobs[4]

Abstract

Background: To understand the oral health promotion practices (OHPPs) in Florida licensed childcare centers (CCCs), we surveyed the childcare center directors (CCCDs) employed at these centers. We determined if CCC's affiliation with Early Head Start/Head Start (EHS/HS) programs was associated with the number of OHPPs implemented.

Methods: For this cross-sectional study we emailed a pretested 45-item online survey to unduplicated email addresses of 5142 licensed CCCDs as listed in the publicly available Florida Department of Child and Family services database. Univariate and bivariate analyses were conducted. In addition, a Poisson regression model predicting higher numbers of OHPPs implemented was conducted.

Results: A response rate of 19.4% was estimated. CCCDs reporting to implement a higher number of OHPPs in their CCCs were more likely to have longer work experience (b = 0.006, 95% CI: 0.001,0.012 $p = 0.03$), work in EHS/HS affiliated centers (b = 0.7, 95%CI: 0.48,0.91) $p < 0.001$, and have more positive attitudes about pediatric oral health (b = 0.08, 95%CI: 0.05, 0.10) $p < 0.001$. CCCDs with more self-perceived barriers reported implementing a lower number of OHPPs (b = − 0.046, 95% CI: -0.09, − 0.003 $p = 0.035$) compared to their counterparts.

Conclusions: A significant association between a CCC's affiliation with EHS/HS programs and the number of OHPPs implemented was observed. In addition, CCCD's years of experience, attitudes towards oral health, and self-perceived barriers in implementing OHPPs were also associated with the number of OHPPs implemented.

Keywords: Oral health, Health promotion, Day care, Child care centers, Dental caries, Prevention, Head start, Early head start

Background

The number of child care facilities in the U.S. rose from 262,511 in 1987 to 766,401 in 2007, indicating an increasing trend in the establishment of such facilities [1]. There were 32.7 million children in 'out-of-home' child care facilities in year 2011, of which most (20.2 million) were aged 5–14 years; while the remaining 12.5 million were aged 0 to 4 years [2]. Preschoolers of employed and non-employed mothers spent approximately 36 h and 21 h respectively per week in these facilities [2]. Because a significant proportion of children spend so much time in these facilities, health intervention and promotion programs can be implemented in these settings to promote the health of the enrolled children.

One significant public health problem is an ongoing epidemic of dental caries in the U.S. children. The 2011–2012 National Health and Nutrition Examination Survey data showed that at least 40% of 2 to 8 year old children experienced dental caries in their primary teeth, with at least 14% having untreated tooth decay, suggesting that despite needing dental care, it was not received [3]. Approximately 21% of children ages 6 to 11, and 53% of adolescents aged 12 to 19 years had experienced dental caries [3]. This national data suggests that children develop dental caries all through their childhood.

Since many children spend a portion of their day in CCCs, centers provide an ideal setting to adopt measures to prevent dental caries, especially since most

* Correspondence: Vinodh.Bhoopathi@temple.edu
[1]Department of Pediatric Dentistry and Community Oral Health Sciences, Temple University Maurice H. Kornberg School of Dentistry, 3223 N Broad Street, Philadelphia, PA 19140, USA
Full list of author information is available at the end of the article

children enrolled in CCCs fall into the susceptible age range for dental caries. CCCs and childcare center directors (CCCDs) could take an active role to prevent dental diseases and promote oral health of all children enrolled in these centers by educating children and their parents about the importance of maintaining proper oral health, and adopting good oral health promotion practices (OHPPs) [4].

The American Academy of Pediatric Dentistry (AAPD) recognizes the importance and impact of oral health promotion within CCCs, based on children's increased utilization of and time spent in these facilities for daily care [5]. The AAPD released a set of oral health guidelines addressing dental disease prevention and oral health promotion in out-of-home child care settings targeting CCCs, pediatric dentists, other health care professionals, legislators and policy makers [5]. This policy encourages CCCs to implement oral health promotion practices (OHPPs) to reduce a child's risk of acquiring early childhood caries and the risk of dental trauma within their centers.

Very few studies have assessed the oral health related policies and regulations in daycare or childcare centers in the U.S. [6–8]. Little is known about licensed CCCs in the state of Florida, and the type of OHPPs implemented within these centers. Florida CCCs provide a unique opportunity to explore oral health promotion practices because children in Florida experience poorer oral health and lack adequate dental care access compared to children in many other states [9]. Therefore our study surveyed child care center directors (CCCDs) employed in Florida licensed CCCs to determine which of the 8 selected AAPD recommended OHPPs were already implemented, and the factors associated with a higher number of OHPPs implemented. Because evidence [10] shows that children in CCCs affiliated with Head Start [HS] programs are significantly more likely to receive health care screenings and consultations compared to non-HS programs, we tested if there was any association between number of OHPPs implemented and the CCC's affiliation with Early Head Start/ Head start (EHS/HS) programs. EHS/HS programs are federal programs that promote school readiness among low-income children 0 to 5 years of age. These programs offer comprehensive early child hood education, health care services, nutrition, and parental involvement services. Many EHS/HS programs are based in preschools, and others are located in licensed childcare centers or family childcare homes.

Methods
Study sample
This cross sectional study was approved by the Nova Southeastern University Health Professions Division Institution Review Board (IRB) (Protocol number: CGG2013–19). The target population for this study was CCCDs working in licensed CCCs within the State of Florida. A publicly available database comprising of unduplicated names and email address of Florida CCCDs ($n = 5142$) was retrieved from the Florida Department of Children and Families website in January 2014. Eight hundred and seventy seven CCCDs responded, 53 opted out, and 631 email addresses were invalid. The overall survey response rate was estimated at 19.4% (877/4511).

Survey instrument
The authors developed the 45-item survey by adapting questions from previously tested and validated surveys [11–13]. AAPD oral health policies for CCCs [5] were also used to construct questions to assess OHPPs implemented in the CCCs. A group of five pediatric dentists provided detailed feedback on the structure and content of the first draft of the survey. The second draft of the modified survey was pretested with 10 CCCDs in Broward county, Florida. The survey was pilot tested through cognitive interviews using the concurrent think aloud method with probes [14]. These procedures we believe improved the content and face validity of the survey.

Data collection
The pilot tested survey was uploaded on the Survey Monkey® online platform (www.surveymonkey.com). We used Dillman's guidelines such as: 1) repeated contacts, 2) varying messages across reminders, 3) caution to minimize spam, and 4) testing the compatibility of the online surveys on different devices and softwares, to contact the CCCDs and boost the responses. [15]. For repeated contact, we included: (1) an introductory email informing the CCCDs about the upcoming survey; (2) an email with a message about the intent of the survey, why they were selected to be part of the study, and the importance of their participation; and (3) reminder emails, sent every 2 weeks intervals (a total of 3 reminders), on early Monday morning hours with personalized links, to both partial and non-respondents over a 6-week period. We varied the content of the email message with all reminders to vary the stimulus across email contacts. To minimize the likelihood of the online survey being flagged as spam we used plain text messages, instead of HTML messages. And finally, we tested the online survey on iphones, androids, desktops, and different software and hard ware configurations. The online version of the survey was also tested for operational and typological issues. The survey was initially sent to the sample in January 2014, and was kept open until the end of March 2014.

Independent variables

Demographic variables Questions were asked about (but not limited to) CCCDs age, gender, race, ethnicity, highest form of education completed, annual income, years of experience as a CCCD, and if they had a child of their own.

Pediatric oral health knowledge (knowledge) Three questions/statements assessing the CCCD's knowledge about pediatric oral health, were adapted from a previous study [11]. The first statement specified that the parents should start cleaning a child's mouth at the age of 1 (True or False response). The correct answer to this question was False, because cleaning children's teeth should begin as soon as the first tooth erupts. The second True/False statement indicated that a child's first dental visit should be at 2 years. The correct answer is False because children should have a first dental office visit at the age of 1. The third statement asked the respondents to correctly choose the most common chronic childhood disease for children younger than 7 years old from four possible responses (Asthma, Hay Fever, Tooth decay, and Chicken Pox). The correct answer for this question was tooth decay. Correct answers were assigned a score of 1 and were summed to create a composite knowledge score (range 0 to 3). Higher composite scores indicated that CCCDs had a higher level of pediatric oral health knowledge.

Attitudes towards pediatric oral health (attitudes) A 5-point Likert scale (Strongly Agree to Strongly Disagree; coded as 1 to 5) was used to rate the following attitude-based statements: 1) Cleaning baby teeth is not important because they fall out anyway; 2) My center has too many activities to devote any time to dental health; 3) Teaching children younger than 3 years about dental health is too difficult; and 4) I don't believe that the activities that we provide in the center will prevent cavities [12]. A composite attitude score (range 0 to 20) was derived by summing the answers with higher scores indicating positive attitudes towards promoting children's oral health. An acceptable internal consistency (Cronbach's alpha = 0.706) was estimated for the likert scales measuring attitudes.

Self-perceived barriers (barriers) Possible barriers to implementing OHPPs were listed with a check box option. CCCDs could check any of the items that apply. The list of barriers were: 1) Insufficient funding to promote pediatric oral health; 2) Parents' negative attitudes towards child safety and oral health; 3) Parental cultural/religious barriers; 4) Parents' language barriers; 5) Insufficient training of center staff about oral health

promotion topics; 6) Insufficient space to implement OHPPs; 7) Inadequate time to implement OHPPs; 8) Infection control concerns; and 9) other (open response). All checked responses (coded as 1) were summed together to derive a composite SPB score (ranging from 0 to 9), with higher scores indicating that CCCDs had greater difficulty implementing OHPPs in their centers.

Affiliation with EHS/HS programs (main independent variable) CCCDs were asked using a check box option to choose if their center was affiliated with EHS/HS programs or not. A checked response meant that CCCD was at a center affiliated with EHS/HS programs.

Main outcome variable

Oral health promotion practices (OHPPs) CCCs implementation of OHPPs, as recommended by the AAPD's "Policy on Oral Health in Child Care Centers" [5] was measured by asking 8 binary option (yes/ no) questions. In order to accommodate the time constraints and to prevent potential overlap between OHPPs, researchers developed questions for only 8 out of a possible 14 AAPD recommended OHPPs. The decision to include only 8 of the 14 AAPD recommended OHPPs was made based on the feedback received from 5 pediatric dentists who provided feedback on the content and structure of the survey. The questions asked the CCCDs whether the center he/she was employed at: 1) had an oral health consultant; 2) regularly maintained dental records for enrolled children; 3) had training or educational programs for staff about traumatic dental injuries 4) had an onsite dental emergency manual; 5) regularly distributed oral health promotion materials to parents; 6) provided optimally fluoridated water for the children; 7) promoted the dental home concept to parents; and 8) encouraged children to brush their teeth after meals or snacks. All "yes" responses were considered positive responses, and were given a score of 1, while "no" responses were coded as 0. The responses were summed to derive a composite OHPS score (Score range: 0 to 8) with higher scores indicating more OHPS implemented by CCCs.

Analyses

Data analyses were performed using the version 9.3 of the SAS statistical analysis software (SAS Institute, Inc. Cary, N.C.). Alpha coefficients were performed to test reliability between items included in the attitude-based questions. We conducted descriptive statistics to understand the characteristics of the study sample. The following variables were described through frequencies and percentages: CCCD's age, gender, ethnicity, race, education, annual income, having a child of their own (being a parent), and the center's affiliation with EHS/HS programs. The following variables were described through means and standard deviation: CCCD's age, years of experience working at a CCC, knowledge, attitudes, barriers, and the self-reported number of OHPPs implemented in their center. Bivariate comparisons were conducted using chi-square tests and independent student t-tests to understand differences in the proportion of CCCDs reporting OHPPs implementation, and the overall number of OHPPs implemented in CCCs. One Poisson regression model was created which predicted the number of OHPPs implemented in Florida CCCs. We included all independent variables explained above as covariates. Multi-collinearity diagnostic analysis was performed to assess collinearity between the predictor variables that were included in the regression model, and none was detected. To assess the fit of the poisson regression model, we used the goodness-of-fit chi-squared test.

Results

The mean age of the CCCD respondents was 48.5 ± 10.5 years and they had mean years of experience of 11.6 ± 9.3 years. A majority of the study participants were women (96%) and belonged to the White race (74%). Approximately 19% of the sample was Hispanics. The majority (65%) reported having a college degree or higher. More than 60% reported earning an annual income of less than $50,000, with just over 20% reporting an income of $50,000 and above. Only 5% of the responding CCCDs reported that their center was affiliated with EHS/HS programs.

On average, participants answered only one knowledge question out of 3 correctly [Knowledge score: 1.3 ± 0.8 (mean ± SD)]. When asked if age 1 was the correct age to initiate cleaning a child's teeth, only 1 in 5 correctly answered "False". Only 2 in 5 CCCDs correctly answered that the child's first dental visit should not be at 2 years. However, an overwhelming 85% of the respondents correctly identified that tooth decay or cavities is the most common childhood disease.

The mean attitude score (16.8 ± 2.7) suggested that CCCDs had positive attitudes towards pediatric oral health. Most of the respondents (94%) believed that cleaning baby teeth was very important. Only 9% felt that that there were too many activities at the center to devote any time to children's dental health. Most (87%) felt that teaching children younger than 3 about the importance of oral health was not difficult. More than 65% believed that providing oral health promotion activities in CCCs will prevent dental caries.

CCCDs did not perceive that there were too many barriers to implementing OHPPs in their centers (mean SPB score: 1.55 ± 1.64). Funding issues (38.5%) and lack of oral health promotion training for staff (32.7%) were the most frequently reported self-perceived barriers by CCCDs. Less frequent barriers were lack of time to address oral health (24.7%), infection control issues (15.2%), lack of space to promote adequate oral health (14.1%), and negative parental attitudes (11.6%). Few CCCDs perceived parent's language barriers (6.6%), cultural issues (5.4%), or other issues (2.5%) to be significant barriers to providing OHPPs in their center.

Figure 1 illustrates the percentage of respondents reporting about the implementation of 8 OHPPs in their centers. Slightly more than half of CCCDs reported that they promote the dental home concept to parents (53%) and provide optimally fluoridated water to children (53%), while the least implemented OHPPS were having an oral health emergency manual on site (8%) and maintaining children's dental records (5%). On average, CCCDs reported implementing only 2.1 ± 1.6 (mean ±

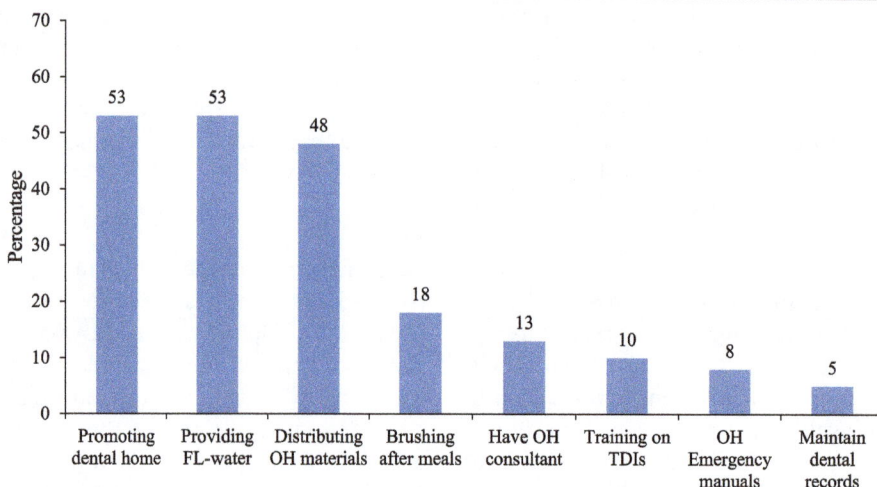

Fig. 1 Percentage of childcare directors reporting implementation of certain oral health promotion practices in their centers

SD) out of 8 possible AAPD recommended OHPPs in their CCCs.

Bivariate analysis

Tables 1 compares the differences in number of OHPPs implemented by selected characteristics of CCCDs. No significant differences in OHPPs implemented were observed by ethnicity, income, and having a child of their own. Male CCCDs reported a significantly higher number of OHPPs implemented compared to female CCCDs ($p = 0.02$). Those belonging to a non-White racial background ($p = 0.001$), and those with a college degree ($p = 0.03$) and above reported implementing a significantly higher number of OHPPs compared to their counterparts. Table 2 compares CCCs affiliated with EHS/HS programs to unaffiliated centers. More EHS/HS affiliated CCCDs consistently reported implementing 7 OHPPs compared to their counterparts, with the exception of one OHPP. Directors in EHS/HS affiliated centers were as likely (52%) to report providing clean optimally fluoridated water throughout the day as directors in centers that are not affiliated (47%). Overall, the directors in centers affiliated with EHS/HS programs reported to have implemented a significantly higher mean number (5.1 ± 2.3) of OHPPs compared to those in centers not affiliated (1.9 ± 1.8).

Table 1 Mean differences in OHPPs implemented by selected CCCD characteristics

Variable	OHPPs (mean ± SD)	p-value
Gender		
Male	2.79 ± 2.2	0.02
Female	2.04 ± 1.6	
Race		
White	1.95 ± 1.5	0.001
Non-White	2.39 ± 1.9	
Ethnicity		
Hispanics	2.24 ± 1.7	0.15
Non-Hispanics	2.02 ± 1.6	
Income		
> =50,000	2.04 ± 1.5	0.92
< 50,000	2.03 ± 1.6	
Education		
College degree and above	2.16 ± 1.7	0.03
< College degree	1.89 ± 1.4	
Have Child Of your own		
Yes	2.04 ± 1.6	0.9
No	2.06 ± 1.7	

Poisson regression analysis

The adjusted Poisson regression model predicting higher number of OHPPs implemented in Florida licensed CCCs is shown in Table 2. CCCDs employed at a center affiliated with EHS/HS programs reported implementing a higher number of OHPPs compared to CCCDs at centers not affiliated with EHS/HS programs (b = 0.7, 95%CI: 0.48,0.91) $p < 0.001$. The results also confirmed that CCCDs reporting higher number of OHPPs implemented in their centers were more likely to have longer work experience (b = 0.006, 95% CI:0.001, 0.012 $p = 0.03$), and have more positive attitudes about pediatric oral health (b = 0.08, 95%CI: 0.05, 0.10) $p < 0.001$. CCCDs who had more self-perceived barriers in implementing OHPPs reported that their centers had implemented significantly lower number of OHPPs (b = – 0.046, 95% CI: -0.09, – 0.003 $p = 0.035$). The goodness of fit test proved that the Poisson regression model fit the data reasonably well because the test was not statistically significant ($p = 0.094$).

Discussion

Understanding the oral health promotion practices in Florida licensed CCCs is important because these centers can be utilized as alternate non-traditional settings to promote optimal oral health of children. So we conducted a survey of CCCDs in Florida licensed CCCs to examine whether their center implemented any OHPPs, and if their center's affiliation with EHS/HS programs affected the number of OHPPs implemented.

Of the 8 OHPPs assessed, our findings indicate that, on average, CCCDs reported implementing very few OHPPs in their centers, suggesting that OHPPs may not adequately practiced in these centers. More than 80% of the CCCDs reported that their enrollees did not brush after meals, their center lacked an oral health consultant and oral health emergency manuals, the staff were not trained in traumatic dental injuries, and did not maintain children's dental records. This indicates that, based on the CCCDs' reports, AAPD recommended oral health prevention and promotion activities were not frequently practiced in licensed Florida CCCs. In fact, a substantial number of children younger than 5 years old were enrolled in these centers at the time of our study (more than 80%), which is problematic because this age group has high dental caries risk and oral health promotion should already be initiated. At least in this study, we did not find any association between CCCD's oral health knowledge and the number of OHPPs implemented. However, possessing correct oral health knowledge and high oral health literacy is important for CCCDs to practice appropriate OHPPs not only for themselves but also to implement into that childcare system that will benefit the enrolled children. Therefore Florida CCCDs need more education about the importance of implementing

Table 2 Factors predicting higher number of oral health promotion practices implemented in Florida child care centers

Variable	Parameter estimate	95% CI	p-value
Age	0.006	(−0.001, 0.013)	0.95
Years of experience (Higher number)	0.006	(0.0006, 0.012)	*0.03*
Gender (Male versus Female)	0.093	(−0.224, 0.41)	0.57
Race (White versus Non-Whites)	−0.08	(−0.218, 0.057)	0.25
Have a Child of your own (Yes Versus No)	0.074	(−0.073, 0.22)	0.33
Income (< 50,000 versus > = 50,000)	−0.009	(−0.15, 0.132)	0.90
Education (college degree and above versus Less than college degree)	0.033	(−0.103, 0.17)	0.64
Type of Center (Early Head Start Versus Non-Early Head Start)	0.7	(0.48, 0.914)	*<.0001*
Oral Health Knowledge (Higher number)	0.001	(−0.08, 0.08)	0.98
Attitudes (Higher number)	0.08	(0.05, 0.103)	*<.0001*
Barriers (Higher number)	−0.046	(− 0.09, − 0.003)	*0.035*

OHPPs within their CCCs, along with the long-term impact it can have on a child's overall health and well-being. However, it was encouraging to find that most participants (67%) reported that they might implement OHPPs in the upcoming year.

To test our hypothesis and to determine factors associated with more implemented OHPPs in Florida CCCs, we conducted an adjusted Poisson regression model that yielded interesting results. Our study found that CCCDs working in EHS/HS affiliated centers implemented more OHPPs compared to their counterparts (*p* < 0.001). We conclude that there was a significant association between the number of OHPPs implemented and the center's affiliation with EHS/HS programs. Literature supporting this result exists, with HS centers promoting health considerably more frequently than non-HS centers [10]. In a multi-state survey a higher proportion of responding CCCDs in HS centers reported consulting health professionals and screening for health problems in enrolled children, compared to their counterparts. This is due to greater awareness about pediatric health, and CCCDs in HS centers may attach greater importance to children's health issues [10]. More experienced CCCDs may have been more confident and efficacious compared to inexperienced CCCDs, and therefore may have implemented more OHPPs. CCCDs with positive pediatric oral health promotion attitudes were more likely to report implementing OHPPs in their centers. Evidence suggests that those with more positive attitudes about health maintenance are more likely to adopt and practice healthy behaviors for their own well-being [16]. Prior research supports the idea that more barriers (perceived and real) impede prevention program implementation [17]. The most frequently reported barriers to implementing OHPPs by study participants were: 1) insufficient funding to implement oral health programs, 2) insufficient staff training about oral health promotion, and 3)

insufficient staff time for pediatric oral health promotion. Previous literature has shown that these three elements are critical to the success of any health promotion or disease prevention programs in CCCs. Therefore we recommend that CCCDs identify strategies to overcome these three barriers to health promotion. Additional open-ended responses provided insights into other potential barriers faced by CCCDs when implementing OHPPs including: dentists rarely treating and educating children younger than 3 years, few community dentists, and there is no need to enforce oral health promotion at the center because it is not required for Florida's licensure.

Ours is the first study to survey CCCDs in Florida on relevant OHPPs in their centers. Therefore our study highlights for the first time, the status of licensed CCCs in Florida and the lack of adequate oral health promotion in these settings. Limitations of this study include but are not limited to low response rate, use of a convenience sample, and induced bias due to selective participation. Therefore our study results should be interpreted with caution. Only 5% of the respondents reported working in EHS/HS affiliated centers compared to their counterparts (95%). A previous study showed very similar findings, with only 10% of the responding CCCDs reporting to work at HS affiliated centers [10]. We did not find information about the proportion of licensed CCCs in Florida that were affiliated with EHS/HS programs and therefore we were unable to determine if non-EHS/HS CCCDs were more or less likely to participate in the survey compared to their counterparts. A very small proportion of the respondents were males. Other types of childcare facilities, such as non-licensed CCCs, group childcare homes or family child care homes, were not explored because we did not have access to these facilities. Understanding the demographic differences between respondents and non-respondents could not be accomplished because the researchers did not manually track the participants as deemed by the IRB guidelines. Due to the limited funds to execute this study, postal surveys were not economically feasible.

Because the EHS/HS affiliated centers implement more OHPPs, we believe that EHS/HS programs may serve as a model that can be integrated into non-EHS/HS affiliated programs. Because many children receive daycare in CCCs, it is imperative that policy makers and State Departments of Health focus on policies and regulations that will improve the integration of OHPPs into these settings. For example, in the State of Florida, the child care licensing program is a component of the services provided by the Department of Children and Families. This program through regulations and consultation ensures that licensing requirements are met by the childcare facilities thus preventing operation of substandard childcare programs. Such departments can add mandatory regulations related to maintaining certain oral health standards in CCCs. By doing so, optimal oral health in children can be achieved by all CCCs. Child care centers are non-traditional alternate settings where new disease prevention and health promotion programs can be implemented to improve the health of enrolled children. These settings are excellent resources to apply oral health intervention programs, provided there are few barriers.

Conclusions

We conclude that affiliation with EHS/HS programs is associated with the number of OHPPs implemented licensed Florida licensed CCCs. In addition, CCCDs years of experience, attitudes towards oral health, and self-perceived barriers in implementing OHPPs were also associated with number of OHPPs implemented.

Abbreviations

AAPD: American Academy of Pediatric Dentistry; CCCDs: Child care center directors; CCCs: Child care centers; EHS/HS: Early Head Start/ Head Start; HS: Head Start; IRB: Institution Review Board; OHPPs: Oral health promotion practices

Acknowledgements
We thank all the child care center directors who participated in this study.

Funding
This study was supported by funding from the Nova Southeastern University Health Professions Division. Grant #335548. The funding agency did not contribute to the design of the study, collection, analysis, and interpretation of data, and in writing the manuscript.

Authors' contributions
VB: Conceptualization, study design, data collection and analysis, writing manuscript, critical editing of the manuscript for important intellectual content. AJ: Data collection, manuscript writing, critical editing of the manuscript. RO: Study design, manuscript writing, critical editing of the manuscript. RJ: Study design, data analysis, and critical editing of the manuscript for important intellectual content. All authors read and approved the final manuscript.

Authors' information
Dr. Vinodh Bhoopathi, was an Assistant Professor at Nova Southeastern University College of Dental Medicine, and the thesis committee chair for Dr. Joshi's thesis when this study was conducted. Currently Dr. Bhoopathi is an Assistant Professor at the Temple University Maurice H Kornberg School of Dentistry, Philadelphia, PA. Dr. Ajay Joshi was a pediatric dental resident at Nova Southeastern University College of Dental Medicine when this thesis study was conducted. Currently he is an Assistant Clinical Professor at Indiana University School of Dentistry and maintains his private practice in Marion, IN. Dr. Romer Ocanto is Associate Professor, and Chair of Pediatric Dentistry at Nova Southeastern University. Dr. Robin J. Jacobs is Associate Professor at Nova Southeastern University College of Osteopathic Medicine at the time of the study. Currently she is an Associate Professor at Baylor College of Medicine. Address correspondence to Dr. Bhoopathi. E-mail: Vinodh.Bhoopathi@temple.edu

Competing interests
Dr. Bhoopathi is an Associate Editor of the BMC Oral Health Editorial Board. Other author(s) declare no competing interests.

Author details
[1]Department of Pediatric Dentistry and Community Oral Health Sciences, Temple University Maurice H. Kornberg School of Dentistry, 3223 N Broad Street, Philadelphia, PA 19140, USA. [2]Pediatric Dentistry Department, Indiana University School of Dentistry, 1121 W. Michigan Street, Indianapolis, IN 46202, USA. [3]Department of Pediatric Dentistry, Nova Southeastern University College of Dental Medicine, 3200 S University Drive, Fort Lauderdale, FL 33328, USA. [4]Department of Family and Community Medicine – Research Programs, Baylor College of Medicine, 3701 Kirby Drive, Suite 600, Houston, TX 77098, USA.

References
1. United States Census Bureau. Demand for Child Care and the Distribution of Child Care Facilities in the United States: 1987–2007. Available at http://www.census.gov/library/working-papers/2013/econ/2013_child_care.html Accessed 20 May 2017.
2. United States Census Bureau. Child Care an Important Part of American Life. How do we know? Available at: https://www.census.gov/content/dam/Census/library/visualizations/2013/comm/child_care.pdf . Accessed 17 Apr 2017.
3. Dye BA, Thornton-Evans G, Li X, Iafolla TJ. Dental caries and sealant prevalence in children and adolescents in the United States, 2011–2012. NCHS data brief, no 191. Hyattsville: National Center for Health Statistics; 2015.
4. Kim J, Kaste LM. Associations of the type of childcare with reported preventive medical and dental care utilization for 1- to 5-year-old children in the United States. Community Dent Oral Epidemiol. 2013;41:432–40.
5. Policy on Oral Health in Child Care Centers. Pediatr Dent. 2012;34:33–4.
6. Kranz AM, Rozier RG. Oral health content of early education and child care regulations and standards. J Public Health Dent. 2011;71:81–90.
7. Kim J, Kaste LM, Fadavi S, et al. Are state child care regulations meeting national oral health and nutritional standards? Pediatr Dent. 2012;34:317–24.
8. Scheunemann D, Schwab M, Margaritis V. Oral health practices of state and non-state-funded licensed childcare centers in Wisconsin, USA. J Int Soc Prev Community Dent. 2015;5:296–301.
9. The Pew Center of States. 2011. The State of Children's Dental Health: Making Coverage Matter. The Pew Charitable Trusts. Available at http://

www.pewtrusts.org/~/media/legacy/uploadedfiles/wwwpewtrustsorg/
reports/state_policy/childrensdental50statereport2011pdf.pdf .

10. Gupta RS, Pascoe JM, Blanchard TC, Langkamp D, Duncan PM, Gorski PA, Southward LH. Child health in child care: a multi-state survey of head start and non-head start child care directors. J Pediatr Health Care. 2009;23:143–9.

11. Akpabio A, Klausner CP, Inglehart MR. Mothers'/guardians' knowledge about promoting children's oral health. J Dent Hyg. 2008;82:12.

12. Mathu-Muju KR, Lee JY, Zeldin LP, Rozier RG. Opinions of early head start staff about the provision of preventive dental services by primary medical care providers. J Public Health Dent. 2008;68:154–62.

13. Joshi A, Ocanto R, Jacobs RJ, Bhoopathi V. Florida child care center directors' intention to implement oral health promotion practices in licensed child care centers. BMC Oral Health. 2016;16(1):100.

14. DeMaio TL, Rothgeb J, Hess J. Improving survey quality through pretesting. Washington, DC: U.S. Bureau of the Census; 1998. Retrieved March 5, 2018 from http://www.census.gov/srd/papers/pdf/sm98-03.pdf.

15. Dillman DA, Smyth JD, Christian LM. Mail and internet surveys: the tailored design method. 3rd ed. New York: John Wiley and Sons; 2009.

16. Lino S, Marshak HH, Herring RP, Belliard JC, Hilliard C, Campbell D, Montgomery S. Using the theory of planned behavior to explore attitudes and beliefs about dietary supplements among HIV-positive black women. Complement Ther Med. 2014;22:400–8.

17. Sigman-Grant M, Christiansen E, Fernandez G, Fletcher J, Johnson SL, Branen L, Price BA. Child care provider training and a supportive feeding environment in child care settings in 4 states, 2003. Prev Chronic Dis. 2011;8:A113.

8

An in vitro study evaluating the effect of ferrule design on the fracture resistance of endodontically treated mandibular premolars after simulated crown lengthening or forced eruption methods

Qingfei Meng[1,2], Qian Ma[2*], Tianda Wang[2] and Yaming Chen[2]

Abstract

Background: The purpose of this study was to evaluate the effect of ferrule design on the fracture resistance of endodontically treated mandibular first premolars after simulated crown lengthening and orthodontic forced eruption methods restored with a fiber post-and-core system.

Methods: Forty extracted and endodontically treated mandibular first premolars were decoronated to create lingual-to-buccal oblique residual root models, with a 2.0 mm height of the lingual dentine wall coronal to the cemento-enamel junction, and the height of buccal surface at the cemento-enamel junction. The roots were divided randomly into five equal groups. The control group had undergone incomplete ferrule preparation in the cervical root, with 0.0 mm buccal and 2.0 mm lingual ferrule lengths (Group F0). Simulated surgical crown lengthening method provided ferrule preparation of 1.0 mm (Group CL/F1) and 2.0 mm (Group CL/F2) on the buccal surface, with ferrule lengths of 3.0 mm and 4.0 mm on the lingual surface, respectively. Simulated orthodontic forced eruption method provided ferrule preparation of 1.0 mm (Group OE/F1) and 2.0 mm (Group OE/F2) on the buccal surface and ferrule lengths of 3.0 mm and 4.0 mm on the lingual surface, respectively. After restoration with a glass fiber post-and-core system and a cast Co-Cr alloy crown, each specimen was embedded in an acrylic resin block to a height on the root 2.0 mm from the apical surface of the crown margin and loaded to fracture at a 135° angle to its long axis in a universal testing machine. Data were analyzed statistically using two-way ANOVA with Tukey HSD tests and Fisher's test, with $\alpha = 0.05$.

Results: Mean fracture loads (kN) for groups F0, CL/F1, CL/F2, OE/F1 and OE/F2 were as follows: 1.01 (S.D. = 0.26), 0.91 (0.29), 0.73 (0.19), 0.96 (0.25) and 0.76 (0.20), respectively. Two-way ANOVA revealed significant differences for the effect of ferrule lengths ($P = 0.012$) but no differences for the effect of cervical treatment methods ($P = 0.699$). The teeth with no buccal ferrule preparation in control group F0 had the highest fracture resistance. In contrast, the mean fracture loads for group CL/F2 with a 2.0-mm buccal and 4.0-mm lingual ferrule created by simulated crown lengthening method were lowest ($P = 0.036$).

Conclusions: Increased apically complete ferrule preparation resulted in decreased fracture resistance of endodontically treated mandibular first premolars, regardless of whether surgical crown lengthening or orthodontic forced eruption methods been used.

Keywords: Ferrule, Surgical crown lengthening, Orthodontic forced eruption, Fracture resistance, Residual root

* Correspondence: qianma1981@126.com
[2]College of Stomatology, Nanjing Medical University, 136 Hanzhong Road, Nanjing 210029, Jiangsu Province, China
Full list of author information is available at the end of the article

Background

When endodontically treated teeth are restored with a post-and-core system, the prognosis can be affected by the following factors: the remaining amount of residual tooth [1–4], ferrule design [3, 5–8], post material [3, 5, 6], the tooth fracture mode and its severity [9, 10], and so on. According to previous studies [1–4], the amount of residual tooth structure has been considered the most important factor with regard to the fracture resistance of endodontically treated teeth. If adequate supragingival tooth structure could be conserved and greater than a 1.0-mm complete ferrule could be achieved, the fracture resistance would increase significantly and the long-term success of post-and-core restorations could be expected [7, 8].

However, because of severe dental caries, wedge-shaped defects, trauma or other reasons, teeth were broken obliquely in some cases, starting at the crown and extending longitudinally through the pulp chamber to the cervical line or subgingival area, with one or more dentine walls lost and only an incomplete ferrule prepared in the residual cervical root. Mangold et al. had evaluated the fracture resistance of endodontically-treated residual teeth in this particular condition and found that the fracture loads of such obliquely broken teeth decreased proportionally with the loss of dentine walls [11–13]. Moreover, the position of the lost dentine wall would still affect the long-term success of oblique endodontic root restorations [14, 15]. According to previous studies [14, 15], the fracture resistance of anterior upper teeth having a 2.0-mm lingual ferrule (labial dentine wall was lost) was better than those with a 2.0-mm labial ferrule (lingual dentine wall was lost). The lowest fracture resistance was found in residual roots with no ferrule or only a labial ferrule. The long-term prognosis for such residual roots appears to be poor after post-and-core restorations.

The surgical crown lengthening method (SCLM) and orthodontic forced eruption method (OFEM) have been recommended for restoring subgingival roots [16–20]. SCLM reestablishes the dentogingival junction at a more apical level on the root to accommodate the junctional epithelium and the connective tissue attachment in a relatively short time frame [16–18]. In contrast, continued, slow, passive or active OFEM at approximately 2 mm per month allows the periodontal ligament to repair and the alveolar bone to remodel by orthodontic adjustments [19, 20]. Both cervical treatment methods can provide sound tooth structure over the bone crest for the complete ferrule preparation. OFEM has been shown to provide greater fracture resistance and better clinical outcome for post-and-core restored roots than SCLM [4, 8]. However, whether SCLM or OFEM is supportive for residual roots with an oblique fracture is still unclear.

The purpose of this in vitro study was to investigate the effect of ferrule length on the fracture resistance of obliquely-fractured (with buccal tooth structure lost) endodontically treated mandibular premolars, which were treated with simulated SCLM or OFEM to provide a complete ferrule and restored with a prefabricated fiber post and core system. The null hypotheses were that the fracture resistance of endodontically-treated residual roots would not be affected by the ferrule length, nor by the cervical treatment methods (SCLM or OFEM).

Methods

Specimen preparation

Forty healthy human mandibular first premolars recently-extracted for orthodontic reasons from patients aged 20–30 years who lived in the same locality without water fluoridation were used for this study. Written informed consent was obtained under a protocol approved by the Ethics Committee of Affiliated Stomatology Hospital of Nanjing Medical University. After cleaning and the removal of attached soft tissues, the teeth were examined stereoscopically at 10× magnification to exclude those already cracked before being stored in 0.9% saline solution at 4 °C for no longer than 2 weeks [8]. Diamond disks were used to section the natural crowns transversely, 2 mm occlusal to the buccal cemento-enamel junction (CEJ) with an average root length of 15.0 ± 1.0 mm to simulate endodontically treated roots (Fig. 1). All the roots were assigned randomly into five equal groups (F0, CL/F1, CL/F2, OE/F1 and OE/F2), according to a table of random numbers. The root dimensions including the root lengths, the cross-sectional widths of the canal walls at the mesial, buccal, distal and lingual root face sites and the mesiodistal and buccolingual diameters of the roots were measured to 0.02 mm with a vernier caliper (Vernier Caliper Model 93,218–0654, Harbin Measuring & Cutting Tool Group Co. Ltd., Harbin, PR China). The roots had similar dimensions among the five groups, as shown in Table 1.

The root canals were prepared with hand files (K-files, Dentsply-Maillefer, Ballaigues, Switzerland) and

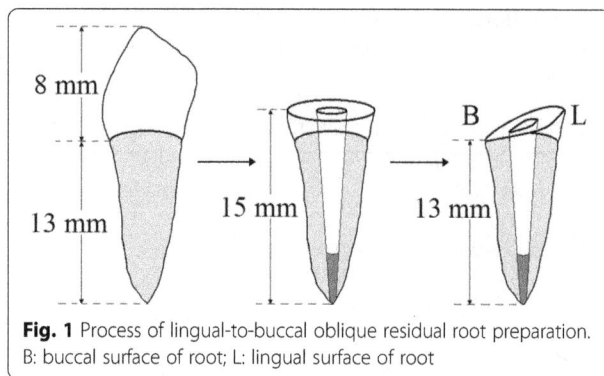

Fig. 1 Process of lingual-to-buccal oblique residual root preparation. B: buccal surface of root; L: lingual surface of root

Table 1 Mean dimensions (mm) of randomly assigned mandibular first premolar roots in each group

Group (N = 40)	Root Length[a]	Width of canal wall sites, and roots, at root face[a]					
		Mesial	Buccal	Distal	Lingual	M-D	B-L
F0	15.12 (0.36)	2.19 (0.30)	2.55 (0.15)	2.17 (0.41)	2.36 (0.26)	6.18 (0.97)	8.16 (0.73)
CL/F1	15.16 (0.35)	2.04 (0.41)	2.40 (0.43)	1.92 (0.19)	2.43 (0.20)	5.66 (0.58)	7.88 (0.63)
CL/F2	15.18 (0.27)	2.47 (0.54)	2.63 (0.37)	2.12 (0.33)	2.60 (0.34)	6.40 (0.77)	8.25 (0.52)
OE/F1	15.12 (0.26)	2.06 (0.37)	2.47 (0.27)	2.00 (0.42)	2.52 (0.38)	5.89 (0.96)	8.07 (0.70)
OE/F2	15.19 (0.42)	2.18 (0.30)	2.65 (0.30)	2.11 (0.33)	2.66 (0.36)	6.26 (0.60)	8.13 (0.35)
1-way ANOVA	$F = 0.083$ $P = 0.987$	$F = 1.502$ $P = 0.223$	$F = 0.823$ $P = 0.519$	$F = 0.691$ $P = 0.603$	$F = 1.2$ $P = 0.328$	$F = 1.140$ $P = 0.354$	$F = 0.412$ $P = 0.799$

Group F0: glass fiber post-core with 0.0 mm buccal and 2.0 mm lingual ferrule lengths, as control; Group CL/F1: glass fiber post-core with simulated crown lengthening and 1.0 mm buccal and 3.0 mm lingual ferrule lengths; Group CL/F2: glass fiber post-core with simulated crown lengthening and 2.0 mm buccal and 4.0 mm lingual ferrule lengths; Group OE/F1: glass fiber post-core with simulated orthodontic forced tooth eruption and 1.0 mm buccal and 3.0 mm lingual ferrule lengths; Group OE/F2: glass fiber post-core with simulated orthodontic forced tooth eruption and 2.0 mm buccal and 4.0 mm lingual ferrule lengths
[a]Mean (Standard Deviation); M-D: mesiodistal root width; B-L: buccolingual root width

size 4 Gates-Glidden drills (Dentsply-Maillefer) for the purpose of standardized canal forms [8], rinsed with 2. 5% sodium hypochlorite solution, dried with paper points, and then applied with a thin layer of sealer (AH Plus, Dentsply Detrey, Konstanz, Germany). The cold laterally-condensed gutta percha points (Dentsply International Inc., York, PA, USA) were placed to obturate the canals. After endodontic treatment, all the residual roots were cut as lingual-to-buccal obliquely-broken root models, starting at the middle point of the lingual section and extending longitudinally to the middle point of the buccal CEJ, with the height of buccal dentine wall 2.0 mm lower than that of the lingual position in the section area (Fig. 1). Each root was restored with prefabricated glass fiber post-and-core system. Post space was prepared to 10 mm deep for No. 2 glass fiber post (#2, R.T.D., France), using matching drills with a slow speed contra angle handpiece, according to the manufacturer's instructions. The prepared root wall was first etched with 32% phosphoric acid gel (UNI-ETCH, BISCO, Inc., Schaumburg, IL, USA) for 15 s and then rinsed thoroughly with an air-water spray and dried lightly with paper points. A resin-based adhesive (ONE-STEP PLUS, BISCO, Inc) was applied twice as a thin layer over the walls of the root wall and once over the surfaces of a prefabricated glass fiber post. After thinning lightly with dry oil-free air, the adhesive was light-cured for 10 s at 600 mW/cm^2 (Variable Intensity Polymerizer Junior, BISCO, Inc). The post-hole was filled completely by injecting resin luting cement (DUAL-LINK luting cement, BISCO, Inc) into which the fiber post was inserted. This was followed by light-curing for 40 s from a coronal direction. A resin composited core (Light-Core™, Bisco, Inc) was built up around the post and light-cured again for 40 s.

Cores, 6.0–8.0 mm high with a 6° convergence angle, were prepared using a milling machine (F3/Egro, Degussa AG, Dusseldorf, Germany) with flat-ended tapered carbide

burs, leaving a 0.8 mm wide encircling shoulder in dentine. The incomplete ferrule was designed with no ferrule on the buccal surface and 2.0 mm-high ferrule on the lingual surface in the control group (Group F0), which had a 6.0 mm high core. Simulated SCLM resulted in nonuniform circumferential ferrule preparation of 1.0 mm length (Group CL/F1) and of 2.0 mm length (Group CL/F2) in the buccal surface, with the ferrule prepared 3.0 and 4.0 mm length respectively in the lingual surface of the oblique residual roots, which increased the height of the core to 7.0 mm and 8.0 mm, respectively. Simulated OFEM resulted in complete ferrule preparation of 1.0 mm (Group OE/F1) and 2.0 mm (Group OE/F2) on the buccal surface, with the ferrule length at 3.0 and 4.0 mm, respectively, on the lingual surface, while maintaining the 6.0 mm height of the core (as shown in Fig. 2).

After 24 h in the isotonic saline storage medium, a standardized Cobalt-Chromium (Co-Cr) alloy (BEGO Bremer Goldschlägerei Wilh. Herbst GmbH & Co. KG, Germany) crown fabricated in the dental laboratory for each of the prepared teeth was cemented with glass-ionomer cement (Glasionomer, Shofu Inc., Kyoto, Japan). The teeth were kept in the storage medium at all time except during experimental testing.

Each root was coated with a 0.1–0.2 mm thin vinyl polysiloxane silicone layer (modulus of elasticity 0. 3 MPa) (Aquasil, Dentsply International Inc) to simulate the periodontal ligament before being embedded, from 2.0 mm apical to the crown preparation margins, in a block of self-cured acrylic resin (Shanghai Dental Materials Manufacture Co., Shanghai, PR China) (Fig. 3).

Fatigue resistance testing

A 1,200,000-times dynamic load of 0–50 N, which simulated the oral masticating condition, was applied to the buccal cusp of the Co-Cr alloy crown, at an angle of 135° from the long axis of the root, using a cylindrical Ni-Cr alloy rod (4.0 cm long × 1.2 cm diameter) in a

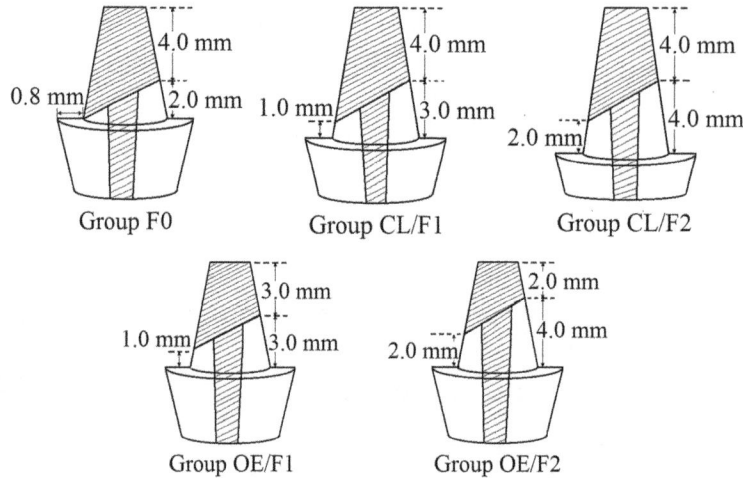

Fig. 2 Preparation designs. F0: with 0.0 mm buccal and 2.0 mm lingual ferrule lengths, as control; CL/F1: with simulated crown lengthening and 1.0 mm buccal and 3.0 mm lingual ferrule lengths; CL/F2: with simulated crown lengthening and 2.0 mm buccal and 4.0 mm lingual ferrule lengths; OE/F1: with simulated orthodontic forced tooth eruption and 1.0 mm buccal and 3.0 mm lingual ferrule lengths; OE/F2: with simulated orthodontic forced tooth eruption and 2.0 mm buccal and 4.0 mm lingual ferrule lengths

universal load-testing system (MTS810, MTS Systems Co., USA), with the frequency of 1.6 Hz [3]. The failed specimens were recorded and the failure site pattern noted.

Fracture resistance testing

A unidirectional static load was then applied to the buccal cusp of the Co-Cr alloy crown of the specimen that had passed fatigue testing without failure, with the same load-testing machine (MTS810, MTS Systems Co., USA)

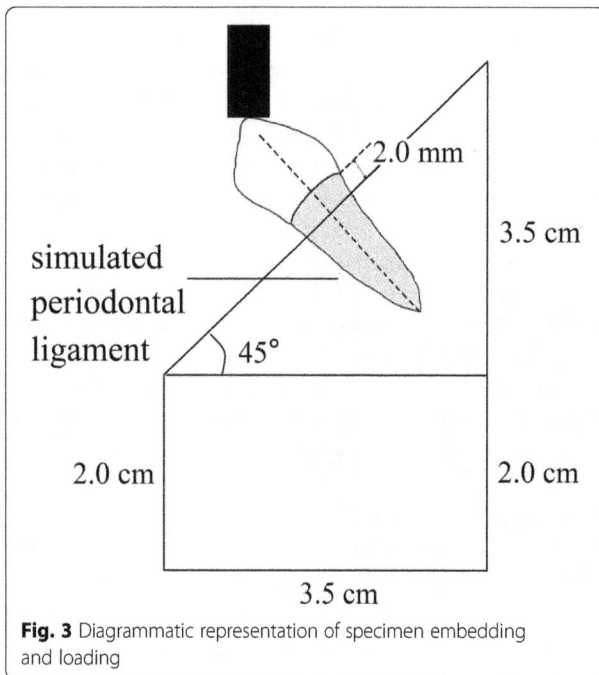

Fig. 3 Diagrammatic representation of specimen embedding and loading

and the same load angle at a cross-speed of 0.5 mm/minute (Fig. 3). The force (kilonewton, kN) for initial root fracture was recorded and the failure pattern noted. The fracture modes were divided in repairable (less severe fractures located at or above the cervical third of the roots and potentially repairable) and irrepairable (catastrophic fractures, such as vertical or oblique root fracture located below the cervical third of the roots), according to the root fracture sites.

Statistical analysis

Statistical analysis was performed using SPSS 21.0 for Windows (SPSS Inc., Chicago, IL, USA). Two-way ANOVA with the Tukey HSD test and Fisher's exact test were used to detect any significant differences between the groups. The probability level for statistical significance was set at $\alpha = 0.05$.

Results

No specimen failed during the fatigue resistance testing. The mean forces required to fracture the restored teeth and the specimen fracture patterns in each group are shown in Table 2. For fracture resistance, 2-way ANOVA revealed a statistically significant difference in the effect of ferrule length (F = 4.955, $P = 0.012$) but no significant differences in the effect of cervical treatment methods (F = 0.152, $P = 0.699$) or interactions between the two sources of variation (F = 0.043, $P = 0.958$) were discerned (Table 3).

For the simulated SCLM and OFEM, no significant differences were found in fracture resistance between groups CL/F1 and CL/F2 and between groups OE/F1 and OE/F2 ($P > 0.05$). Only the fracture loads of group

Table 2 Mean force (kN) required to fracture the tooth roots and the root fracture sites, in each group

Groups	Fatigue testing	Fracture strength (kN)[a]	Root fracture sites[b]	
			At or above cervical 1/3	Below cervical 1/3
F0	0/8	1.01(0.26)	7	1
CL/F1	0/8	0.91 (0.29)	6	2
CL/F2	0/8	0.73 (0.19)	8	0
OE/F1	0/8	0.96 (0.25)	6	2
OE/F2	0/8	0.76 (0.20)	7	1

Group codes are defined in Table 1
[a]Mean (Standard Deviation)
[b]Failed roots were classified repairable (the fracture sites located at or above cervical one-third), and irrepairable (the fracture sites below cervical one-third)

CL/F2 were significantly lower than that of the control group (Group F0) ($P = 0.036$) (Table 4). The control group F0 had the highest fracture resistance, and the fracture loads of the obliquely-broken residual roots decreased along with the increasing ferrule lengths regardless of whether SCLM or OFEM had been used.

Almost all the fracture lines were found at or above the cervical one-third of the roots (Table 2). No statistically significant differences in fracture modes were found among the groups by Fisher's exact test ($P = 1.00$).

Discussion

Specimen preparation and fracture strength testing

Mandibular first premolars were selected for this study as these teeth were vulnerable to oblique root fracture because of wedge-shaped defect and following endodontic treatment [21]. The teeth were collected for orthodontic reasons from young adults who lived in the same area, and had very similar root forms and dimensions, as shown in Table 1. Gross destruction of coronal tooth structure was simulated by using standardized root-face preparations. The obliquely broken teeth may also need SCLM [16–18] or OFEM [19, 20], which facilitates placement of a long complete ferrule to potentially improve the fracture resistance of the residual roots [3, 5–8]. All the cores and ferrule preparations were machined by the same person (Q-F M) using the same milling device, to decrease the personal error at a minimum.

The roots of the restored teeth were coated with silicone rubber and embedded in acrylic resin. The moduli of elasticity of these materials approximated those of the

viscoelastic periodontal ligament and the alveolar bone, respectively [22, 23]. The in vitro dynamic loading testing and the following unidirectional static loading forces were both used in this and many other studies of teeth fractures, in order to closely simulate the complex oral mastication [3, 11]. The oblique force applied at 135° from the long axis of the mandibular premolar was employed to simulate functional working-side buccal cuspid loading [24].

Fracture resistance of restored premolars

The effective clinical crown length (Ce) to embedded root length (Rb) ratio of the restored mandibular premolar with its root embedded in acrylic resin, is defined as "the physical relationship between the portion of the tooth not in the alveolar bone and the portion within the alveolar bone, as determined radiographically" [25]. When the oblique force applied to the buccal cuspid of the premolar, the tooth with its root embedded in the acrylic resin could be considered as a Class I lever, with the fulcrum in the cervical portion [26]. The fracture resistance of endodontically treated teeth is dependent on the level of surrounding supporting alveolar bone and the reduction of alveolar bone height may lead to an increased risk of tooth failure [27, 28]. SCLM increases the effective clinical crown length of the lever (effort arm) during the cervical ferrule preparation, with the embedded root length (resistance arm) decreased. Thus, the Ce/Rb ratio for groups CL/F1 and CL/F2 in this study were 1.10 and 1.33 (20.9 and 46. 2% greater than the control group F0), and the mean fracture resistance were 9.9 and 27.7% lower than that for the control group F0, respectively (Table 2 and Fig. 4). OFEM

Table 3 ANOVA table representing effective decomposition of main variables and their interaction

Source	Sum of Squares	df	Mean Square	F	P
Ferrule	0.580	2	0.290	4.955	0.012[a]
Treatment method	0.009	1	0.009	0.152	0.699
Interaction	0.005	2	0.003	0.043	0.958
Error	2.460	42	0.059		

[a]Statistically significant

Table 4 Statistical comparisons between groups using Tukey HSD tests

Buccal Ferrule length	Simulated crown lengthening	Simulated forced eruption
0.0 mm/1.0 mm	$P = 0.457$	$P = 0.712$
0.0 mm/2.0 mm	$P = 0.036$[a]	$P = 0.052$
1.0 mm/2.0 mm	$P = 0.154$	$P = 0.107$

[a]Statistically significant

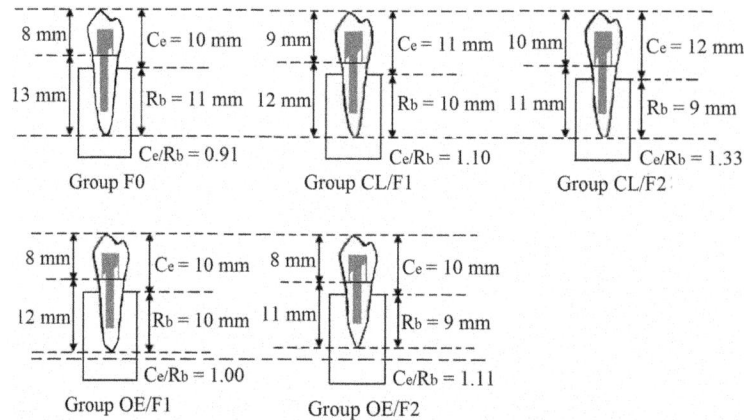

Fig. 4 Effective crown length (Ce) to root length in bone (Rb) ratios (Ce/Rb) for restored teeth: group codes are defined in Fig. 1

only decreases the embedded root length of the tooth, remaining the height of the crown portion the same as that in control group F0. However, with an increase in ferrule height prepared in the cervical portion and the reduction of root length embedded in bone, the diameter and dentine bulk of the residual root was decreased towards the root apex because of the root taper. Thus, the mean fracture resistance for group OE/F1 and OE/F2 were 5.0 and 24.8% lower than that for the control group, respectively (Table 2).

The crown-to-root ratio is one of the main variables in evaluating the suitability of a tooth as an abutment for a fixed partial denture [4, 29, 30]. Shillingburg suggested 1:1 as a minimum ratio for a prospective abutment under normal circumstances [30]. In this study, the crown-to-root ratio was defined as the effective clinical crown length (Ce) to embedded root length (Rb) ratio (Ce/Rb). As shown in Fig. 4, the Ce/Rb ratio for the control group F0 was 0.91, which was less than the minimum suggested. In contrast, the Ce/Rb ratios for groups CL/F1, CL/F2, OE/F1 and OE/F2 were 1.10, 1.33, 1.00 and 1.11 respectively, all of which were equal to, or more than, 1:1 (the acceptable minimum ratio), which may be another reason for the variable trend of fracture resistance in this study (Table 2 and Fig. 4). The relationship between the crown-to-root ratio and the fracture resistance of the endodontically treated teeth was also supported by other in vitro study [31], but further more researches being needed for in the future.

In this in vitro study, the combination of cervical treatment methods (SCLM or OFEM) and a complete ferrule preparation decreased the fracture resistance of endodontically-treated obliquely-fractured mandibular premolar. Therefore, the null hypothesis that the fracture resistance of endodontically treated residual roots would not be affected by the ferrule length, was rejected; however, that the fracture resistance would not be affected by the cervical treatment methods, was accepted.

Conclusions

Within the limitations of this in vitro study, the following conclusions were drawn:

1. The fracture resistance of endodontically treated premolar with a lingual-to-buccal oblique fracture and an incomplete ferrule preparation were highest.
2. The combination of cervical treatment methods (SCLM or OFEM) and a complete ferrule preparation decreased the fracture resistance of endodontically-treated mandibular premolar.

Abbreviations
Ce/Rb: The effective clinical crown length (Ce) to embedded root length (Rb) ratio; CEJ: Cemento-enamel junction; kN: Kilonewton; OFEM: Orthodontic forced eruption method; SCLM: Surgical crown lengthening method

Acknowledgements
The authors thank Shanghai Dental Lab for their support with the milling machine and the State Key Laboratory of the China University of Mining and Technology for their support with the fracture test.

Funding
This research was supported by Jiangsu Provinicial medical youth talent (grant number QNRC-2016391). The authors declare that the funding body played no role in the design of the study and collection, analysis, and interpretation of data and in writing the manuscript.

Authors' contributions
QF-M participated in the research design of the study, data analysis and wrote the manuscript. Q-M participated in the testing process and in the design of the study. TD-W participated in the research design and data analysis, and YM-C participated in the design of the study and reviewed the article. All authors read and approved the final manuscript.

Competing interests
The authors declare that they have no competing interests.

Author details

[1]Department of Stomatology, Xuzhou Central Hospital, Xuzhou 221009, Jiangsu Province, China. [2]College of Stomatology, Nanjing Medical University, 136 Hanzhong Road, Nanjing 210029, Jiangsu Province, China.

References

1. Yang A, Lamichhane A, Xu C. Remaining coronal dentin and risk of fiber-reinforced composite post-core restoration failure: a meta-analysis. Int J Prosthodont. 2015;28:258–64.

2. Santana FR, Castro CG, Simamoto-Júnior PC, Soares PV, Quagliatto PS, Estrela C, et al. Influence of post system and remaining coronal tooth tissue on biomechanical behavior of root filled molar teeth. Int Endod J. 2011;44:386–94.

3. Zicari F, Van Meerbeek B, Scotti R, Naert I. Effect of ferrule and post placement on fracture resistance of endodontically treated teeth after fatigue loading. J Dent. 2013;41:207–15.

4. Mekayarajjananonth T, Chitcharus N, Winkler S, Bogert MC. The effect of fiber dowel heights in resin composite cores on restoration failures of endodontically treated teeth. J Oral Implantol. 2009;35:63–9.

5. Santos-Filho PC, Veríssimo C, Soares PV, Saltarelo RC, Soares CJ, Marcondes Martins LR. Influence of ferrule, post system, and length on biomechanical behavior of endodontically treated anterior teeth. J Endod. 2014;40:119–23.

6. Roscoe MG, Noritomi PY, Novais VR, Soares CJ. Influence of alveolar loss, post type, and ferrule presence on the biomechanical behavior of endodontically treated maxillary canines: strain measurement and stress distribution. J Prosthet Dent. 2013;110:116–26.

7. Juloski J, Radovic I, Goracci C, Vulicevic ZR, Ferrari M. Ferrule effect: a literature review. J Endod. 2012;38:11–9.

8. Meng QF, Chen LJ, Meng J, Chen YM, Smales RJ, Yip KH. Fracture resistance after simulated crown lengthening and forced tooth eruption of endodontically-treated teeth restored with a fiber post-and-core system. Am J Dent. 2009;22:147–50.

9. Naumann M, Preuss A, Rosentritt M. Effect of incomplete crown ferrules on load capacity of endodontically treated maxillary incisors restored with fiber posts, composite build-ups, and all-ceramic crowns: an in vitro evaluation after chewing simulation. Acta Odontol Scand. 2006;64:31–6.

10. Kutesa-Mutebi A, Osman YI. Effect of the ferrule on fracture resistance of teeth restored with prefabricated posts and composite cores. Afr Health Sci. 2004;4:131–5.

11. Mangold JT, Kern M. Influence of glass-fiber posts on the fracture resistance and failure pattern of endodontically treated premolars with varying substance loss: an in vitro study. J Prosthet Dent. 2011;105:387–93.

12. Ferrari M, Vichi A, Fadda GM, Cagidiaco MC, Tay FR, Breschi L, et al. A randomized controlled trial of endodontically treated and restored premolars. J Dent Res. 2012;91(7 Suppl):72S–8S.

13. Hou QQ, Gao YM, Sun L. Effects of residual coronal walls on the fracture resistance under dynamic loading in fiber post-core and crown system. J Modern Stomatol. 2013;27:129–32.

14. Ng CC, Dumbrigue HB, Al-Bayat MI, Griggs JA, Wakefield CW. Influence of remaining coronal tooth structure location on the fracture resistance of restored endodontically treated anterior teeth. J Prosthet Dent. 2006;95:290–6.

15. Liu SM, Liu YH, Lu X, Xu YX, Xu J. Influence of incomplete ferrule on stress distribution of post and core restored maxillary premolar. Chin J Stomatol. 2012;47:162–6.

16. Levine DF, Handelsman M, Rayon NA. Crown lengthening surgery: a restorative driven periodontal procedure. J Calif Dent Assoc. 1999;27:143–51.

17. de Oliveira PS, Chiarelli F, Rodrigues JA, Shibli JA, Zizzari VL, Piattelli A, et al. Aesthetic surgical crown lengthening procedure. Case Rep Dent. 2015;2015:437412.

18. Parwani SR, Parwani RN. Surgical crown lengthening: a periodontal and restorative interdisciplinary approach. Gen Dent. 2014;62:e15–9.

19. Patil PG, Nimbalkar-Patil SP, Karandikar AB. Multidisciplinary treatment approach to restore deep horizontally fractured maxillary central incisor. J Contemp Dent Pract. 2014;15:112–5.

20. Rokn AR, Saffarpour A, Sadrimanesh R, Iranparvar K, Saffarpour A, Mahmoudzadeh M, et al. Implant site development by orthodontic forced eruption of nontreatable teeth: a case report. Open Dent J. 2012;6:99–104.

21. Wu MK, van der Sluis LW, Wesselink PR. Comparison of mandibular premolars and canines with respect to their resistance to vertical root fracture. J Dent. 2004;32:265–8.

22. Watanabe MU, Anchieta RB, Rocha EP, Kina S, Almeida EO, Freitas AC Jr, Basting RT. Influence of crown ferrule heights and dowel material selection on the mechanical behavior of root-filled teeth: a finite element analysis. J Prosthodont. 2012;21:304–11.

23. Bourauel C, Freudenreich D, Vollmer D, Kobe D, Drescher D, Jäger A. Simulation of orthodontic tooth movements. A comparison of numerical models. J Orofac Orthop. 1999;60:136–51.

24. Sherfudhin H, Hobeich J, Carvalho CA, Aboushelib MN, Sadig W, Salameh Z. Effect of different ferrule designs on the fracture resistance and failure pattern of endodontically treated teeth restored with fiber posts and all-ceramic crowns. J Appl Oral Sci. 2011;19:28–33.

25. The glossary of prosthodontics terms. J Prosthet Dent. 1999;81:63.

26. Wilson TG, Kornman KS. Fundamentals of periodontics. 2nd ed. Chicago: Quintessence; 2003. p. 531–9.

27. Naumann M, Rosentritt M, Preuss A, Dietrich T. The effect of alveolar bone loss on the load capability of restored endodontically treated teeth: a comparative in vitro study. J Dent. 2006;34:790–5.

28. Luo Z, Zhang LL, Zhang Y, Liu YH, Xu J. Influence of alveolar bone heights on fracture resistance and pattern of post and core restored maxillary premolars. J Peking Univ (Health Sci). 2014;46:62–6.

29. Grossmann Y, Sadan A. The prosthodontic concept of crown-to-root ratio: a review of the literature. J Prosthet Dent. 2005;93:559–62.

30. Shillingburg HT, Sather DA, Wilson EL, CainJR MDL, Blanco LJ, Kessler JC. Fundamentals of fixed prosthodontics. 4th ed. Chicago: Quintessence; 2012. p. 99–130.

31. Meng QF, Chen LJ, Meng J. In vitro study evaluating the effect of different subgingival root exposure methods and ferrule designs on fracture resistance of residual root. Hua Xi Kou Qiang Yi Xue Za Zhi. 2014;32:75–9.

9

A novel in vivo method to evaluate trueness of digital impressions

Emad A. Albdour[1,2], Eman Shaheen[1], Myrthel Vranckx[1], Francesco Guido Mangano[3], Constantinus Politis[1] and Reinhilde Jacobs[1,4]* [iD]

Abstract

Background: Intraoral scanners are devices for capturing digital impressions in dentistry. Until now, several in vitro studies have assessed the trueness of digital impressions, but in vivo studies are missing. Therefore, the purpose of this study was to introduce a new method to assess trueness of intraoral scanners and digital impressions in an in vivo clinical set-up.

Methods: A digital impression using an intraoral scanner (Trios® 3 Cart wired, 3Shape, Copenhagen, Denmark) and a conventional alginate impression (Cavex Impressional®, Cavex, Haarlem, the Netherlands) as clinical reference were made for two patients assigned for full mouth extraction. A total of 30 teeth were collected upon surgery after impressions making. The gypsum model created from conventional impression and extracted teeth were then scanned in a lab scanner (Activity 885®, SmartOptics, Bochum, Germany). Digital model of the intraoral scanner (DM), digital model of the conventional gypsum cast (CM) and those of the extracted natural teeth (NT) were imported to a reverse engineering software (3-matic®, Materialise, Leuven, Belgium) in which the three models were registered then DM and CM were compared to their corresponding teeth in NT by distance map calculations.

Results: DM had statistically insignificant better trueness when compared to CM for total dataset ($p = 0.15$), statistically insignificant better trueness for CM when mandibular arches analyzed alone ($p = 0.56$), while a significantly better DM trueness ($p = 0.013$) was found when only maxillary arches were compared.

Conclusions: Our results show that digital impression technique is clinically as good as or better than the current reference standard for study models of orthognathic surgery patients.

Keywords: Intraoral scanners, Digital impression, Conventional impression, Trueness

Background

Conventional impression taking for dental cast preparation is still the clinical reference standard for replicating the intraoral situation [1]. Yet, such conventional approaches are considered cumbersome, bearing in mind the obstacles and challenges for both patient and dentist, including discomfort, nausea, unsatisfactory taste, time consumption, remakes in case of air bubble inclusion, forceful removal of highly retentive impressions with a risk for potential damage [2].

To overcome the drawbacks of conventional methods in dentistry, digital virtual models were introduced by Computer Aided Design/Computer Aided Manufacturing (CAD/CAM) solutions [3, 4]. Digital models can be created by indirect or direct approaches where indirect method uses laser optical scanning or computed tomography imaging of conventional impressions or plaster cast to produce digital virtual models [5, 6]. The direct method uses an intraoral scanning device to capture the patient dentition directly to produce a digital model that can be used to create temporary or final restorations [7–9].

During the last decade the use of intraoral digital impression systems have been steadily increasing. The possibilities and potential of digital impression taking as compared to the conventional approach may be related to its three dimensional representation on the computer,

* Correspondence: reinhilde.jacobs@uzleuven.be
[1]OMFS IMPATH research group, Department of Imaging and Pathology, Faculty of Medicine, University of Leuven and Oral & Maxillofacial Surgery, University Hospitals Leuven, Leuven, Belgium
[4]Department of Dental Medicine, Karolinska Institutet, Stockholm, Sweden
Full list of author information is available at the end of the article

enable its versatile use for diagnostic model fabrication and integrated treatment planning. For clinical use, it is important to gain some idea on time and cost efficiency. These factors were assessed in some studies with a rather promising outcome [1, 2]. Another point is the system accuracy. Accuracy assessment has been targeted by several studies [10–13]. Yet, it is important to mention that accuracy is most often determined by standardized quality control measures using an in vitro set-up for assessment of precision and trueness. Precision expresses the closeness of repeated measurements to each other. Trueness describes the deviation of the measurement from the dimensions of a reference object. A higher precision means a more predictable measurement, while high trueness means less deviation from the reference object dimensions [9]. So far most accuracy studies mention low error levels, obtained via in vitro methodological set-ups. However, it should be indicated that all those studies start from laboratory testing or an in vitro model approach. A crucial point may however be the performance and accuracy in the clinic, as compared to the reference standard being conventional impression taking. There are a number of potential advantages, favouring digital impression taking to be implemented in daily dental practice. It is therefore crucial to also obtain information on the accuracy of such systems during in vivo use. It is indeed important to evaluate precision and trueness in a clinical environment in the presence of the patient, the operator and related factors that might affect accuracy such as blood and saliva in the mouth, patient movement, operator movement, obstructions by cheek and tongue, reflection of light by intraoral structures and restrictions of space inside the patient's mouth [14]. Studying precision in the clinical set up can be done by repeating the scan of the same dentition intraorally multiple times and measure the deviations among these impressions [12, 15]. Assessing clinical trueness is more challenging, since the dimensions of the natural dental structure for which the digital or conventional impressions are made need to be captured accurately to be used as a reference model for comparison [16].

Focusing on study models made for orthognathic surgery patients, the aim of this study was to introduce a new method to validate the trueness of digital impressions of teeth scanned with an intraoral scanner and conventional impression (clinical standard) when compared to the corresponding natural teeth after extraction and scanned with a high resolution scanner (gold standard) in an in vivo clinical set-up.

Methods

Patient selection

Two patients who required full teeth extraction from Oral and Maxillofacial Surgery department (University Hospitals of Leuven, Belgium) were included in this study which was approved by the Ethical Review Board of the University Hospitals Leuven (S55619 ML9535, University Hospitals Leuven), signed informed consents were obtained from participants.

Impressions and collecting teeth protocols

Before the surgical procedure, the upper and lower dentitions of each patient were digitally captured in the dental office with a chair-side intraoral scanner (Trios® 3 Cart wired, 3Shape, Copenhagen, Denmark) one time by a single experienced operator (first author) according to the manufacturer instructions for full arch scanning. For the mandible, one continuous motion starting on occlusal surfaces of posterior teeth starting from one side to the other with alternating movement on the anterior buccolingual area. Followed by scanning the lingual surfaces of all teeth from one side to the other. Finally rolling to buccal side and scan buccal surfaces of all teeth. For the maxilla, the same procedure was repeated except scanning the buccal surfaces of teeth before palatal ones and ending with scanning the palate.. A digital model (DM) was created and exported in stereolithographic (STL) format for each jaw.

One upper and one lower Conventional alginate (Cavex impressional®, Cavex, Holland) impressions in best fitting trays were made for each patient by the same operator and sent to the dental lab to create plaster casts. These plaster casts were digitized via high resolution optical scanner (Activity 885®, SmartOptics, Bochum, Germany), with an accuracy of 4 μm as provided by the manufacturer. Data was exported in STL format and referred to as conventional model (CM).

During surgery, 30 extracted teeth which had full anatomic crowns or minor defects not affecting the dimensions of the crowns were collected from the patients to be used as reference models. All teeth with major defects or loose were excluded. After cleaning from blood and soft tissue residues, each tooth crown was scanned separately by the same lab scanner Activity 885˙. Each tooth was fixed during scanning using a custom made gypsum base with a hole in the middle filled with modeling wax (Fig. 1a) by inserting the root into the wax and keeping the crown clear for scanning (Fig. 1b). Data were exported as natural teeth (NT) in STL format.

Evaluation protocol

All the STL files of the DM, CM and NT for each patient were imported into a reverse engineering software (3-matic®, Materialise, Leuven, Belgium) to evaluate the trueness of DM and CM to its corresponding NT model. The steps are summarized in the flow chart in Fig. 2 and described as follows:

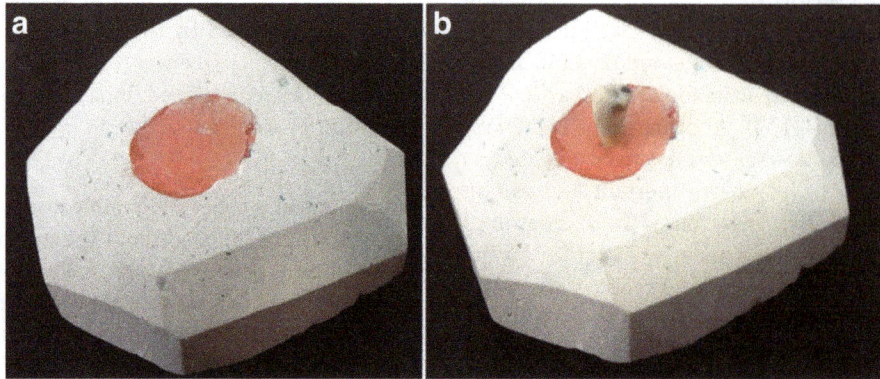

Fig. 1 a Custom made gypsum base used to fix the teeth during scanning. **b** Each tooth was fixed by inserting its root into wax to keep the crown clear for scanning

(1) Register CM on DM using surface based registration (best fit alignment method).
(2) Register each NT model onto its corresponding DM using surface based registration.
(3) Isolate each tooth group using cutting planes which are parallel to the teeth.
(4) Remove soft tissue from isolated CM and DM models due to lack of soft tissue in NT and to guarantee matched equal borders.
(5) Calculate the distance maps (Euclidean distances) between surfaces using unsigned part comparison in 3-matic software providing a color-coded map. These distance maps were calculated between CM - NT and DM - NT separately provided that NT was used as the reference gold standard model in both cases.

The Root Mean Square deviation (RMS) was used to quantify and report degree of conformity of CM and DM compared to NT. RMS is a frequently used measure of the individual difference between values of a model and the values observed from the original object being modelled. RMS aggregates these individual differences into a single measure of predictive power.

Statistical analysis

Statistical analysis was done using a dedicated statistical software (MedCalc version 16.4°, Ostend, Belgium). Normality of distribution was tested by the Shapiro-Wilk Normality test for CM and DM (maxilla, mandible and both jaws). Non-parametric Wilcoxon matched pairs test was used to compare degree of trueness between CM and DM to NT for maxillary, mandibular and both jaws, level of significance was set at $P < 0.05$.

Results

Table 1 shows median, inter quartile range (IQR), mean and standard deviation (STD) for RMS values for CM and DM when compared with NT.

CM exhibited a total (maxilla and mandible) mean discrepancy and deviation of 133 ± 45 µm (range 10 -250 µm), while DM showed a total mean discrepancy of 119 ± 48 µm (range 60 -280 µm). Figure 3 shows a box-plot for deviations of CM and DM for both arches.

Results of Wilcoxon Matched Pairs Test for comparing CM and DM are reported in Table 2, statistically insignificant better trueness for DM compared to CM ($P = 0.15$) was found when total dataset was analyzed, statistically insignificant better trueness for CM when mandibular arches analyzed alone ($p = 0.56$). While a statistically significant difference was found between DM and CM for maxillary arches alone, favoring DM ($P = 0.013$).

Visual assessment of color-coded deviation maps for teeth showed maximum positive deviations concentrated mainly in two areas: cervical and proximal regions in both CM and DM (Fig. 4), and occlusal surface only in CM (Fig. 5).

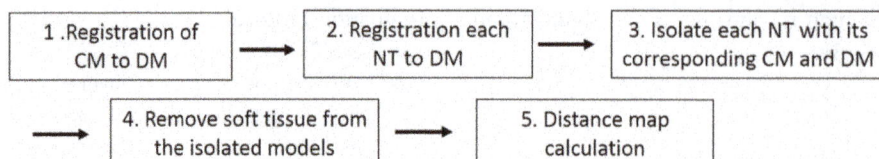

Fig. 2 Evaluation protocol flaw chart

Table 1 Descriptive statistics of RMS values for CM and DM compared to NT

Model	Arch	Teeth (N)	Median µm	Inter quartile range µm	Mean µm	Standard deviation µm
CM	Maxilla	14	151	70	154	45
	Mandible	16	121	45	120	45
	Total	30	130	68	133	45
DM	Maxilla	14	113	65	106	37
	Mandible	16	118	53	133	57
	Total	30	118	38	119	48

Discussion

In this study, we presented a new in vivo method to evaluate the trueness of intraoral scanner by comparing conventional and digital impressions to the corresponding natural teeth after extraction.

DM using the former intraoral scanner showed better trueness values (119 µm) than CM (133 µm) when both arches were compared. Maxillary arches were significantly higher for DM than CM, while mandibular arches showed insignificant deviations between both methods with higher trueness for CM.

Cervical (buccal, lingual or proximal) deviation areas for CM can be caused by variable thickness or deficiency of impression materials between neighboring teeth, especially for alginate which has low tear resistance affecting the accuracy of gypsum model (Fig. 4 *left*) [2, 17–20]. While in DM, this can be caused by light reflection of saliva in interproximal areas as well as the difficulty of scanner light to penetrate these areas (Fig. 4 *right*) [21] affecting their accuracy in the mandible were saliva has higher concentrations. Another possible effect would be the proximity to gingival tissues which has different light reflective capabilities than tooth structure which might cause potential distortion of light transmitted by intraoral scanner in these areas. Anna et al. [22] found the same area to be affected, it was mentioned that best fit method used for comparison would cause an axial movement of the point-cloud for the model being compared, and such adjustment would cause positive distortions in the margin with reduced distortions at occlusal surface.

The second area with deviations was only shown in CM on the occlusal surfaces of posterior teeth and palatal (lingual) on anterior teeth. No specific pattern of distribution was detected. This might be attributed to unavoidable trapped air bubbles on the surface of alginate impression which are duplicated on gypsum cast surface and appear as local deviations (Fig. 5 *left*).

Less saliva content in upper arches, more flexibility and space for scanner tip movement and less movement of maxillary arches compared to mandibular ones could explain significantly better trueness for DM in maxillary arches.

Trueness of intraoral scanners has been examined in few studies, some by taking digital or conventional impressions for industrial manufactured models in controlled lab set-up [23], where the absence of in vivo set-up with its intraoral factors mentioned earlier might affect reported trueness results. Other studies used conventional and digital impressions taken for patients to be compared together using one of them as a reference [24]. These studies neglected the presence of inherited errors in this reference impression or the model created from it leading to less trueness and trusted results. On the other hand, there are studies that used marginal and internal fit of final crown and bridge restorations constructed using digital and conventional impressions to

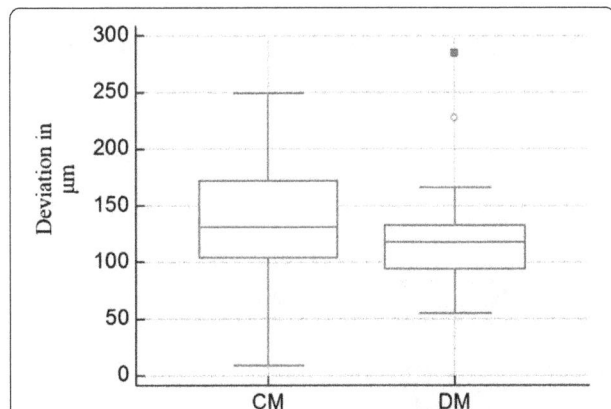

Fig. 3 Boxplot of trueness deviations for CM and DM for total dataset (maxilla and mandible). The box represents the range of 50% of the difference measurements. The bar within the box represents the median trueness of CM and DM using the 25–75 percentile value. Square represents outlier difference measurements (more than 1.5 times the interquartile range). Circle represents extreme values (more than 3 times the interquartile range)

Table 2 Trueness level of CM and DM to NT

Model	Arch	N(Teeth)	P-level
CM - DM	Maxilla	14	0.013*
	Mandible	16	0.56
	Total	30	0.15

*indicates significant difference (P < 0.05)

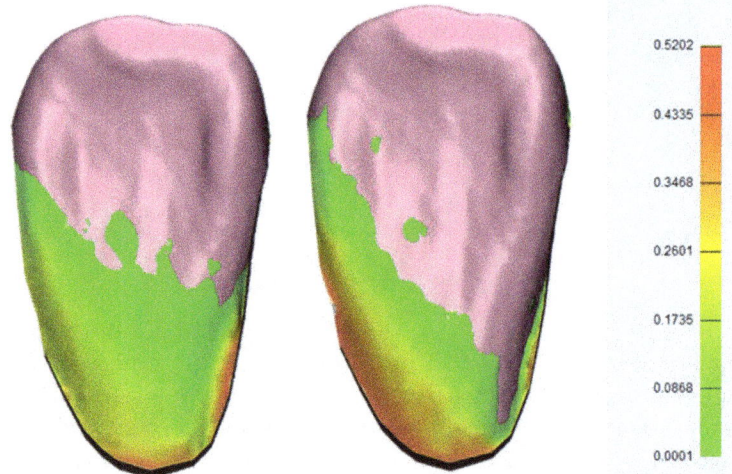

Fig. 4 Color deviation map shows positive deviations in proximal and cervical areas. CM (left), DM (right). A positive value (red) in the color deviation map indicates that the CM and DM are larger than NT in these specific areas

assess the trueness level [21]. In fact, this method involved the trueness of all steps in manufacturing final restoration, and not only the trueness level of impression itself [25].

Intraoral scanners have many advantages which include and not limited to better accuracy values as shown in our results, easy to use, patients' comfort, physical storage space not needed, impressions can be sent directly to milling machine to finalize restorations in minutes, reduced labor work and fast with cost efficient implementation [26, 27], which encourage replacement of conventional impressions by digital ones for many cases of surgical planning and splints manufacturing in maxillofacial surgeries and orthodontic treatments.

In our study, all factors affecting trueness values were neutralized, up to the authors knowledge it was not mentioned in literature that digital and conventional impressions where made in vivo and compared to the same original intraoral structures captured in these impressions. Evaluation was limited to teeth as soft tissue could not be cropped with those teeth (NT) for comparison. Moreover, each tooth was separately evaluated as it is impossible to extract all the teeth and preserve their position accurately on a gypsum base as they are in the patient mouth to be examined for trueness as complete arch.

The use of only one intraoral scanner was another limitation of this study. However, this Trios scanner allows exporting STL files that are compatible with multiple CAD/CAM software. In addition, it supports a powder free, colored scans, ultrafast optical sectioning technique and confocal microscopy scanning technology

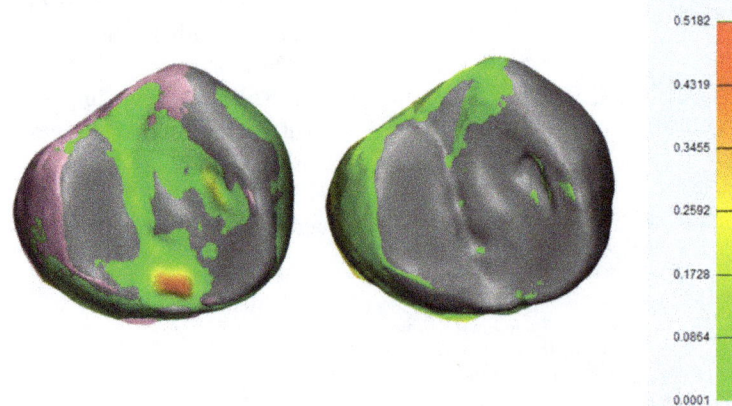

Fig. 5 Positive localized deviations on the surface of CM (left) which are absent on the same surface in DM (right). A positive value (red) in the color deviation map indicates that CM is larger than NT in these specific areas

[6, 28, 29]. Moreover, this study focused on the introduction of a new method to evaluate the accuracy of intraoral scanners in terms of trueness and not to compare several scanners.

Nevertheless the current results show that the digital impressions technique is clinically as good as or better than the current reference standard used for orthognathic surgery patients. Optimally clinical and digital impression taking for prosthetic work should yield error values of around 25 μm [30].

It is recommended to conduct more studies using other types of impression materials and commercial intraoral scanners and include more patient data to report on clinical accuracy rather than technical factory accuracy.

Conclusions

Direct digital impression methods using intraoral scanning have many advantages over conventional impressions with accurate in vivo results. Yet the present clinical study indicates that the variability in scanner output is still large, with error levels somewhat around or below the conventional impression method.

Abbreviations
CAD/CAM: Computer Aided Design/Computer Aided Manufacturing; CM: Conventional gypsum cast model; DM: Digital model of the intraoral scanner; IQR: Inter quartile range; NT: Natural extracted teeth model; RMS: Root Mean Square deviation; STD: Mean and standard deviation; STL: Standard Tessellation or Stereolithographic File

Funding
The present study was self-funded, and it was not supported by any grant; therefore, the authors have no conflict of interest related to the present work.

Authors' contributions
All authors made substantial contributions to the present study. EAA, ES, MV and RJ contributed to conception and design, acquisition of data, analysis and interpretation of data; they were, moreover, involved in writing and editing the manuscript. Together, EAA, ES, CP and RJ were the major contributors in preparing and writing the manuscript. FGM and RJ revised the manuscript before submission. All authors read and approved the final manuscript.

Competing interests
The authors declare that they have no competing interests in relation to the present work. Francesco Mangano is a Section Editor for BMC Oral Health.

Author details
[1]OMFS IMPATH research group, Department of Imaging and Pathology, Faculty of Medicine, University of Leuven and Oral & Maxillofacial Surgery, University Hospitals Leuven, Leuven, Belgium. [2]Department of Prosthodontics, Royal Medical Services, Jordanian Armed Forces, Amman, Jordan. [3]Department of Medicine and Surgery, Dental School, University of Varese, Varese, Italy. [4]Department of Dental Medicine, Karolinska Institutet, Stockholm, Sweden.

References
1. Gjelvold B, Chrcanovic BR, Korduner EK, Collin-Bagewitz I, Kisch J. Intraoral digital impression technique compared to conventional impression technique. A randomized clinical trial. J Prosthodont. 2016;25(4):282–7.
2. Patzelt SBM, Lamprinos C, Stampf S, Att W. The time efficiency of intraoral scanners. An in vitro comparative study J Am Dent Assoc. 2014;145(6):542–51.
3. Otto T, De Nisco S. Computer-aided direct ceramic restorations: a 10-year prospective clinical study of Cerec CAD/CAM inlays and onlays. Int J Prosthodont. 2002;15(2):122–8.
4. Mörmann WH. The evolution of the CEREC system. J Am Dent Assoc. 2006; 137 Suppl(September):7S-13S.
5. Güth JF, Keul C, Stimmelmayr M, Beuer F, Edelhoff D. Accuracy of digital models obtained by direct and indirect data capturing. Clin Oral Investig. 2013;17(4):1201–8.
6. Fasbinder DJ. Computerized technology for restorative dentistry. Am J Dent. 2013;26(3):115–20.
7. Beuer F, Schweiger J, Edelhoff D. Digital dentistry: an overview of recent developments for CAD/CAM generated restorations. Br Dent J. 2008;204(9):505–11.
8. Mangano F, Gandolfi A, Luongo G, Logozzo S. Intraoral scanners in dentistry: a review of the current literature. BMC Oral Health. 2017;17(1):149.
9. Ender A, Mehl A. Accuracy of complete-arch dental impressions: a new method of measuring trueness and precision. J Prosthet Dent. 2013; 109(2):121–8.
10. Rödiger M, Heinitz A, Bürgers R, Rinke S. Fitting accuracy of zirconia single crowns produced via digital and conventional impressions—a clinical comparative study. Clin Oral Investig. 2017;21(2):579–87.
11. Cho SH, Schaefer O, Thompson GA, Guentsch A. Comparison of accuracy and reproducibility of casts made by digital and conventional methods. J Prosthet Dent. 2015;113(4):310–5.
12. Imburgia M, Logozzo S, Hauschild U, Veronesi G, Mangano C, Mangano FG. Accuracy of four intraoral scanners in oral implantology: a comparative in vitro study. BMC Oral Health. 2017;17(1):92.
13. Mangano FG, Veronesi G, Hauschild U, Mijiritsky E, Mangano C. Trueness and precision of four intraoral scanners in oral implantology: a comparative in vitro study. PLoS One. 2016;11(9):e0163107.
14. Luthardt RG, Walter MH, Weber A, Koch R, Rudolph H. Clinical parameters influencing the accuracy of 1- and 2-stage impressions: a randomized controlled trial. Int J Prosthodont. 2007;21:322–7.
15. Flügge TV, Schlager S, Nelson K, Nahles S, Metzger MC. Precision of intraoral digital dental impressions with iTero and extraoral digitization with the iTero and a model scanner. Am J Orthod Dentofac Orthop. 2013;144(3):471–8.
16. Ender A, Mehl A. Accuracy in dental medicine, a new way to measure trueness and precision. J Vis Exp. 2014;86:e51374.
17. DeLong R, Knorr S, Anderson GC, Hodges J, Pintado MR. Accuracy of contacts calculated from 3D images of occlusal surfaces. J Dent. 2007; 35(6):528–34.
18. Endo T, Finger WJ. Dimensional accuracy of a new polyether impression material. Quintessence Int. 2006;37(1):47–51.
19. Chen SY, Liang WM, Chen FN. Factors affecting the accuracy of elastometric impression materials. J Dent. 2004;32(8):603–9.
20. Ceyhan JA, Johnson GH, Lepe X, Phillips KM. A clinical study comparing the three-dimensional accuracy of a working die generated from two dual-arch trays and a complete-arch custom tray. J Prosthet Dent. 2003;90(3):228–34.
21. Boeddinghaus M, Breloer ES, Rehmann P, Wöstmann B. Accuracy of single-tooth restorations based on intraoral digital and conventional impressions in patients. Clin Oral Investig. 2015;19(8):2027–34.
22. Persson ASK, Odén A, Andersson M, Sandborgh-Englund G. Digitization of simulated clinical dental impressions: virtual three-dimensional analysis of exactness. Dent Mater. 2009;25(7):929–36.

23. Vecsei B, Joós-Kovács G, Borbély J, Hermann P. Comparison of the accuracy of direct and indirect three-dimensional digitizing processes for CAD/CAM systems – an in vitro study. J Prosthodont Res. 2017;61(2):177–84.
24. Gan N, Xiong Y, Jiao T. Accuracy of intraoral digital impressions for whole upper jaws, including full dentitions and palatal soft tissues. PLoS One. 2016;11(7):1–15.
25. Seelbach P, Brueckel C, Wöstmann B. Accuracy of digital and conventional impression techniques and workflow. Clin Oral Investig. 2013;17(7):1759–64.
26. Patzelt SBM, Vonau S, Stampf S, Att W. Assessing the feasibility and accuracy of digitizing edentulous jaws. J Am Dent Assoc. 2013;144(8):914–20.
27. Patzelt SBM, Emmanouilidi A, Stampf S, Strub JR, Att W. Accuracy of full-arch scans using intraoral scanners. Clin Oral Investig. 2014;18(6):1687–94.
28. Hack GD, SBM P. Evaluation of the Accuracy of Six Intraoral Scanning Devices. An in-vitro Investigation. 2015;10(4):1–5.
29. Franceschini G. A comparative analysis of intraoral 3d digital scanners for restorative dentistry. Internet J Med Technol. 2011;5(1):1–18.
30. Hamalian TA, Nasr E, Chidiac JJ. Impression materials in fixed prosthodontics: influence of choice on clinical procedure. J Prosthodont. 2011;20(2):153–60.

10

E-learning or educational leaflet: does it make a difference in oral health promotion?

Susan Al Bardaweel[*] and Mayssoon Dashash

Abstract

Background: The early recognition of technology together with great ability to use computers and smart systems have promoted researchers to investigate the possibilities of utilizing technology for improving health care in children. The aim of this study was to compare between the traditional educational leaflets and E-applications in improving oral health knowledge, oral hygiene and gingival health in schoolchildren of Damascus city, Syria.

Methods: A clustered randomized controlled trial at two public primary schools was performed. About 220 schoolchildren aged 10–11 years were included in this study and grouped into two clusters. Children in Leaflet cluster received oral health education through leaflets, while children in E-learning cluster received oral health education through an E-learning program. A questionnaire was designed to register information related to oral health knowledge and to record Plaque and Gingival indices. Questionnaire administration and clinical assessment were undertaken at baseline, 6 and at 12 weeks of oral health education. Data was analysed using one way repeated measures ANOVA, post hoc Bonferroni test and independent samples t-test.

Results: Leaflet cluster (107 participants) had statistically significant better oral health knowledge than E-learning cluster (104 participants) at 6 weeks ($P < 0.05$) and at 12 weeks ($P < 0.05$) (Leaflet cluster:100 participants, E-learning cluster:100 participants). The mean knowledge gain compared to baseline was higher in Leaflet cluster than in E-learning cluster. A significant reduction in the PI means at 6 weeks and 12 weeks was observed in both clusters ($P < 0.05$) when compared to baseline. Children in Leaflet cluster had significantly less plaque than those in E-learning cluster at 6 weeks ($P < 0.05$) and at 12 weeks ($P < 0.05$). Similarly, a significant reduction in the GI means at 6 weeks and 12 weeks was observed in both clusters when compared to baseline ($P < 0.05$). Children in Leaflet cluster had statistically significant better gingival health than E-learning cluster at 6 weeks ($P < 0.05$) and 12 weeks ($P < 0.05$).

Conclusions: Traditional educational leaflets are an effective tool in the improvement of both oral health knowledge as well as clinical indices of oral hygiene and care among Syrian children. Leaflets can be used in school-based oral health education for a positive outcome.

Keywords: Health education, Knowledge, Oral health promotion, E-learning, Leaflets, Schoolchildren, Syria

* Correspondence: susan.bardaweel@hotmail.co.uk
Department of Paediatric Dentistry, Faculty of Dentistry, Damascus University, Damascus city, Syria

Background

Due to the tremendous increase in the use of new technologies, it is thought that younger generations think and process information in a different manner than their predecessors [1]. Technology has changed the way we see the world [2]. There are many definitions of E-learning, one of these definitions is the use of "Internet technologies to deliver a broad array of solutions that enhance knowledge and performance" [3]. However, E-learning is a broad term that includes any use of computers to support learning process, whether online or offline [4].

School age is influential in people's lives. It is a time when lifelong sustainable oral health related behaviors, beliefs and attitudes are being instilled. During this stage, children are more receptive; in addition, earlier establishment of habits produces a longer lasting impact. Therefore, schools can be considered an ideal environment for promoting oral health [5].

Dental caries has been considered to be a major public health problem for Syrian children. Despite a significant increase in the number of dentists in Damascus city, epidemiological data did not indicate any decrease in the dmft (decayed, missing and filled primary teeth) or DMFT (decayed, missing and filled permanent teeth) values for any age group. Additionally, no decrease in the percentage of untreated dental caries is detected [6]. Moreover, many challenges can be faced in providing access and delivering oral health care to children in Syria. Therefore, it is thought wise to increase preventative care in the form of school-based health education programs aiming at children.

Researchers have measured the effectiveness of E-learning in different areas. However, there are no previous studies that compare the effects of two different educational methods (E-learning versus leaflets) on oral health promotion geared for school children. Our intention was to enhance the application of evidence so, to minimize contamination, the unit of randomization was the school. The present study aimed to determine if E-learning instructions improve the acquisition of oral health knowledge and skills when compared to traditional educational leaflets in children aged 10–11 years living in Damascus city. Also, to consequently determine which educational method can better direct the child towards practicing appropriate oral health care.

Methods
Study design

A clustered randomized controlled trial at two public primary schools of Damascus city, Syria, was conducted. Using a list of the public schools in the city of Damascus, two schools were randomly selected by simple random sampling method using the table of random numbers; geographic location was taken into consideration in order to minimize any unintentional spillover effect of the assigned intervention. For allocation of the schools, simple randomization through flipping a coin was used by an investigator with no clinical involvement in the trial. The two schools were randomly allocated into two clusters: Leaflet cluster included 110 children, who received oral health education through leaflets, and E-learning cluster included 110 children who received oral health education through an E-learning program. The whole study was carried out for a period of 3 months (February 2016–April 2016).

Sample

An estimate of 100 subjects per cluster was calculated to detect a difference between the two clusters with a two-tailed, α of 0.05 and a (1-β) of 0.80. Common occurrences such as loss to follow-up, missing data and withdrawals from the experiment were anticipated and additional subjects were recruited into each cluster. Initially 247 children from two public primary schools were asked to participate in the study. Informed consent was obtained from the parents of 220 with 110 children in each cluster who were initially included in the study, and then sample diminished through the recall visits due to children having moved to other schools or being absent the day of the examination. Thus the final sample included 200 with 100 children in each cluster (91 boys and 109 girls) aged 10–11 year old.

Inclusion criteria

All healthy children who accepted to take part in this study, who did not receive any previous dental educational program, had internet access connection and ability to browse and use the internet, were included in this study.

Exclusion criteria

The following groups were excluded: children outside the age range of the study; children currently under the regular care of an oral health care provider; children who have access to oral health education through a different and separate source than our intervention; children with acute dental issues (e.g.: dental abscess); mentally or physically compromised children and finally children whose parents did not provide consent for participation in our study.

Ethical considerations

Ethical Approval was obtained from the ethics committee of the Faculty of Dentistry in Damascus University, Syria. In addition, a formal permission was obtained from the Ministry of Education in order to get access to schools and perform the required examinations on children. A written informed consent was obtained from all parents of the study participants.

Educational tools

Leaflets: A colorful and attractive leaflet in the form of a short story named "Adnan likes the dentist" was designed by a graphic designer (Figs. 1 and 2). The leaflets were designed with particular emphasis on creating interest amongst the children. These educational papers included information related to proper brushing technique and frequency; introduced the regular use of dental floss; emphasized regular dental visits as well as provided basic demonstration of dental plaque and the implications of not removing it. The leaflets also contained nutritional guidelines in regards to minimizing caries risk, and finally the role of fluoride in caries control.

E-learning program

An E-learning program was designed by an expert in artificial intelligence. The program was full of colorful images, videos, interactive quizzes and age-related developmental tasks in the quest to deliver the information in an interactive, entertaining and simple manner. The E-learning program included the same information of the leaflet; only the way in which the content is conveyed to the children was different.

Questionnaire design

Several issues were considered essential in designing the questionnaire for the children aged 10–11 years. The developmental age of children was the key in order to provide them with age–related developmental tasks that can offer educational opportunities and tools for health promotion and encourage children to use and maintain their oral health. Therefore, a panel of experts from the Faculties of Education and Dentistry were consulted in order to design the questionnaire.

Information related to oral health and nutrition was included. A pilot study which included 25 children was undertaken to identify any ambiguous or unclear terms, and to assess the time required for filling the questionnaire.

The final draft of the designed questionnaire included demographic data such as name, age and school name. It also included charts for recording Plaque and Gingival indices and simple Arabic questions to assess knowledge, practices of oral health and diet (Additional file 1).

Study procedures

The two selected schools were randomly allocated into two clusters: Children in Leaflet cluster received oral health education through leaflets, and children in E-learning cluster received oral health education through an E-learning program. Only one trained investigator (S.B) clinically examined all children in their classroom using mirror, probe and artificial light. This was performed without informing children about oral examination and intervention dates. Dental Plaque was assessed using Plaque Index (PI) for Silness and Löe [7]. Gingival health was assessed using Gingival Index (GI) for Löe and Silness [7].

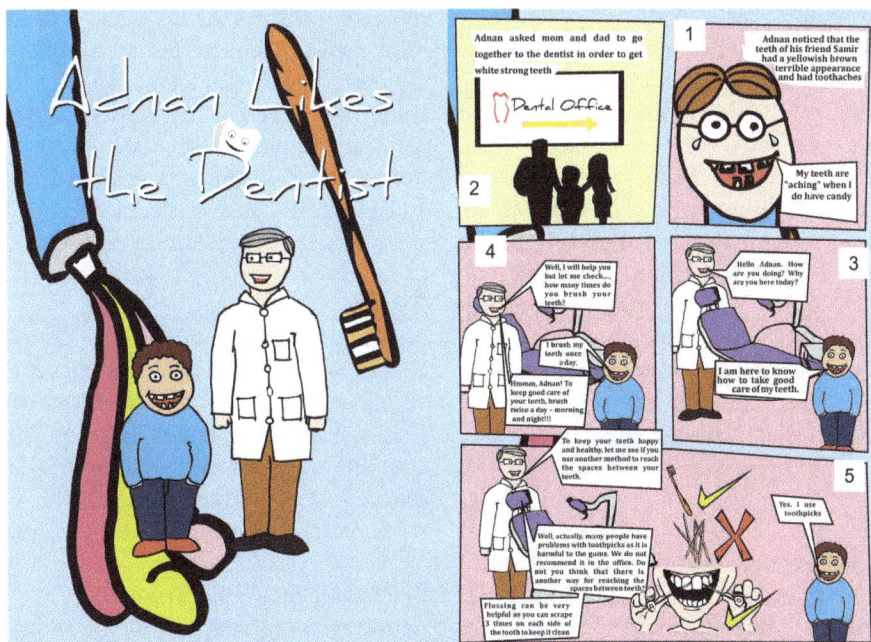

Fig. 1 Shows the first part of the educational leaflet

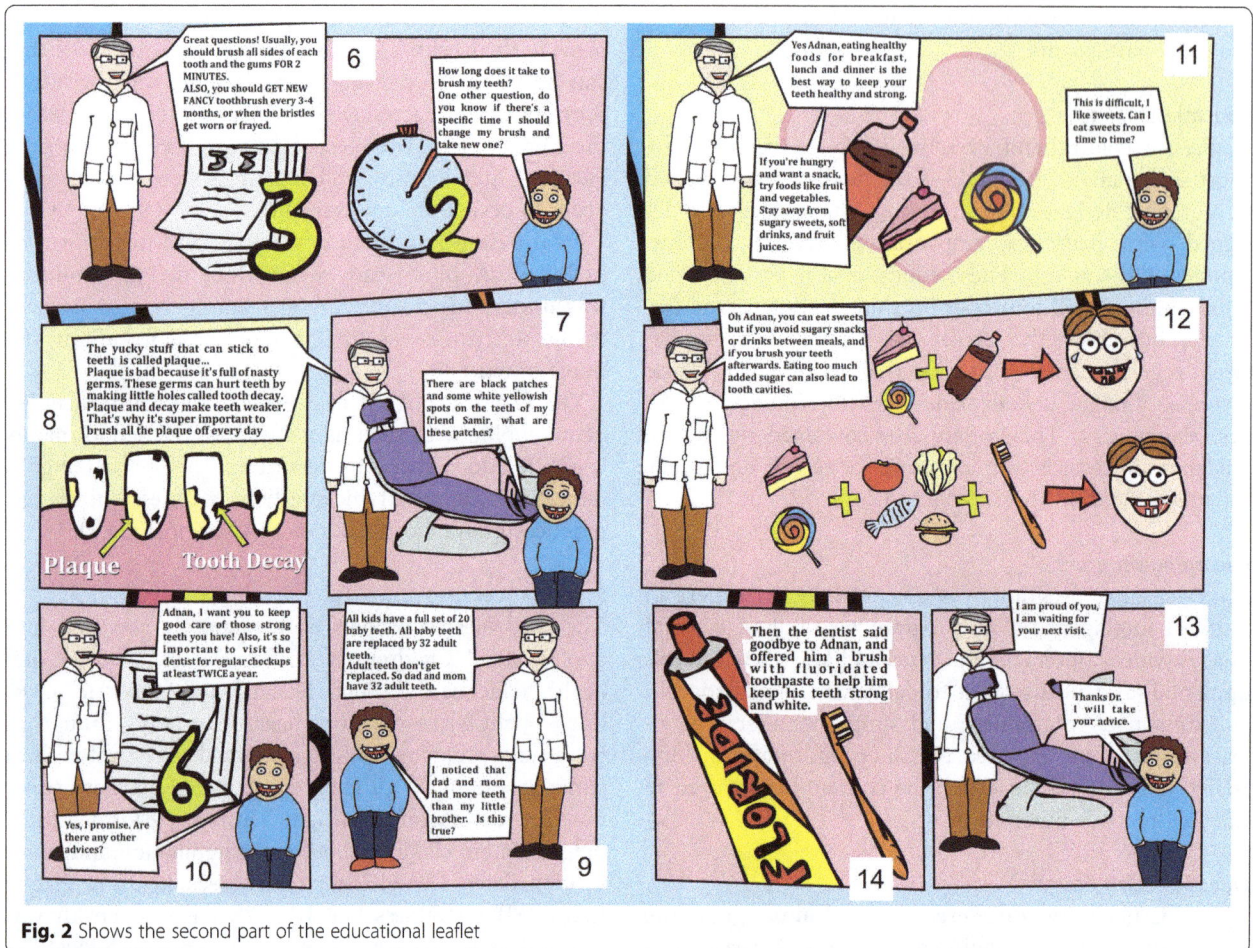

Fig. 2 Shows the second part of the educational leaflet

Blinding of the intervention was not possible, because it's obvious to the investigator (S.B) who examined the children which cluster they were in. Realistically, it was going to be difficult to hide this information from children too.

After collecting the baseline data, oral health educational tools were provided to subjects in which leaflets were given to children in Leaflet cluster, whilst children in E-learning cluster were provided with CDs which contained instructions on how to access the website via the link www.oralhealthforchildren.com. The level of oral health knowledge, plaque accumulation and gingival status were also re-evaluated after a period of six weeks and also after twelve weeks by the same examiner. The period of experiment was limited by the length of the school trimester in Syria which lasts 3 months (Fig. 3).

Statistical analysis

The primary outcome was a change in oral health knowledge during the 12 weeks of the study in the two clusters. Secondary outcomes included changes in plaque accumulation and gingival health during the period of the study in the clusters. Data was entered in Microsoft Excel 2010, and statistically analyzed using the software SPSS 19.0.

Descriptive statistical analysis was carried out. One way repeated measures ANOVA and post hoc Bonferroni test were used to compare the mean differences of study parameters (Oral health knowledge, PI scores and GI scores) within the same cluster. Between the two clusters, independent samples t-test was used to compare the mean differences of parameters evaluated at baseline, 6 weeks and 12 weeks. Level of significance and confidence interval were set at 5 and 95%, respectively.

Results

About 220 schoolchildren aged 10–11 years were included in this study, and then there was a drop-out of 20 subjects. A total of 200 children (91 boys and 109 girls) were then included in the study in which, 100 children allocated to Leaflet cluster and the other 100 were grouped in E-learning cluster. The mean age for the study population was 10.74 ± 0.44 (Table 1).

Oral health knowledge scores

At the start of the study, the mean knowledge scores of children in the two clusters did not present any statistical significant differences ($P = 0.73$) (Table 2). After the

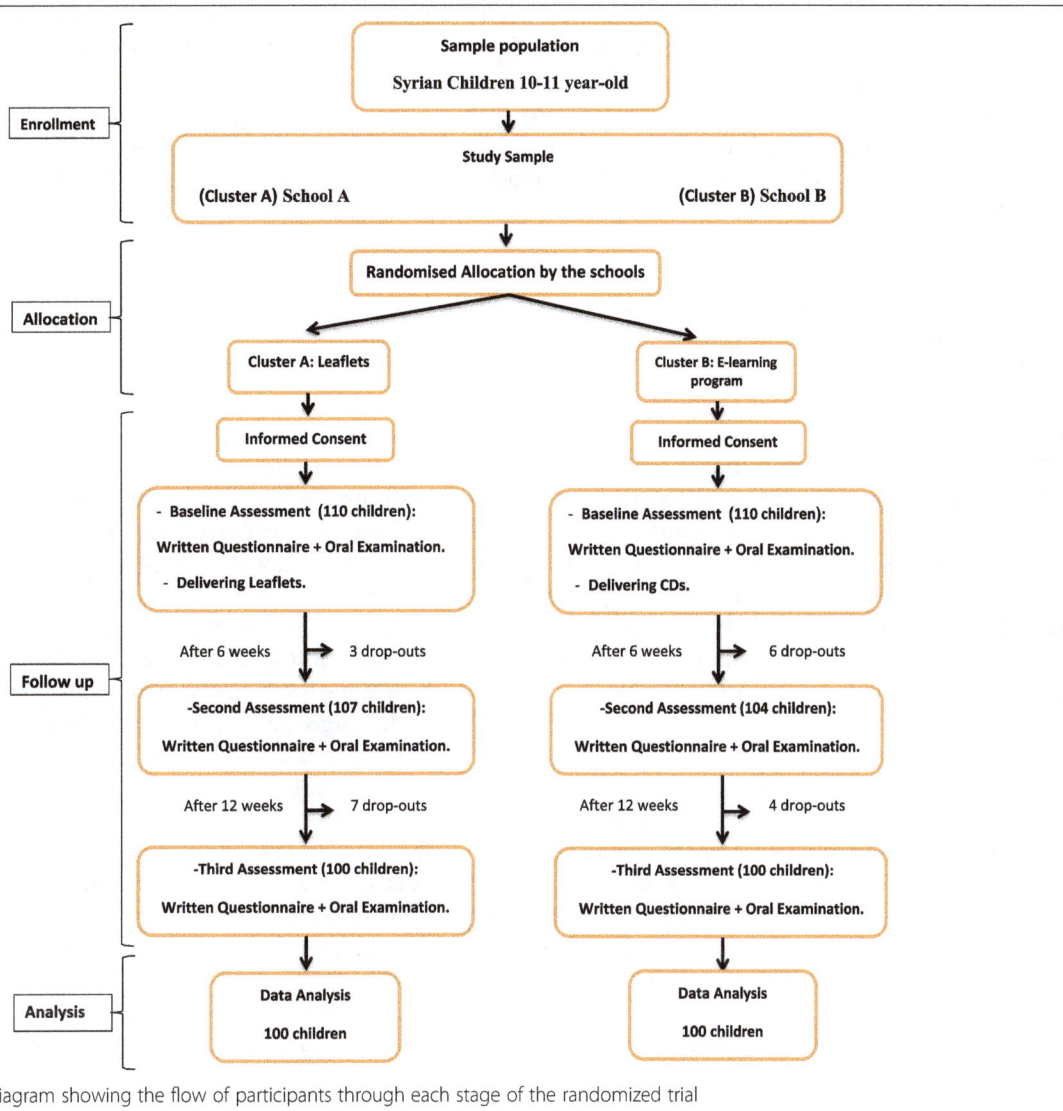

Fig. 3 CONSORT diagram showing the flow of participants through each stage of the randomized trial

intervention, the mean knowledge score was 82.87 ± 10.69 at 6 weeks and 89.12 ± 8.16 at 12 weeks in Leaflet cluster, while E-learning cluster showed values of 72.16 ± 10.25 at 6 weeks and 74.66 ± 8.98 at 12 weeks. Comparison of the baseline values with their respective post-intervention knowledge scores illustrated a statistically significant ($P < 0.05$) increase in knowledge for both clusters (Table 2). However, children in Leaflet cluster had significantly better knowledge than those in E-learning

Table 1 Age and gender distribution of children studied

Cluster	Gender		Total N (%)	Age Mean ± SD
	Male N (%)	Female N (%)		
Leaflet Cluster	43 (43)	57 (57)	100 (50)	10.69 ± 0.47
E-learning Cluster	48 (48)	52 (52)	100 (50)	10.80 ± 0.40
Total	91 (45.5)	109 (54.5)	200 (100)	10.74 ± 0.44

Table 2 The intracluster and intercluster comparison of oral health knowledge score between the two clusters

Cluster	Knowledge score Mean ± SD			P value
	Baseline	6 weeks	12 weeks	
Leaflet Cluster	54.94 ± 12.74	82.87 ± 10.69	89.12 ± 8.16	F = 665.67; P < 0.001*
E-learning Cluster	55.50 ± 9.93	72.16 ± 10.25	74.66 ± 8.98	F = 223.39; P < 0.001*
Significance	t = −0.35; P = 0.73**	t = 7.24; P < 0.001**	t = 11.92; P < 0.001**	

*One way repeated measures ANOVA was applied to compare the mean differences of knowledge score within the same cluster
**Independent samples t-test was applied to compare the mean differences of knowledge score between the two clusters at baseline, 6 weeks and 12 weeks

cluster at 6 weeks ($P < 0.001$) and at 12 weeks ($P < 0.001$) (Table 2). Further analysis using independent samples t-test revealed that the difference in knowledge gain was statistically significant between the two clusters, and that the increase was higher in Leaflet cluster than in E-learning cluster (34.19 ± 11.35 versus 19.60 ± 9.75, respectively, $P < 0.001$).

PI scores

PI scores in the two clusters were similar with no statistically significant difference at baseline ($P = 0.17$) (Table 3). After the oral health education, the mean PI score was 1.06 ± 0.33 at 6 weeks and 0.85 ± 0.35 at 12 weeks in Leaflet cluster. On the other hand, in E-learning cluster it was 1.31 ± 0.39 and 1.21 ± 0.40 at 6 weeks and 12 weeks, respectively.

Within the cluster comparisons using one way repeated measures ANOVA, a significant improvement of oral health with decreased PI scores in both clusters was observed (Table 3). As for the intercluster comparison using independent samples t-test, Leaflet cluster had significantly lower PI scores than E-learning cluster at 6 weeks ($P < 0.001$) and at 12 weeks ($P < 0.001$) (Table 3).

GI scores

At baseline, the differences in the mean GI scores between Leaflet cluster and E-learning cluster were not statistically significant ($P = 0.12$) (Table 4). After the intervention, the mean GI scores were 0.88 ± 0.25 at 6 weeks and 0.74 ± 0.22 at 12 weeks in children in Leaflet cluster. The mean GI scores in children related to E-learning cluster were 1.17 ± 0.25 at 6 weeks and 1 ± 0.25 at 12 weeks. Comparison between the baseline values (1.76 ± 0.36 in Leaflet cluster versus 1.83 ± 0.34 in E-learning cluster) and their respective post-intervention GI scores, revealed a statistically significant decrease in GI scores in both clusters (Table 4). Also, the independent t-test for intercluster comparison showed that Leaflet cluster had lower GI scores than E-learning cluster, and this difference was statistically significant at 6 weeks ($P < 0.001$) and at 12 weeks ($P < 0.001$) (Table 4).

Due to the educational nature of the intervention, no untoward effects were anticipated nor observed.

Table 3 The intracluster and intercluster comparison of plaque index score between the two clusters

Cluster	PI score Mean ± SD			P value
	Baseline	6 weeks	12 weeks	
Leaflet Cluster	2.25 ± 0.43	1.06 ± 0.33	0.85 ± 0.35	$F = 733.57$; $P < 0.001*$
E-learning Cluster	2.33 ± 0.38	1.31 ± 0.39	1.21 ± 0.40	$F = 427.62$; $P < 0.001*$
Significance	$t = -1.39$; $P = 0.17**$	$t = -4.81$; $P < 0.001**$	$t = -6.82$; $P < 0.001**$	

*Test applied: One way repeated measures ANOVA
**Test applied: Independent samples t-test

Table 4 The intracluster and intercluster comparison of gingival index score between the two clusters

Cluster	GI score Mean ± SD			P value
	Baseline	6 weeks	12 weeks	
Leaflet Cluster	1.76 ± 0.36	0.88 ± 0.25	0.74 ± 0.22	$F = 803.33$; $P < 0.001*$
E-learning Cluster	1.83 ± 0.34	1.17 ± 0.25	1 ± 0.25	$F = 441.12$; $P < 0.001$
Significance	$t = -1.57$; $P = 0.12**$	$t = -8.34$; $P < 0.001**$	$t = -7.92$; $P < 0.001**$	

*Test applied: One way repeated measures ANOVA
**Test applied: Independent samples t-test

Discussion

To our knowledge, this study is the first of its kind to investigate the role of E-learning instructions in improving oral health in children, and to compare it with the traditional educational leaflets in school children in Syria. The results of this school-based educational intervention were found to be effective for short term improvement of oral health knowledge, gingival health and in decreasing plaque levels in primary school children.

The target group for the specific oral health education was the primary school children because of their consumption of large amounts of sugars and soft drinks. Children aged 10–11 years were selected since they can, at this age, do logic thoughts, can realize the cause-result interaction, and explore everything. Younger children possibly would not be able to present those skills [8].

Since the semester in Syrian school lasts for three months, it was necessary to follow up children at 6 weeks and 12 weeks of oral health education. In addition, the amount of time and frequency with which children were exposed to the two different educational tools were similar to previous works [9–12].

Results of the present study suggest that baseline knowledge scores, the mean plaque index and mean gingival index scores in the two clusters were almost similar with no statistical differences, since the children included were in the same age group, similar socioeconomic status and did not receive any previous dental educational program. However, a statistically significant increase in knowledge score was seen in the two clusters after health education programs. This improvement can be attributed to the health messages delivered interactively to children as a short story, in simple language, with colorful images, quizzes as well as videos, so the children could get useful information in an easy and entertaining way. In addition, the study sample expressed a desire to discover the new educational materials provided to them, either through leaflets or E-program. The results of the present study were in accordance with other studies [10, 13–19] aiming at improving knowledge and health behavior. The findings of this study were also consistent with a study that claimed that using educational printed materials and websites had a significantly positive effect on the acquisition of knowledge [20]. In our study, after the educational program, better results in knowledge score were found in Leaflet cluster as compared to E-learning cluster at 6 weeks and 12 weeks. This finding can be attributed to the fact that introduction of web-based educational programs to disseminate health education among school children, is still in its embryonic stage in Syria, where parents and children still depend on textbooks, TV programs, lectures or leaflets as sources of health awareness. The idea of introducing internet-based health education to schools appeared to be a new and unfamiliar approach to children and their parents. Consequently, some children were not computer-literate to gain access to the website, and some children found difficulties in using smart phones to access the entire contents of the website. Moreover, children in E-learning cluster were hampered by the slow connection speeds when using sound, graphics and video files, and other technical problems were also reported. Due to these challenges, this study can be considered as a baseline study in which future work could be undertaken after a period of time to evaluate the development of knowledge in the field of technology and its implementation in improving oral health care. On the other hand, leaflets were able to reach a large segment of school children regardless of the frequency of dental visits, socioeconomic status, possession of computers and internet network at their homes, and other technical problems related to using website as an educational method to disseminate information among school children in Damascus city. These findings were in accordance with previous study [21] which found that leaflets are a cost-effective way to spread awareness about prevention of dental caries. This is particularly true in developing countries where budgetary allocations are restricted and resources to disseminate electronic educational materials are limited and often hindered with technical difficulties. In agreement with our results, previous studies reported that leaflets are good educational method that can raise awareness and deliver health messages to members of the community [22, 23]. In contrast, our findings were different from another study conducted in Germany which found that web-based multimedia program was more effective than traditional print-based self-study by medical students [24].

As for the oral hygiene status, the mean PI and GI scores were significantly lower in both clusters, and this could be attributed to the fact that the use of animated colorful pictures, videos and quizzes in the E-learning program, similarly, the style of short story in simple language and pictorial sketches in the leaflet can help children to understand the concepts of oral health better. Besides emphasizing some immediate gains from good oral hygiene such as fresh breath, clean and white teeth and attractive appearance, were key aspects for motivating these children and creating an interest to modify their behavior. Results of the present study were comparable with many studies [9, 11, 13, 25–27] depicting the impact of school dental health education programs which resulted in significant improvement in oral hygiene of school children after imparting dental health education. Another study found no significant reduction in plaque scores of the children after short-term dental health education program [28].

In comparing the two clusters, highest improvement in oral hygiene status was seen in Leaflet cluster. A reason for notable lack of improvement of oral hygiene in E-learning cluster may be that children in this cluster were hampered by many difficulties that mentioned earlier, and consequently they had not achieved a notable behavior change related oral hygiene. Consistent with our findings, other previous studies found that children in the leaflets group showed positive results reflected on their daily oral health practices compared with other study groups [12, 29]. In accordance with interventions in Iran [11] and Brazil [21], the present results bring to light the importance of educational leaflets in improving oral health status and behavior of school children. This is especially true in countries with a developing oral health care system, where the need is to find a suitable educational program without relying upon costly professional input.

This study provides valuable insight regarding the effectiveness of dental health education among Damascus City's school-aged children. However, there are some limitations. The length of the study was limited to a time frame of 3 months, which may be considered a relatively short period, so the permanence of the impact requires more longitudinal research. Additionally, the present study has been conducted in a small geographic area, and its results will be better validated via multicenter studies. However, the study was conducted at public schools which represent the largest segment of schools in Damascus city, and that will make it more generalizable.

Conclusions

From the results observed, it can be concluded that short term oral health education programs may be useful in improving oral hygiene practices in children. Educational instructional leaflets are appropriate effective economic tools for improving oral and gingival health among Syrian children when compared to E-learning program, and they can be suggested as educational tools in school-based oral health education programs with more fruitful outcomes. How long the benefit will be retained is an important question in all health education programs. Further longitudinal studies to study the retention of knowledge and oral hygiene practices are therefore required and crucial.

Abbreviations

CD: Compact disc; CONSORT: Consolidated Standards of Reporting Trials; DMFT: Decayed missing filled permanent teeth; dmft: Decayed, missing, filled primary teeth; GI: Gingival index; PI: Plaque index; SD: Standard deviation

Acknowledgments

The authors would like to thank Mr. Khaled Omar for his effort to develop and design the E-learning program, Mr. Habib Hanna who assisted in designing this program and Mr. Ammar Alassafeen who designed the educational instructional leaflets. The authors wish to express their gratitude to all the children and staff of the schools who made this project possible.

Funding

The project was funded by Damascus University, Syria which is a public University. The University provided financial support for all printing materials, leaflets, website design, and other IT costs, transportations and data analysis.

Authors' contributions

SAB carried out the clinical examinations, acquired and statistically analyzed data and drafted the manuscript. MD supervised the study, participated in its design, helped in the interpretation of data and revised the paper to its final version. Both authors read and approved the final manuscript.

Competing interests

The authors declare that they have no competing interests.

References

1. Rennie F, Morrison T. E learning and social networking handbook: resources for higher education. 2nd ed. New York: Routledge; 2013.
2. Mishra P, Koehler MJ. Technological pedagogical content knowledge: a framework for teacher knowledge. TCRecord. 2006;108(6):1017–54.
3. Ruiz JG, Mintzer MJ, Leipzig RM. The impact of e-learning in medical education. Acad Med. 2006;81(3):207–12.
4. Piccoli G, Ahmad R, Ives B. Web based virtual learning environments: a research framework and a preliminary assessment of effectiveness in basic it skills training. Mis Quart. 2001;25(4):401–26.
5. Kwan SYL, Petersen PE, Pine CM, Borutta A. Health promoting schools: an opportunity for oral health promotion. Bull World Health Organ. 2005;83(9):677–85.
6. Dashash M, Blinkhorn A. The dental health of 5 year-old children living in Damascus, Syria. Community Dent Health. 2012;29(3):209–13.
7. Löe H. The gingival index, the plaque index and the retention index systems. J Periodontol. 1967;38(Suppl):610–6.
8. Jackson L, Caffarella RS, Caffarella RS. Experiential learning: a new approach. San Fransisco: Jossey-Bass; 1994.
9. Alwayli H, Mosadomi HA, Alhaidri E. The impact of a school based oral hygiene instruction program on the gingival health of middle school children in Riyadh: Saudi Arabia. Saudi J Oral Sci. 2015;2(2):99–102.
10. Ajithkrishnan CG, Thanveer K, Sudheer H, Abhishek S. Impact of oral health education on oral health of 12 and 15 year old schoolchildren of Vadodara city, Gujarat state. J Int Oral Health. 2010;2(3):15–20.
11. Yazdani R, Vehkalahti MM, Nouri M, Murtomaa H. School-based education to improve oral cleanliness and gingival health in adolescents in Tehran, Iran. Int J Paediatr Dent. 2009;19(4):274–81.
12. Saied-Moallemi Z, Virtanen JI, Vehkalahti MM, Tehranchi A, Murtomaa H. School-based intervention to promote preadolescents'gingival health: a community trial. Community Dent Oral Epidemiol. 2009;37(6):518–26.
13. Hebbal M, Ankola AV, Vadavi D, Patel K. Evaluation of knowledge and plaque scores in school children before and after health education. Dent Res J. 2011;8(4):189–96.
14. Sanadhya YK, Thakkar JP, Divakar DD, Pareek S, Rathore K, Yousuf A, et al. Effectiveness of oral health education on knowledge, attitude, practices and oral hygiene status among 12-15 year old schoolchildren of fishermen of Kutch district, Gujarat, India. Int Marit Health. 2014;65(3):99–105.
15. Conrado CA, Maciel SM, Oliveira MR. A school based oral health educational program: the experience of Maringa-PR, Brazil. J Appl Oral Sci. 2004;12(1):27–33.
16. Angelopoulou MV, Kavvadia K, Taoufik K, Oulis CJ. Comparative clinical study testing the effectiveness of school based oral health education using experiential learning or traditional lecturing in 10 year-old children. BMC Oral Health. 2015; https://doi.org/10.1186/s12903-015-0036-4.
17. Nakre PD, Harikiran AG. Effectiveness of oral health education programs: a systematic review. J Int Soc Prev Communit Dent. 2013;3(2):103–15.
18. Worthington HV, Hill KB, Mooney J, Hamilton FA, Blinkhorn AS. A cluster randomized controlled trial of a dental health education program for 10-year-old children. J Public Health Dent. 2001;61(1):22–7.
19. Gauba A, Bal IS, Jain A, Mittal HC. School based oral health promotional intervention: effect on knowledge, practices and clinical oral health related parameters. Contemp Clin Dent. 2013; https://doi.org/10.4103/0976-237X.123056.
20. Rezvani E, Ketabi S. On the effectiveness of using web and print based materials in teaching grammar to Iranian EFL learners. Procedia Soc Behav Sci. 2011;15:376–81.
21. Azevedo MS, Romano AR, Correa MB, Santos I, Dos DS, Cenci MS. Evaluation of a feasible educational intervention in preventing early childhood caries. Braz Oral Res. 2015;29(1):1–8.
22. Bester N, Di Vito SM, McGarry T, Riffkin M, Kaehler S, Pilot R, et al. The effectiveness of an educational brochure as a risk minimization activity to communicate important rare adverse events to health care professionals. Adv Ther. 2016;33(2):167–77.
23. Wao H, Aluoch M, Wright J, Rodriguez C. Using brochures as educational tools to promote routine HIV testing in youth. Austin J pediatr. 2014;1(2):7.
24. Grundman JA, Wigton RS, Nickol D. A controlled trial of an interactive, web-based virtual reality program for teaching physical diagnosis skills to medical students. Acad Med. 2000;75(Suppl 10):47-9.
25. Haque SE, Rahman M, Itsuko K, Mutahara M, Kayako S, Tsutsumi A, et al. Effect of a school-based oral health education in preventing untreated dental caries and increasing knowledge, attitude, and practices among adolescents in Bangladesh. BMC Oral Health. 2016; https://doi.org/10.1186/s12903-016-0202-3.
26. Shenoy RP, Sequeira PS. Effectiveness of a school dental education program in improving oral health knowledge and oral hygiene practices and status of 12 to 13 year old school children. Indian J Dent Res. 2010;21(2):253–9.
27. D' Cruz AM, Aradhya S. Impact of oral health education on oral hygiene knowledge, practices, plaque control and gingival health of 13 to 15 year old school children in Bangalore city. Int J Dent Hyg. 2013;11(2):126–33.
28. Biesbrock AR, Walters PA, Bartizek RD. Short term impact of a national dental education program on children's oral health and knowledge. J Clin Pediatr Dent. 2004;15(4):93–7.
29. Redmond CA, Hamilton FA, Kay EJ, Worthington HV, Blinkhorn AS. An investigation into the value and relevance of oral health promotion leaflets for young adolescents. Int Dent J. 2001;51(3):164–8.

11

Association of mastication and factors affecting masticatory function with obesity in adults

Akio Tada[1*] and Hiroko Miura[2]

Abstract

Background: A substantial number of adults suffer from obesity, that is caused by the risk factor, masticatory dysfunction. The association between mastication and obesity, however, is inconclusive. This systematic review aims to provide literature regarding the association between mastication and factors affecting masticatory function, and obesity in adults.

Methods: Four electronic databases (PubMed, EMBASE, Cochrane Library, and Web of Science) were used to search for publications that met the following criteria: published between 2007 and 2016, written in English, and assessed the associations between mastication and obesity among the population aged ≥18 years. The included publications were analyzed based on the study design, main conclusions, and strength of evidence identified by the two authors who screened all the abstracts and full-text articles and, abstracted data, and performed quality assessments by using a critical appraisal tool, the Critical Appraisal Skills Programme Cohort Studies Checklists.

Results: A total of 18 articles (16 cross-sectional, 1 cohort studies, and 1 randomized controlled trial [RCT]) met our inclusion criteria and were evaluated. Poorer mastication was associated with obesity in 12 out of 16 cross-sectional studies. One cohort study showed that the obesity group displayed higher tooth loss than the normal weight group. One RCT demonstrated that gum-chewing intervention for 8 weeks significantly decreased waist circumference.

Conclusions: Most studies revealed a positive association between mastication and obesity among adults. Nonetheless, most of them are cross-sectional studies, which are insufficient to demonstrate a causal relation. Further advancement requires RCT, especially an intervention of improvement of mastication and obesity needed to confirm this association.

Keywords: Mastication, Obesity, Overweight, Adults

Background

Globally, the prevalence of obesity has increased and is expected to reach around 20% by 2025 if trends in the mean body mass index (BMI), which characterizes its population distribution continue [1]. Obesity causes various health issues. In obese individuals, there is an increased risk of developing type 2 diabetes [2], dyslipidemia [2], hypertension [2], cardiovascular disease [3], fatty liver disease [4], certain types of cancer [5], dementia [6], obstructive sleep apnea [7] and so on. Increases in being overweight and obese reduced life expectancy by 5–13 years [8], increases health care expenditures by 50–200% [9], and dramatically alters quality of life [10]. Increased obesity is a big concern for a person's medical care and health.

Obesity and being overweight are caused by an energy imbalance between calories consumed and expended [11]. An increased intake of high calorie foods and decreased physical activity due to the increasingly sedentary occupation, and development of transportation are major factors causing energy imbalance. Furthermore, recent obesity has been associated with various factors such as sleeping and smoking [12].

In the last couple of decades, the association between obesity and masticatory function has been noticed, because masticatory function affects nutritional intake [13, 14]. Masticatory function means the objective capacity of a

* Correspondence: atada@hyogo-dai.ac.jp
[1]Department of Health Science, Hyogo University, 2301 Shinzaike Hiraoka-cho, Kakogawa, Hyogo 675-0195, Japan
Full list of author information is available at the end of the article

person to tear solid food into pieces or the subjective response of a person to questions concerning chewing food [15]. Objective masticatory function is defined as masticatory performance, which assesses the particle size distribution of food when chewed for a given number of strokes [16] and therefore its impact on obesity is of great concern. However, due to difficulty and variety of objective measurements for mastication, little information is available on the association between masticatory function and obesity. Objective masticatory function has been strongly associated with factors such as the number of remaining teeth, number of missing teeth, and use of prostheses [17–23]. These factors affecting masticatory function have been studied on the association with obesity. Taking this situation into consideration, to review studies for associations both between objective masticatory function and obesity and between factors affecting masticatory function (FAM) and obesity is considered to provide more extensive assessment for the impact of mastication on obesity.

No systematic review article has been published that conducts an overview of a wide range of literature describing this association. Further progression of studies in this field requires an overview of the literature.

In this review article, we provide a literature overview on the association of obesity with objective masticatory function and FAM.

Methods
Literature search
The investigation was conducted by searching four electronic databases (PubMed, EMBASE, Cochrane Library, and Web of Science), using the following terms: ("chewing" OR "number of teeth" AND "obesity"), ("mastication" OR "number of teeth" AND "obesity") and ("masticatory performance" AND "obesity"). Two authors (AT and HM) independently assessed each retrieved document for eligibility by examining the titles and abstracts, based on the inclusion and exclusion criteria shown in Table 1. Since subjective masticatory function includes adaptive and psychological factors, the range of mastication was limited to objective masticatory function. We defined the FAM as dentition and salivary flow rate, which follows the criteria written in a review article previously reported [15].

Table 1 Inclusion and exclusion criteria used in this review

	Inclusion criteria	Exclusion criteria
Sample	Subjects aged 18 years or older,	Subjects who received oral and maxillofacial surgery or, radiotherapy Subjects who have systemic illness
Language	Written in English	Not written in English
Analysis	Any association between mastication and obesity	Descriptive studies, review, or studies with no analyses investigating the association between mastication and obesity

Epidemiological studies that investigated the association between mastication and obesity in adults published between 2007 and 2016 were included. Additional inclusion criteria were (1) studies in adult subjects (age ≥ 18 years); (2) studies written in English. The papers were excluded from the systematic review if (1) studies that were conducted in subjects who received oral and maxillofacial surgery or radio therapy; (2) studies that were conducted in people with systemic illness; (3) descriptive studies, review, or studies with no analyses investigating the association between mastication and obesity.

Quality assessments
The Critical Appraisal Skills Programme Cohort Studies Checklists [24] was used for quality assessment. The checklist for cohort studies was modified for application to cross-sectional studies (e.g. Question 2, "Was the cohort recruited in an acceptable way?" was modified to "Was the sample recruited in an acceptable way?", and questions regarding follow-up of participants were excluded). For each study, the strength and weaknesses were calculated based on the relevant checklist items and a grade of "low", "moderate," or "high" was assigned with the two authors' (AT and HM) approval.

Data extraction
Two authors extracted information independently, and disagreements were resolved by consensus. The following data were extracted from each eligible study: first author, year of publication, country where the study conducted, study type, study period, number of cases, confounding factors, and both adjusted odds rate (95% CI).

Results
Literature searches and study characteristics
Our initial search identified a total of 634 publications, as shown in flow chart (fig. 1). After removal of duplication and title and abstract screening, 46 articles were selected for full-text screening. The full-text articles of the 46 potentially relevant references were reviewed, 28 of which did not fit the inclusion criteria and were consequently excluded. Finally, 18 publications (16 cross-sectional studies, 1 cohort studies, and 1 randomized controlled trial [RCT]) were selected as the "key articles", that would subsequently be scrutinized for the study design.

Of the 18 included studies, except the RCT, 7 studies evaluated masticatory function (masticatory performance) [25–31], 10 factors affecting masticatory function (the number of teeth, number of missing teeth, use of prostheses, chewing-gum-stimulated saliva flow) [32–41]. In this article, we systematically review the published findings on the associations of obesity with masticatory function and FAM.

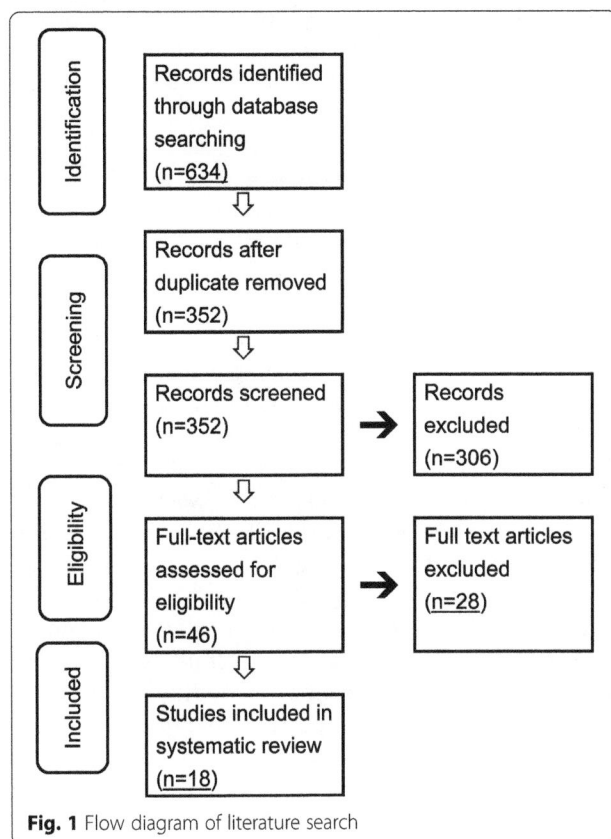

Fig. 1 Flow diagram of literature search

With regard to obese and overweight criteria, 16 studies measured BMI, 8 waist circumference (WC) and 5 waist-to-hip ratio (WHR).

Quality of studies

Additional file 1: Table S1 presents the results of the critical appraisal assessment. Recurrent strengths of the evidence included the following: (1) addressing a clearly focused issue ($n = 18$; 100%); (2) recruiting subjects in an acceptable manner (cross-sectional $n = 14$ [87.5%], cohort $n = 1$ [100%], and RCT n = 1; [100%]); (3) measuring exposure to minimize bias (cross-sectional $n = 15$ [93.8%], cohort $n = 1$ [100%], and RCT $n = 1$; [100%]), and (4) measuring outcome to minimize bias ($n = 18$; 100%).

The most common issue for critical appraisal that was observed across studies was not adjusting all potential confounding factors. Only three studies adequately adjusted their analyses for all the potential confounders, such as the socio-demographic and, socioeconomic factors, and health habits including physical activity for obesity [32, 33, 41].

Overall, the quality of the included articles were "High" (4 studies: 2 cross-sectional, 1 cohort, and 1 RCT) to "Moderate" (11 cross-sectional) with only 3 studies judged

as being "Low" (2 cross-sectional studies for masticatory function, 1 cross-sectional study for FAM).

Impact of mastication on obesity

Additional file 1: Table S2 describes the findings regarding the association between mastication and obesity from the studies.

Cross-sectional studies for masticatory function

Seven cross-sectional studies investigated the association between masticatory function and obesity [25–31]. All studies used BMI as an obesity indicator. Three studies demonstrated that participants with lower masticatory function had significantly higher BMI [25, 27, 30]. One study showed that the obese group exhibited worse masticatory function than other anthropometric groups in men but not in women [28]. However, three showed no association [26, 29, 31].

Cross-sectional studies for FAMs

Nine studies analyzed the associations between FAM and obesity [32–40]. The findings from five of these studies showed a significant association between the number of teeth / missing teeth and BMI [32, 36, 37, 39, 40]. One study showed no association between the number of teeth and BMI [33]. Five studies showing higher number of teeth had lower WC/WHP [32, 33, 35, 36, 38]. One study examined the associations between the masticatory ability evaluated using a chewing-gum-stimulated salivary flow rate and anthropometric indices [34].

Longitudinal studies for masticatory function and FAM

One cohort study and one RCT showing the relationship between mastication and obesity were found. One prospective cohort study showed that tooth loss was higher among men and women with the third tertile of WHR (Men: IRR = 1.37, 95% CI = 1.04 to 1.80; Women: IRR = 1.53, 95% CI = 1.14 to 2.05) [41]. It is discussed that periodontal disease is involved in the association between tooth loss and obesity. One RCT showed that an intervention of gum-chewing and printed nutrition information for 8 weeks significantly decreased the WC [42]. However, the control group which received only printed nutrition information presented a little decrease in WC. A significant effect might not be obtained only by gum-chewing.

Discussion

Quality assessment of the studies

One important finding of this review is the use of objective indicators for mastication and obesity in almost all studies. One study used the self-reported number of missing teeth [36]. Since subjective measurements yield much more optimistic results than practitioner's measurements do [43], there is a possibility that self-reported number attenuated the accuracy of the data.

Cut-off values of the number of teeth for categorization were differential and likely depend on ethnicity, with ≥20/21 versus < 20/21 for European [32, 40] and ≥ 8/10 versus < 8/10 for Brazilian people [36, 39]. This difference may be due to the consideration of the level of oral health in each country. Since the number of teeth does not have any international standard like BMI (25 for overweight, 30 for obese) [44], its cut-off values in key articles differ widely among studies. Therefore, an international standard to categorize oral health with regard to the number of teeth will be beneficial for oral epidemiological studies.

With regard to masticatory function, five key articles used particle size [26–29, 31], and one chewing mixing method [25]. Other than these methods, masticatory function assessments generally used questionnaires, kinematics, and video recording, as indirect methods, and chewing activity, and maximum bite force, as direct methods. These different methods make comparison of the masticatory function levels among studies difficult.

Cut-off values of BMI used in key articles were ≥ 25 [25, 39], ≥25 and ≥ 30 [40] and ≥ 30 [33, 37], which follow the WHO standards [44]. Studies conducted in the Japanese population used ≥25 as the cutoff value, based on the criteria established by the Japan Society for obesity [45]. In general, a smaller percentage of Japanese have a BMI of ≥30. Careful attention is necessary when comparing the associations between Japanese people and other ethnic population. Cut-off values of WC used were > 102 cm for men and > 88 cm for women [33, 36], > 94 cm for men and > 80 cm for women [35, 38], and > 88 cm for both [32]. Although WC is influenced by ethnicity, four articles investigated Brazilians. Although detailed information on ethnicity in these studies are not available, double standards in one country may affect the outcome.

The majority of obesity cases are thought to be explained by a combination of excessive food energy intake and lack of physical activity [46]. Furthermore, other possible factors have been identified to contribute to the recent increase of obesity [12]. Although socio-demographic factors were used in 12 of the 17 studies, lifestyle variables, including physical activity were employed in only six studies. Energy intake was adjusted for by only one key article probably due to the need for professional staff during evaluation. Moreover, five key articles did not adjust for confounding factors [26, 28–30, 37]. The lack of adjustment of these factors would possibly lead to overestimation or underestimation of the relationship between mastication and obesity.

Relationship between mastication and obesity

The association between tooth loss/ edenturism and obesity was reviewed previously [47]. Our study has a strength to review studies concerning association between masticatory function and obesity in addition to that between tooth loss/ edenturism and obesity. Most key articles in our studies evaluating the number of teeth and obesity showed significant association. This result is consistent with observation in Nascimento's systematic review [47]. However, four out of eight studies failed to observe the association between masticatory function and obesity [26, 28, 29, 31]. These studies investigated participants aged ≤40 yrs. Almost all studies including participants aged ≥50 showed significant associations between masticatory function or factors affecting masticatory function and obesity. The influence of mastication on obesity may not be significant in younger population because they have higher physical activity and basal metabolic than older population do. However, there is one study that failed to find this association in older people [48]. Furthermore, since the significant association disappeared by stringent adjustments in some key articles, the significance of association might not be necessarily great.

One prospective cohort study revealed that obese group had higher tooth loss than normal group does [41], suggesting that obesity causes tooth loss. However, another causal relationship showing that decreased mastication causes obesity should be investigated. Prospective cohort studies that observe and compare changes in the body weight among participants with differential masticatory function are necessary. Although RCT is necessary to reveal causal relationship, only one has been available in this association. More intervention studies should be conducted to verify the impact of mastication on obesity. Especially, intervention studies that examine the body weight changes in participants who are provided prosthetics and experience restoration of mastication will provide beneficial information to determine the causal relationship between obesity and chewing status.

Of the three key articles that measured both BMI and WC, two found higher odds ratio for the associations between the number of teeth and WC than those with BMI [33, 36], but one displayed similar odds ratio for both [32]. The participants of the former were Brazilian and those of the latter were Germans. The difference might be explained by ethnicity, but it needs more studies conducted in differential ethnic. Since abdominal obesity is related to metabolic syndrome [49], further research regarding relationship between mastication and obesity (general and abdominal obesity) is of great concern.

There are two possible reasons which explain the association between mastication and obesity (fig. 2). One is that people with poor masticatory function tend to have smaller consumption of vegetable and fruit, and higher consumption of high energy food than those with adequate mastication [50–53], which causes obesity. Another is that less chewing leads to obesity-causing-phenomena (decrease in diet induced thermogenesis and inactivation of neuronal histamine) [54–56]. Small number of chewing strokes decreases the effect of chewing to prevent obesity. Diet with soft food due to decreased masticatory ability decrease the number of chewing cycle. Other than that, quickly eating, although being a problem of eating behavior, decreases number of chewing cycle. Several cross-sectional studies [57–59] showed that people who tend to eat quickly have increased BMI than those who ate slowly. Yamane et al. demonstrated this association in a longitudinal prospective study [60]. One cohort study showed that the lowest group in the number of chewing cycles during meals had a significantly higher rate of incremental increases in body weight than the highest group [61]. Moreover, this association was reviewed in a systematic review [62]. Robinson argued that a slower eating rate was associated with lower energy intake in comparison to a faster eating rate in a systematic review [63]. These studies support that lower number of chewing cycle is associated with obesity. On the other hand, there were reports showing that chewing rate and eating behavior did not differ between people with high and normal BMI [64, 65]. A study reported that anthropometric status affect energy intake after chewing, which makes association between mastication and obesity complex [66].

Findings of key articles is considered to be responsible for these mechanisms. The former mechanism is assumed to give considerable influence on the studies in this review with subjects of older adults.

Association among obesity, mastication and periodontal disease

Periodontal disease is an essential factor for considering the association between mastication and obesity because it is strongly linked to mastication and obesity. Obesity is considered one of the factors that cause incidence and progression of periodontal disease [67]. Proinflammatory adipocytokines such as TNF-α, which is produced, primarily in the abdominal adipose tissue, induces the breakdown of alveolar bones, in turn periodontal tissue degradation [68, 69]. Periodontal disease is one of the major causes of tooth loss because it destroys the tissue supporting the teeth, which deteriorate masticatory function. Most elderly people with decreased mastication are considered to have periodontitis. The key articles observed a significant association between masticatory function and obesity in younger populations in which severe periodontal disease are supposed to be less prevalent, suggesting that mastication influenced obesity independent of the presence of periodontal disease [25, 27]. Given that decreased mastication increases obesity, the following vicious circle is hypothesized in elderly people (Fig. 3). Obesity causes periodontal disease progression, subsequently, in turn, leading to deterioration of mastication caused by tooth loss. Furthermore, decreased mastication progresses obesity. Moreover, it is guessed that the association between periodontitis and obesity is bidirectional [70–72]. Endotoxin from Gram negative bacilli have been reported to be responsible for body weight gain and diabetes [73] which suggests the possibility of induction of obesity by endotoxin of periodontal pathogens. There may be complicated cascades among mastication, periodontal disease and obesity. In a study by Meisel et al., inflammatory materials are discussed to mediate the association between tooth loss and obesity [41]. Analysis of the influence of oral health on obesity will need approaches from both mastication perspective and periodontal perspective.

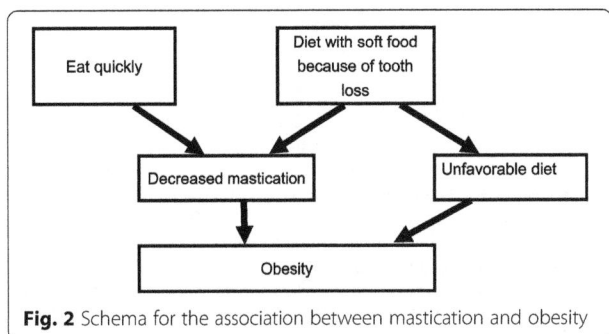

Fig. 2 Schema for the association between mastication and obesity

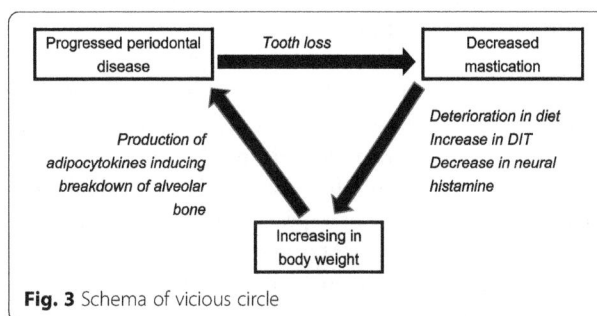

Fig. 3 Schema of vicious circle

Limitation

There are several limitations in this study. First, only a small number of intervention and cohort studies were found. These longitudinal studies, particularly intervention study, are necessary to analyze the causal relationships. Second, less than half studies used the masticatory function as indicator of mastication. Although a low number of natural teeth has been reported to be associated with a poor chewing function [74, 75], it does not necessarily show a close relation with mastication [76]. This can be explained by the fact that chewing efficiency differs depending on the location of the missing teeth among individuals with the same number of teeth. Third, although obesity is strongly related to physical activity and energy intake, more than half of studies did not adjust these factors in calculating the odds ratio for the association between mastication and obesity, or did not even do adjustment any factors. This insufficient adjustment prevents accurate assessment of the association. Finally, many studies were conducted in Japan or Brazil, preventing generalization of the results. Therefore, since mastication is influenced by the dietary culture, integrated evaluation of results from various areas is necessary.

Future direction

More intervention studies are necessary to elucidate the association between mastication and obesity. In particular, prospective cohort and intervention studies are necessary to analyze if decreased mastication leads to obesity and investigate if provision of prosthesis will work to improve obesity, respectively.

Cross sectional and cohort studies revealing the association between mastication and obesity should be analyzed by adjusting the energy intake and physical activity. Studies regarding the relationship between mastication and dietary/nutrient intake have been published [14, 77–79]. Adding obesity measurement in these investigations would be possible.

Since mastication is the process of crushing and grounding the food using the teeth, it should be evaluated using functional parameters such as masticatory function rather than the number of anatomically present teeth. The measurement of mastication function is desirable to be easy and reliable. Moreover, a unified assessment method should be used to compare these studies. Chewing gum mixing method has made mastication assessment easy and made the evaluation of large-scale participants in a short period of time [80, 81] and its reliability and validity of the color scale to evaluate the chewing ability have been previously reported [82]. It may be used more frequently to evaluate the mastication in large-scale studies to elucidate the impact of mastication on obesity in the future.

In elderly people, progression of periodontal disease facilitates decreased masticatory function, which in turn, increases obesity. Moreover, periodontopathogens have been suggested to induce obesity. Regression models and meditation analysis should be used to elucidate the association among mastication, periodontal disease and obesity.

Conclusion

Most cross-sectional studies show that poor mastication was associated with obesity. Two prospective cohort studies and RCT demonstrated that poorer mastication is one of the risk factor of obesity. These studies suggest that mastication may have close relationship with obesity. Further research, especially involving intervention studies are required to improve our current understanding of the relationship of mastication and obesity.

Acknowledgements

We would like to thank Editage (www.editage.jp) for English language editing.

Funding

This study was supported by Health and Labour Sciences Research Grants, Research on Regional Medicine.

Authors' contributions

Authors AT, and HM contributed to the conception, design of the study, acquisition of data, interpretation of data, and manuscript revisions. Both authors read and approved the final manuscript.

Competing interests

The authors declare that they have no competing interests.

Author details

[1]Department of Health Science, Hyogo University, 2301 Shinzaike Hiraoka-cho, Kakogawa, Hyogo 675-0195, Japan. [2]Department of International Health and Collaboration, National Institute of Public Health, 2-3-6, Minami, Wako, Saitama 351-0197, Japan.

References

1. NCD Risk Factor Collaboration (NCD-RisC). Trends in adult body-mass index in 200 countries from 1975 to 2014: a pooled analysis of 1698 population-based measurement studies with 19·2 million participants. Lancet. 2016; 387(10026):1377–96. https://doi.org/10.1016/S0140-6736(16)30054-X. Review
2. Haslam DW, James WP. Obesity. Lancet. 2005;366:1197–209. Review
3. Global Burden of Metabolic Risk Factors for Chronic Diseases Collaboration (BMI Mediated Effects), Lu Y, Hajifathalian K, Ezzati M, Woodward M, Rimm EB, Danaei G. Metabolic mediators of the effects of body-mass index, overweight, and obesity on coronary heart disease and stroke: a pooled analysis of 97 prospective cohorts with 1·8 million participants. Lancet. 2014; 383(9921):970–83. https://doi.org/10.1016/S0140-6736(13)61836-X. Epub 2013 Nov 22

4. Dibaise JK, Foxx-Orenstein AE. Role of the gastroenterologist in managing obesity. Expert Rev Gastroenterol Hepatol. 2013;7:439–51. https://doi.org/10.1586/17474124.2013.811061. Review.

5. Basen-Engquist K, Chang M. Obesity and cancer risk: recent review and evidence. Curr Oncol Rep. 2011;13:71–6. Review

6. Beydoun MA, Beydoun HA, Wang Y. Obesity and central obesity as risk factors for incident dementia and its subtypes: a systematic review and meta-analysis. Obes Rev. 2008;9:204–18. https://doi.org/10.1111/j.1467-789X.2008.00473.x. Epub 2008 Mar 6. Erratum in: Obes Rev. 2008 May;9(3):267.

7. Poulain M, Doucet M, Major GC, Drapeau V, Sériès F, Boulet LP, et al. The effect of obesity on chronic respiratory diseases: pathophysiology and therapeutic strategies. CMAJ. 2006;174:1293–9. Review

8. Peeters A, Barendregt JJ, Willekens F, Mackenbach JP, Al Mamun A, Bonneux L. Obesity in adulthood and its consequences for life expectancy: a life-table analysis. Ann Intern Med. 2003;138:24–32.

9. Andreyeva T, Sturm R, Ringel JS. Moderate and severe obesity have large differences in health care costs. Obes Res. 2004;12:1936–43.

10. Jia H, Lubetkin EI. The impact of obesity on health-related quality-of-life in the general adult US population. J Public Health. 2005;27:156–64.

11. World Health Organization. Obesity and overweight. Fact sheet Updated June 2016. http://www.who.int/mediacentre/factsheets/fs311/en/.

12. Keith SW, Redden DT, Katzmarzyk PT, Boggiano MM, Hanlon EC, Benca RM, et al. Putative contributors to the secular increase in obesity: exploring the roads less traveled. Int J Obes. 2006;30:1585–94. Epub 2006. Review

13. Moynihan P, Bradbury J. Compromised dental function and nutrition. Nutrition. 2001 Feb;17(2):177–8.

14. Krall E, Hayes C, Garcia R. How dentition status and masticatory function affect nutrient intake. J Am Dent Assoc. 1998 Sep;129(9):1261–9.

15. van der Bilt A. Assessment of mastication with implications for oral rehabilitation: a review. J Oral Rehabil. 2011 Oct;38(10):754–80. https://doi.org/10.1111/j.1365-2842.2010.02197.x. Epub 2011 Jan 17. Review.

16. Bates JF, Stafford GD, Harruson A. Masticatory function-a review of the literature III. Masticatory performance and efficiency. J Oral Rehabil. 1976;3:57–67.

17. Iguchi H, Magara J, Nakamura Y, Tsujimura T, Ito K, Inoue M. Changes in jaw muscle activity and the physical properties of foods with different textures during chewing behaviors. Physiol Behav. 2015 Dec 1;152(Pt A):217–24. https://doi.org/10.1016/j.physbeh.2015.10.004. Epub 2015 Oct 9.

18. Hatch JP, Shinkai RS, Sakai S, Rugh JD, Paunovich ED. Determinants of masticatory performance in dentate adults. Arch Oral Biol. 2001;46:641–8.

19. Yamashita S, Sakai S, Hatch JP, Rugh JD. Relationship between oral function and occlusal support in denture wearers. J Oral Rehabil. 2000;27:881–6.

20. Miura H, Araki Y, Umenai T. Chewing activity and activities of daily living in the elderly. J Oral Rehabil. 1997;24:457–60.

21. Tsuga K, Carlsson GE, Osterberg T, Karlsson S. Self-assessed masticatory ability in relation to maximal bite force and dental state in 80-year-old subjects. J Oral Rehabil. 1998;25:117–24.

22. Wayler AH, Muench ME, Kapur KK, Chauncey HH. Masticatory performance and food acceptability in persons with removable partial dentures, full dentures and intact natural dentition. J Gerontol. 1984;39:284–9.

23. Witter DJ, Cramwinckel AB, van Rossum GM, Käyser AF. Shortened dental arches and masticatory ability. J Dent. 1990;18:185–9. Review

24. Critical Appraisal Skills Programme (CASP) 2014; CASP Checklists. Oxford.

25. Katagiri S, Nitta H, Nagasawa T, Izumi Y, Kanazawa M, Matsuo A, et al. Reduced masticatory function in non-elderly obese Japanese adults. Obes Res Clin Pract. 2011;5:e267–360. https://doi.org/10.1016/j.orcp.2011.03.005.

26. Flores-Orozco EI, Tiznado-Orozco GE, Osuna-González OD, Amaro-Navarrete CL, Rovira-Lastra B, Martinez-Gomis J. Lack of relationship between masticatory performance and nutritional status in adults with natural dentition. Arch Oral Biol. 2016;71:117–21. https://doi.org/10.1016/j.archoralbio.2016.07.008.

27. Sánchez-Ayala A, Campanha NH, Garcia RC. Relationship between body fat and masticatory function. J Prosthodont. 2013;22:120–5. https://doi.org/10.1111/j.1532-849X.2012.00937.x.

28. Isabel CA, Moysés MR, van der Bilt A, Gameiro GH, Ribeiro JC, Pereira LJ. The relationship between masticatory and swallowing behaviors and body weight. Physiol Behav. 2015;151:314–9. https://doi.org/10.1016/j.physbeh.2015.08.006.

29. Frecka JM, Hollis JH, Mattes RD. Effects of appetite, BMI, food form and flavor on mastication: almonds as a test food. Eur J Clin Nutr. 2008;62:1231–48. Epub 2007 Jul 18

30. Zijlstra N, Bukman AJ, Mars M, Stafleu A, Ruijschop RM, de Graaf C. Eating behaviour and retro-nasal aroma release in normal-weight and overweight adults: a pilot study. Br J Nutr. 2011;106:297–306. https://doi.org/10.1017/S0007114511000146.

31. Carvalho PM, Castelo PM, Carpenter GH, Gavião MB. Masticatory function, taste, and salivary flow in young healthy adults. J Oral Sci. 2016;58(3):391–9. https://doi.org/10.2334/josnusd.16-0135.

32. Östberg AL, Bengtsson C, Lissner L, Hakeberg M. Oral health and obesity indicators. BMC Oral Health. 2012;20:12–50. https://doi.org/10.1186/1472-6831-12-50.

33. Singh A, Peres MA, Peres KG, Bernardo Cde O, Xavier A, D'Orsi E. Gender differences in the association between tooth loss and obesity among older adults in Brazil. Rev Saude Publica. 2015;49:44. https://doi.org/10.1590/S0034-8910.2015049005590.

34. Maruyama K, Nishioka S, Miyoshi N, Higuchi K, Mori H, Tanno S, et al. The impact of masticatory ability as evaluated by salivary flow rates on obesity in Japanese: The toon health study. Obesity (Silver Spring). 2015;23:1296–302. https://doi.org/10.1002/oby.21071.

35. Peruchi CT, Poli-Frederico RC, Cardelli AA, Fracasso ML, Bispo CG, Neves-Souza RD, Cardoso JR, Maciel SM. Association between oral health status and central obesity among Brazilian independent-living elderly. Braz Oral Res. 2016;30:e116. https://doi.org/10.1590/1807-3107BOR-2016.vol30.0116.

36. Bernardo Cde O, Boing AF, Vasconcelos Fde A, Peres KG, Peres MA. Association between tooth loss and obesity in Brazilian adults: a population-based study. Rev Saude Publica. 2012;46:834–42.

37. Prpić J, Kuis D, Pezelj-Ribarić S. Obesity and oral health–is there an association? Coll Antropol. 2012;36:755–9.

38. De Marchi RJ, Hugo FN, Hilgert JB, Padilha DM. Association between number of teeth, edentulism and use of dentures with percentage body fat in south Brazilian community-dwelling older people. Gerodontology. 2012;29:e69–76. https://doi.org/10.1111/j.1741-2358.2010.00411.x.

39. Hilgert JB, Hugo FN, de Sousa Mda L, Bozzetti MC. Oral status and its association with obesity in southern Brazilian older people. Gerodontology. 2009;26:46–52.

40. Sheiham A, Steele JG, Marcenes W, Finch S, Walls AW. The relationship between oral health status and Body Mass Index among older people: a national survey of older people in Great Britain. Br Dent J. 2002;192:703–6.

41. Meisel P, Holtfreter B, Völzke H, Kocher T. Sex differences of tooth loss and obesity on systemic markers of inflammation. J Dent Res. 2014;93:774–9. https://doi.org/10.1177/0022034514535604.

42. Shikany JM, Thomas AS, McCubrey RO, Beasley TM, Allison DB. Randomized controlled trial of chewing gum for weight loss. Obesity (Silver Spring). 2012; 20:547–52. https://doi.org/10.1038/oby.2011.336.

43. Slagter AP, Olthoff LW, Bosman F, Steen WH. Masticatory ability, denture quality, and oral conditions in edentulous subjects. J Prosthet Dent. 1992;68:299–307.

44. WHO. Preventing and managing the global epidemic. Report of the WHO consultation on obesity. Geneva: WHO; 1997.

45. Examination Committee of Criteria for 'Obesity Disease' in Japan; Japan Society for the Study of Obesity. New criteria for 'obesity disease' in Japan. Circ J. 2002;66:987–92.

46. Lau DC, Douketis JD, Morrison KM, Hramiak IM, Sharma AM, Ur E. Obesity Canada clinical practice guidelines expert panel. 2006 Canadian clinical practice guidelines on the management and prevention of obesity in adults and children [summary]. CMAJ. 2007;176:S1–13. Review

47. Nascimento GG, Leite FR, Conceição DA, Ferrúa CP, Singh A, Demarco FF. Is there a relationship between obesity and tooth loss and edentulism? A systematic review and meta-analysis. Obes Rev. 2016;17(7):587–98. https://doi.org/10.1111/obr.12418. Epub 2016 Apr 29. Review.

48. Ikebe K, Matsuda K, Morii K, Nokubi T, Ettinger RL. The relationship between oral function and body mass index among independently living older Japanese people. Int J Prosthodont. 2006;19(6):539–46.

49. Després JP, Lemieux I. Abdominal obesity and metabolic syndrome. Nature. 2006;444:881–7. Review

50. Tada A, Miura H. Systematic review of the association of mastication with food and nutrient intake in the independent elderly. Arch Gerontol Geriatr. 2014;59:497–505.

51. Tsai AC, Chang TL. Association of dental prosthetic condition with food consumption and the risk of malnutrition and follow-up 4-year mortality risk in elderly Taiwanese. J Nutr Health Aging. 2011;15:265–70.

52. Yoshida M, Kikutani T, Yoshikawa M, Tsuga K, Kimura M, Akagawa Y. Correlation between dental and nutritional status in community-dwelling elderly Japanese. Geriatr Gerontol Int. 2011;11:315–9.

53. Lee JS, Weyant RJ, Corby P, Kritchevsky SB, Harris TB, Rooks R, et al. Edentulism and nutritional status in a biracial sample of well-functioning, community-dwelling elderly: the health, aging, and body composition study. Am J Clin Nutr. 2004;79:295–302.

54. Hamada Y, Kashima H, Hayashi N. The number of chews and meal duration affect diet-induced thermogenesis and splanchnic circulation. Obesity (Silver Spring). 2014;22:E62–9. https://doi.org/10.1002/oby.20715.

55. Morton GJ, Cummings DE, Baskin DG, Barsh GS, Schwartz MW. Central nervous system control of food intake and body weight. Nature. 2006;443: 289–95. Review

56. Sakata T, Yoshimatsu H, Kurokawa M. Hypothalamic neuronal histamine: implications of its homeostatic control of energy metabolism. Nutrition. 1997;13:403–11.

57. Sasaki S, Katagiri A, Tsuji T, Shimoda T, Amano K. Self-reported rate of eating correlates with body mass index in 18-y-old Japanese women. Int J Obes Relat Metab Disord. 2003;27:1405–10.

58. Otsuka R, Tamakoshi K, Yatsuya H, Murata C, Sekiya A, Wada K, et al. Eating fast leads to obesity: findings based on self-administered questionnaires among middle-aged Japanese men and women. J Epidemiol. 2006;16:117–24.

59. Lee KS, Kim DH, Jang JS, Nam GE, Shin YN, Bok AR, et al. Eating rate is associated with cardiometabolic risk factors in Korean adults. Nutr Metab Cardiovasc Dis. 2013;23:635–41. https://doi.org/10.1016/j.numecd.2012.02. 003. Epub 2012 May 26

60. Yamane M, Ekuni D, Mizutani S, Kataoka K, Sakumoto-Kataoka M, Kawabata Y, et al. Relationships between eating quickly and weight gain in Japanese university students: a longitudinal study. Obesity (Silver Spring). 2014;22: 2262–6. https://doi.org/10.1002/oby.20842. Epub 2014 July 10.

61. Fukuda H, Saito T, Mizuta M, Moromugi S, Ishimatsu T, Nishikado S, et al. Chewing number is related to incremental increases in body weight from 20 years of age in Japanese middle-aged adults. Gerodontology. 2013;30: 214–9. https://doi.org/10.1111/j.1741-2358.2012.00666.x.

62. Ohkuma T, Hirakawa Y, Nakamura U, Kiyohara Y, Kitazono T, Ninomiya T. Association between eating rate and obesity: a systematic review and meta-analysis. Int J Obes. 2015;39:1589–96. https://doi.org/10.1038/ijo.2015.96. Epub 2015 May 25. Review.

63. Robinson E, Almiron-Roig E, Rutters F, de Graaf C, Forde CG, Tudur Smith C, et al. A systematic review and meta-analysis examining the effect of eating rate on energy intake and hunger. Am J Clin Nutr. 2014;100:123–51. https:// doi.org/10.3945/ajcn.113.081745. Epub 2014 May 21. Review.

64. White AK, Venn B, Lu LW, Rush E, Gallo LM, Yong JL, Farella M. A comparison of chewing rate between overweight and normal BMI individuals. Physiol Behav. 2015;145:8–13. https://doi.org/10.1016/j.physbeh. 2015.03.028. Epub 2015 Mar 24

65. Spiegel TA, Kaplan JM, Tomassini A, Stellar E. Bite size, ingestion rate, and meal size in lean and obese women. Appetite. 1993;21:131–45.

66. Mattes RD, Considine RV. Oral processing effort, appetite and acute energy intake in lean and obese adults. Physiol Behav. 2013;120:173–81. https://doi. org/10.1016/j.physbeh.2013.08.013. Epub 2013 Aug 15

67. Keller A, Rohde JF, Raymond K, Heitmann BL. Association between periodontal disease and overweight and obesity: a systematic review. J Periodontol. 2015;86:766–76. https://doi.org/10.1902/jop.2015.140589. Review.

68. Graves DT. The potential role of chemokines and inflammatory cytokines in periodontal disease progression. Clin Infect Dis. 1999;28:482–90. Review

69. Page RC. The role of inflammatory mediators in the pathogenesis of periodontal disease. J Periodontal Res. 1991;26:230–42. Review

70. Khosravi R, Ka K, Huang T, Khalili S, Nguyen BH, Nicolau B, Tran SD. Tumor necrosis factor- α and interleukin-6: potential interorgan inflammatory mediators contributing to destructive periodontal disease in obesity or metabolic syndrome. Mediat Inflamm. 2013;2013:728987. https://doi.org/10. 1155/2013/728987. Epub 2013 Aug 28. Review

71. Pischon N, Heng N, Bernimoulin JP, Kleber BM, Willich SN, Pischon T. Obesity, inflammation, and periodontal disease. J Dent Res. 2007;86:400–9. Review

72. Morita T, Yamazaki Y, Mita A, Takada K, Seto M, Nishinoue N, et al. A cohort study on the association between periodontal disease and the development of metabolic syndrome. J Periodontol. 2010;81:512–9. https:// doi.org/10.1902/jop.2010.090594.

73. Cani PD, Amar J, Iglesias MA, Poggi M, Knauf C, Bastelica D, et al. Metabolic endotoxemia initiates obesity and insulin resistance. Diabetes. 2007;56: 1761–72. Epub 2007 Apr 24

74. Tatematsu M, Mori T, Kawaguchi T, Takeuchi K, Hattori M, Morita I, et al. Masticatory performance in 80-year-old individuals. Gerodontology. 2004;21:112–9.

75. Ueno M, Yanagisawa T, Shinada K, Ohara S, Kawaguchi Y. Category of functional tooth units in relation to the number of teeth and masticatory ability in Japanese adults. Clin Oral Investig. 2010;14:113–9.

76. Sato N, Ono T, Kon H, Sakurai N, Kohno S, Yoshihara A, Miyazaki H. Ten-year longitudinal study on the state of dentition and subjective masticatory ability in community-dwelling elderly people. J Prosthodont Res. 2016;60(3):177–84. https://doi.org/10.1016/j.jpor.2015.12.008. Epub 2016 Jan 16

77. Brodeur JM, Laurin D, Vallee R, Lachapelle D. Nutrient intake and gastrointestinal disorders related to masticatory performance in the edentulous elderly. J Prosthet Dent. 1993;70:468–73.

78. Lachapelle D, Brodeur JM, Simard PL, Vallee R, Moisan J. Masticatory ability and dietary adequacy of elderly denture wearers. J Can Diet Assoc. 1992;53:145–50.

79. Laurin D, Brodeur JM, Bourdages J, Vallée R, Lachapelle D. Fibre intake in elderly individuals with poor masticatory performance. J Can Dent Assoc. 1994;60:443–6. 449

80. Weijenberg RA, Lobbezoo F, Visscher CM, Scherder EJ. Oral mixing ability and cognition in elderly persons with dementia: a cross-sectional study. J Oral Rehabil. 2015;42:481–6.

81. Elsig F, Schimmel M, Duvernay E, Giannelli SV, Graf CE, Carlier S, et al. Tooth loss, chewing efficiency and cognitive impairment in geriatric patients. Gerodontology. 2013; https://doi.org/10.1111/ger.12079.

82. Hama Y, Kanazawa M, Minakuchi S, Uchida T, Sasaki Y. Reliability and validity of a quantitative color scale to evaluate masticatory performance using color-changeable chewing gum. Journal of medical and dental sciences. 2014;61:1–6.

12

The prevalence of edentulism and their related factors in Indonesia, 2014/15

Supa Pengpid[1,2] and Karl Peltzer[2,3*] (iD)

Abstract

Background: Little information exists about the loss of all one's teeth (edentulism) among older adults in Indonesia. The aim of this study was to investigate the prevalence of edentulism and associated factors among older adults in Indonesia.

Method: This study examines the self-reported prevalence of edentulism and associated factors among older adults (50 years and older) in a cross-sectional national study using the Indonesia Family Life Survey IFLS-5, 2014/15. The community-based study uses a multi-stage stratified sampling design to interview and assess household members, with a household response rate of over 90%.

Results: The overall prevalence of edentulism was 7.2, 29.8% in 80 years and older and 11.8% in those with no formal education. In adjusted Poisson regression analysis, older age, living in five major island groups and having functional disability were associated with edentulism. In addition, among men, having quit and current tobacco use and among women, having low social capital were associated with edentulism. Further, in adjusted analysis, among men, edentulism was positively associated with hypertension and negatively associated with diabetes, and among women, edentulism was associated with functional disability.

Conclusions: Results suggest that overall and/or among men or women that older age, living in five major island groups, having functional disability, tobacco quitters and users and those with low social capital was associated with edentulism. The identified associated factors of edentulism may be utilized in oral health programmes targeting older adults in Indonesia.

Keywords: Edentulism, Nutrition, Health status, Tobacco use, Older adults, Indonesia

Background

Edentulism (=having lost all of one's natural teeth) is a significant public health problem globally because of its high prevalence (> 10% in individuals 50 years and older) and related disability [1, 2]. The disability-adjusted life-years (DALYs) of oral conditions dramatically increased between 1990 and 2015 (16.9 million years live with disability) [3]. Among oral disorders, edentulism accounted for more than one third (7.6 million DALYs) of the oral disorder disability burden, globally [4]. Monitoring the occurrence of edentulism [5] provides an indication of both popula-tion oral health and oral health care system response [6]. There is a lack of community data on oral health among older adults in low- and middle-income countries [7]. Based on data from the World Health Survey, conducted from 2002 to 2004, the prevalence of self-reported edentulism among persons 50 years and older in countries of the Southeast Asian region were 4.2% in Laos, 22.2% in Malaysia, 2.4% in Myanmar, 14.6% in the Philippines and 5.6% in Vietnam [1]. In a more recent study (2007–2008) among adults 50 years and older, the overall prevalence of edentulism was 11.7% in the six middle-income countries, with India, Mexico, and Russia having higher prevalence rates (16.3–21.7%) than China, Ghana, and South Africa (3.0–9.0%) [2, 8]. In Indonesians aged 65 years or over the prevalence of measured edentulism was 17.6% in 2007 [9].

Using a social determinants of health approach, factors associated with edentulism may include, in addition to caries and periodontal disease [10], sociodemographic

* Correspondence: kpeltzer@hsrc.ac.za
[2]Department of Research & Innovation, University of Limpopo, Turfloop, South Africa
[3]HIV/AIDS/STIs and TB (HAST) Research Programme, Human Sciences Research Council, Private Bag X41, Pretoria 0001, South Africa
Full list of author information is available at the end of the article

factors such as increasing age, female gender, no or lower education, lower economic status and rural residence [2, 8, 11, 12]. Along with socioeconomic factors, health risk behaviours, such as smoking and former smoking remain strong predictors of edentulism [2, 11, 13–16]. Having chronic diseases [17], such as diabetes [18], having underweight [11], arthritis [2, 19], asthma [2, 11], depression [11, 17], reduced physical function [11], functional disability [2, 12], poor self-rated health [12, 17], lack of social support [17] and lack of social capital [20, 21] have also been found to be associated with edentulism. On the other hand, edentulism has been associated with poor health status [12, 22], insufficient fruit and vegetable consumption [22, 23], smoking [24], underweight, poor nutrition [25–27], overweight/obesity [27–29], hypertension [30, 31], angina [32], strokes [33], diabetes [25, 34], rheumatoid arthritis [25], asthma [25], and functional disability [35, 36].

There is a lack of studies on edentulism and associated factors in Indonesia [37, 38]. The aim of this study was to investigate the prevalence of edentulism and associated factors among older adults in Indonesia. The objectives include: (1) to estimate the prevalence of self-reported edentulism in older adults, and (2) to identify possible factors such as sociodemographics and health variables associated with edentulism in Indonesia.

Method
Study design and participants
Secondary data from the fifth wave of the "Indonesia Family Life Survey (IFLS-5) 2014-15" were analysed, being the only of the five surveys that assessed edentulism [39]. The IFLS-5 is a community survey interviewing household members (7994 50 years and older with complete endentulism measurements) selected by multistage stratified sampling representing 83% of the Indonesian population, with a household response rate of over 90%, more details [39, 40].

Measures
Edentulism was assessed with the question, "Have you lost all your teeth?" (Yes, No) [39].

Socio-demographic variables included age, sex, education, area of residence, province, region and subjective socioeconomic background [39, 40].

Social capital was assessed with 4 items related to the past 12 month participation in "1) Community meeting, 2) Voluntary labour, 3), Programme to improve the village/neighbourhood, and 4) Religious activities." Response options, were "yes" or "no" [39]. (Cronbach's alpha 0.59). Those who scored 0 times with "yes" were considered as having low social capital.

Self-reported health status was measured with the item, "In general, how is our health?" (Responses ranged from 1 = Very healthy to 4 = Unhealthy) [39].

Nutrition status. Heights and weights were taken using standard procedures [39], and body mass index (BMI) calculated according to Asian criteria: "underweight (<18.5 kg/m^2), normal weight (18.5 to <23.0 kg/m^2), overweight (23.0 to <25.0 kg/m^2) and 25+ kg/m^2 as obesity" [41].

Functional disability was assessed by 5 items of Activity of Daily Living (ADL) and 6 items of Instrumental Activity of Daily Living (IADL) [42, 43]. A total functional disability score was calculated, with having no difficulty = 0 and one or more ADL/IADL items = 1.

Tobacco use was grouped into never, quitters and current tobacco users, following the questions of ever and current use of various tobacco products [39, 40].

Inadequate fruit and vegetable consumption was defined as eating less than 3 days a week fruits and less than daily vegetables, following questions on the number of days in the past week vegetables (green leafy vegetables and carrots) and fruits (banana, papaya and mango) had been consumed [39, 40].

Chronic condition was measured based on health care provider diagnosed "Diabetes or high blood sugar, High blood pressure, Heart attack, coronary heart disease, angina or other heart problems, Stroke, Arthritis and Asthma" (Yes, No) [39, 40].

Hypertension
Average blood pressure was calculated arithmetically for three averaged measurements of systolic and diastolic blood pressure, assessed by using standard procedures [39]. Hypertension was defined as "SBP ≥140 mm Hg and/or DBP ≥90 mm Hg and/or current use of antihypertensive medication". [44].

The *Centres for Epidemiologic Studies Depression Scale (CES-D: 10 items)* was used to assess depressive symptoms, and scores of 10 or more were classified as having depressive symptoms [45] (Cronbach's alpha = 0.67).

Data analysis
Descriptive statistics were used to describe the variables. Nonparametric tests were used for trend analyses across ordered groups. Associations between key outcomes of edentulism and sociodemographic and health variables were evaluated by calculating prevalence ratios (PR). Poisson regression was used for evaluation of the association of explanatory variables for the outcome of edentulism (binary dependent variable). The Pearson goodness-of-fit test was used. Logistic regression was used to determine the association of edentulism on various health outcome variables. The Hosmer-Lemeshow goodness-of-fit test was used to evaluate multivariable model fit. Potential

multi-collinearity between variables was assessed with variance inflation factors, none of which exceeded critical value. $P < 0.05$ was considered significant. "Cross-section analysis weights were applied to correct both for sample attrition from 1993 to 2014, and then to correct for the fact that the IFLS-1 sample design included over-sampling in urban areas and off Java. The cross-section weights are matched to the 2014 Indonesian population, again in the 13 IFLS provinces, in order to make the attrition-adjusted IFLS sample representative of the 2014 Indonesian population in those provinces." [39] Both the 95% confidence intervals and P-values were adjusted considering the survey design of the study. All analyses were done with STATA software version 13.0 (Stata Corporation, College Station, TX, USA).

Results
Sample characteristics
The total sample included 7994 older adults, 50 years and older (mean age 62.8 years, SD = 9.8, age range of 50–110 years) in Indonesia. The proportion of women was 51.9, 72.2% had no or elementary education, 44.2% described themselves as having medium economic status, 52.0% resided in urban areas, 58.1% were living in Java and 20.8% had low social capital. Regarding health status, 32.9% rated their health as unhealthy, and 31.3% had at least one functional disability. In all, 14.1% of participants were underweight and 21.3% overweight or obese, 33.5% infrequently consumed fruit and vegetables, 33.3% were current tobacco users and 9.8% quit tobacco use. In terms of chronic conditions, 6.3% had diabetes, 58.5% hypertension, 3.6% heart attack, angina or other heart problems, 2.9% had a stroke, 11.8% had arthritis, 11.8% asthma and 17.0% depressive symptoms. The overall prevalence of edentulism was 7.2, 7.6% among women and 6.8% among men, and among those 50 to 59 years 3.1% and those aged 80 years and older 29.8%, and with no education the prevalence of edentulism was 11.8% and those with higher education 2.1% (see Table 1).

Associations with edentulism
In adjusted Poisson regression analysis, older age, living in five major island groups and having functional disability were associated with edentulism. In addition, among men, having quit and current tobacco use and among women, having low social capital were associated with edentulism. In further adjusted age stratified analysis, among 50 to 64 year olds, being male was negatively (Adjusted Prevalence Ratio: APR = 0.60, CI = 0.37, 0.98) and having underweight as positively (APR = 1.85, CI = 1.20, 2.83) associated with edentulism (see Table 2).

Associations between edentulism and health outcomes
In order to estimate the independent association between edentulism and 13 individual health outcomes, 13 separate multivariable models are calculated with edentulism as predictor and each health outcome as dependent variable. In adjusted analysis, among men, edentulism was positively associated with hypertension and negatively associated with diabetes and among women, edentulism was associated with functional disability (see Table 3).

Discussion
The study found in a national community-based survey among individuals 50 years and older, a 7.2% self-reported prevalence of edentulism in 2014/15 in Indonesia, which is similar to a measured survey of 17.6% in 2007 in Indonesia in individuals 65 years and older [7] (in this study 15.7% in the 65 years and older age group) and to what was found previously in China and South Africa [2]. The found prevalence rate of edentulism in Indonesia was higher than previously found in Ghana, Laos, Myanmar and in Vietnam, and lower than in India, Malaysia, Mexico, Philippines and Russia and the global prevalence of 14.0% [1, 2, 15]. The lower than global prevalence rate of edentulism in this study in Indonesia may be attributed to a lower consumption of non-refined carbohydrates and consequently lower dental caries and eventually tooth loss [1, 46]. The study found a significantly higher prevalence of edentulism in the five major island groups (Bali, West Nusa Tenggara, South Kalimantan, and South Sulawesi) than in Java and Sumatra. Reasons for this are not clear. It is possible that in the five major island groups greater gaps in dental care access exists than in Java and Sumatra.

The study found, in agreement with previous studies [2, 15, 47–50], that increasing age and in bivariate analysis having no education were associated with edentulism. It is possible that having no education translates into lower oral health knowledge and lower oral health services utilization where available [46]. Some previous studies [2, 48, 49] found a preponderance of edentulism among women and those living in rural areas, while in this study overall no significant gender and urban-rural differences were found. However, in age stratified analysis, among 50 to 64 year-olds, women had a higher prevalence of edentulism than men. Lower economic status was in this study not associated with edentulism, as found in some previous other studies [2, 48, 51]. This may be because economic status was assessed with a subjective measure, rather than an objective measure. Low social capital was in this study among women associated with edentulism. This finding is consistent with previous studies [20, 52]. It is possible that persons that belong to social networks are more likely to follow

Table 1 Sample characteristics and prevalence rate of edentulism among older adults in Indonesia

	Total sample	Prevalence rate of edentulism	
	N (%)	n	% (95% CI)[a]
Sociodemographics			
All	7994	685	7.2 (6.7, 7.8)
Age in years			
50–59	4024 (52.6)	142	3.1 (2.5, 3.7)
60–69	2226 (27.9)	169	6.4 (5.4, 7.5)
70–79	1251 (14.0)	222	15.9 (13.8, 18.2)
80 or more	493 (5.5)	152	29.8 (25.5, 34.4) P- trend < 0.001
Sex			
Female	4317 (51.9)	392	7.6 (6.8, 8.5)
Male	3677 (48.1)	293	6.8 (6.0, 7.7)
Education			
None	1324 (16.7)	185	11.8 (10.0, 13.8)
Elementary	4308 (55.5)	373	7.3 (6.5, 8.1)
High school	1723 (21.1)	92	4.7 (3.8, 5.8)
Higher education	569 (6.8)	16	2.1 (1.2, 3.7)
Subjective economic background			
Poor	2072 (31.0)	135	6.5 (5.5, 7.7)
Medium	3024 (42.3)	194	6.3 (5.2, 7.5)
Rich	1789 (26.7)	112	6.8 (6.0, 7.8)
Rural	3541 (48.0)	334	7.9 (7.0, 8.9)
Urban	4453 (52.0)	351	6.6 (5.8, 7.4)
Region			
Sumatra	1659 (20.8)	130	6.6 (5.5, 7.8)
Java	4647 (58.1)	309	6.4 (5.7, 7.2)
Main island groups[b]	1688 (21.1)	246	14.8 (13.1, 16.7)
Social capital (low)	1467 (20.8)	134	9.1 (7.8, 10.7)
Health variables			
Self-rated health (Unhealthy)	2849 (32.9)	335	9.9 (8.8, 11.2)
Body mass index			
Normal	2856 (39.0)	258	7.4 (6.4, 8.4)
Underweight	1063 (14.1)	145	11.7 (9.7, 13.9)
Overweight	1177 (15.8)	85	5.6 (4.4, 7.0)
Obese	2355 (31.1)	98	3.8 (3.0, 4.7)
Functional disability	2639 (31.3)	490	12.6 (11.3, 14.0)
Tobacco use			
Never	4663 (56.9)	371	6.6 (5,9, 7.4)
Quit	832 (9.8)	103	11.5 (9.3, 14.0)
Current	2499 (33.3)	211	7.1 (6.1, 8.2)
Diabetes	505 (6.3)	31	5.3 (3.6, 7.7)
Arthritis	1037 (11.8)	108	8.1 (6.6, 10.0)
Asthma	284 (3.4)	34	10.1 (7.0, 14.3)
Depression symptoms	1166 (17.0)	74	6.3 (5.1, 7.9)
Fruit (< 3 days/week) and vegetable consumption (<daily/week)	2119 (33.5)	141	6.7 (5.7, 7.8)

Table 1 Sample characteristics and prevalence rate of edentulism among older adults in Indonesia *(Continued)*

	Total sample	Prevalence rate of edentulism	
	N (%)	n	% (95% CI)[a]
Hypertension	4391 (58.5)	417	9.5 (8.7, 10.4)
Heart attack, coronary heart disease, angina, or other heart problems	299 (3.6)	29	9.1 (6.1, 13.4)
Stroke	243 (2.9)	31	13.2 (9.0, 18.9)

[a]The analysis was adjusted considering the survey design of the study
[b]Major Island groups: Bali, West Nusa Tenggara, South Kalimantan, and South Sulawesi

Table 2 Associations with edentulism estimated by Poisson regression

Variable	All Adjusted Prevalence Ratio[a] (95% CI)	Men Adjusted Prevalence Ratio[a] (95% CI)	Women Adjusted Prevalence Ratio[a] (95% CI)
Sociodemographics			
Age in years			
50–59	1 (Reference)	1 (Reference)	1 (Reference)
60–69	2.21 (1.68, 2.91)***	2.38 (1.55, 3.68)***	2.13 (1.52, 3.00)***
70–79	4.89 (3.65, 6.56)***	4.92 (3.10, 7.79)***	5.05 (3.52, 7.25)***
80 or more	5.94 (3.76, 9.39)***	7.91 (4.27, 14.64)***	4.33 (2.08, 9.01)***
Sex			
Female	1 (Reference)	–	–
Male	0.83 (0.63, 1.10)		
Education			
None	1 (Reference)	1 (Reference)	1 (Reference)
Elementary	1.20 (0.88, 1.64)	1.00 (0.58, 1.72)	1.28 (0.86, 1.78)
High school/Higher education	0.88 (0.59, 1.30)	0.86 (0.46, 1.63)	0.79 (0.48, 1.32)
Subjective economic background			
Poor	1 (Reference)	1 (Reference)	1 (Reference)
Medium	1.12 (0.88, 1.43)	1.12 (0.79, 1.59)	1.15 (0.83, 1.59)
Rich	1.27 (0.95, 1.69)	1.40 (0.91, 2.16)	1.19 (0.82, 1.73)
Urban residence (base = rural)	1.10 (0.88, 1.38)	0.98 (0.70, 1.35)	1.28 (0.94, 1.73)
Region			
Sumatra	1 (Reference)	1 (Reference)	1 (Reference)
Java	0.77 (0.59, 1.00)	1.14 (0.74, 1.75)	0.56 (0.40, 0.79)***
Main island groups	2.08 (1.59, 2.71)***	2.75 (1.79, 4.21)***	1.74 (1.24, 2.45)***
Social capital (low)	1.16 (0.92, 1.47)	1.00 (0.68, 1.47)	1.32 (1.00, 1.79)*
Health variables			
Self-rated health (Unhealthy)	1.07 (0.86, 1.36)	1.17 (0.83, 1.65)	0.97 (0.73, 1.29)
Body mass index (Underweight)	1.23 (0.93, 1.62)	1.26 (0.85, 1.86)	1.18 (0.80, 1.75)
Functional disability	1.34 (1.08, 1.66)**	1.22 (0.89, 1.68)	1.40 (1.05, 1.87)*
Tobacco use			
Never	1 (Reference)	1 (Reference)	1 (Reference)
Quit	1.25 (0.86, 1.82)	1.95 (1.12, 3.39)*	0.73 (0.27, 1.92)
Current	1.17 (0.87, 1.56)	1.64 (1.01, 2.69)*	0.89 (0.51, 1.55)
Diabetes	0.56 (0.31, 1.01)	0.30 (0.09, 1.02)	0.78 (0.40, 1.52)
Arthritis	0.93 (0.69, 1.24)	0.80 (0.47, 1.38)	0.97 (0.69, 1.38)
Asthma	0.89 (0.52, 1.51)	0.45 (0.16, 1.29)	1.26 (0.69, 2.31)
Depression symptoms	0.73 (0.45, 1.16)	0.69 (0.34, 1.39)	0.74 (0.40, 1.39)

CI confidence interval; ***$P < 0.001$; **$P < 0.01$; *$P < 0.05$
[a]Pearson goodness-of-fit test > 0.9 for all models

Table 3 Associations between edentulism and health variables (outcomes) estimated by logistic regression

Health outcome	Men		Women	
	COR	AOR[a,b]	COR	AOR[a,b]
Health status (unhealthy)	2.30 (1.78, 2.97)***	1.18 (0.80, 1.75)	1.98 (1.58, 2.48)***	1.11 (0.80, 1.51)
Functional disability	2.40 (1.83, 3.84)***	1.36 (0.96, 1.92)	3.30 (2.59, 4.20)***	1.43 (1.05, 1.95)*
Underweight (vs. normal weight)	2.11 (1.51, 2.95)***	1.33 (0.83, 2.15)	1.92 (1.37, 2.69)***	1.16 (0.72, 1.88)
Overweigh or obesity (vs. normal weight)	0.48 (0.35, 0.67)***	0.64 (0.40, 1.01)	0.50 (0.38, 0.66)***	0.83 (0.58, 1.17)
Infrequent fruit and vegetable consumption	1.02 (0.74, 1.39)	1.02 (0.71, 1.47)	0.86 (0.64, 1.16)	0.96 (0.68, 1.34)
Current tobacco use	0.89 (0.69, 1.16)	1.15 (0.76, 1.75)	2.16 (1.44, 3.24)***	1.01 (0.55, 1.85)
Hypertension	2.40 (1.81, 3.17)***	1.74 (1.17, 2.57)**	2.00 (1.54, 2.58)***	0.93 (0.62, 1.39)
Heart problems[c]	2.04 (1.07, 3.88)*	1.09 (0.69, 5.17)	1.16 (0.65, 2.07)	1.05 (0.48, 2.31)
Stroke	2.72 (1.43, 5.15)**	0.89 (0.25, 3.18)	2.90 (1.02, 5.19)***	1.35 (0.31, 5.87)
Asthma	2.16 (1.25, 3.72)**	0.58 (0.21, 1.58)	1.40 (0.81, 2.44)	1.35 (0.68, 2.70)
Arthritis	1.29 (0.84, 1.97)	0.88 (0.50, 1.56)	1.58 (1.18, 2.10)**	0.98 (0.66, 1.44)
Diabetes	0.61 (0.29, 1.32)	0.29 (0.09, 0.98)*	1.26 (0.78, 2.03)	0.92 (0.47, 0.82)
Depression	0.56 (0.26, 1.18)	0.68 (0.31, 1.46)	0.70 (0.39, 1.25)	0.67 (0.34, 1.37)

COR crude odds ratio, *AOR* adjusted odds ratio
[a]Adjusted for age, education, socioeconomic status, rural-urban, region, social capital and all other health variables, as shown in this table
[b]Hosmer-Lemeshow goodness-of-fit test between predicted and observed probabilities was for all models $P > 0.05$
[c]Heart attack, coronary heart disease, angina, or other heart problems
***$P<0.001$; **$P<0.01$; *$P<0.05$

health-enhancing behaviours and, hence, have better health and oral health [53–55]. Previous research also showed that the effect of edentulism on facial appearance, eating and speech may decline in social capital due to embarrassment [1, 56].

Previous studies [2, 18, 48, 57] found an association between former and current tobacco use and edentulism, which was confirmed in this study among men. Edentulism was also associated with former smokers in China [15]; China and Indonesia have the highest prevalence of tobacco use among men in the world. Smoking is a known risk factor for periodontitis and tooth loss, meaning that the higher prevalence of edentulism among tobacco users may be directly related to the negative effects of tobacco use on periodontal health [18, 57]. Functional disability was found in this study to be both, a risk factor and a consequence of edentulism, which has also been found in previous studies [2, 12, 35, 36]. It is possible that people with a functional disability are less likely visit dental health care services [12]. Unlike in some previous studies [12, 17, 22], this study did not find an association between poor self-rated health as a risk factor for and consequence of edentulism. Arthritis, asthma, diabetes, angina and depression were in this study not associated with edentulism, as this was found in some previous studies [2, 11, 18, 19].

Among having different chronic conditions, this study found that edentulism was associated with hypertension. Similar results were found in previous studies [30, 31]. It is possible that total tooth loss is a risk factor for developing hypertension, which may be attributed to dietary changes of not be able to consume nutritious foods [30].

Some studies [11, 25–27, 58] found a significant association between undernutrition as a risk factor and consequence of edentulism, both of which were confirmed in this study in bivariate analysis, and in age stratified adjusted analysis, among 50 to 64 year-olds, having underweight was associated with edentulism. In a study among older adults in care homes in Indonesia it was found that individuals who were underweight had a significantly lower number of functional tooth units than those with normal weight [38]. The loss of teeth changes digestive processes and food choices contributing to nutritional deficiencies [38, 58]. Contrary to some previous studies [26–29, 59], this study found that edentulism was negatively associated with overweight or obesity in bivariate analysis. It is possible that edentulism caused individuals in this study to alter their diet, resorting to a diet that is high in fiber and low in saturated fat, reducing the risk of being obese. Contrary to some studies [23, 24], this study did not find that edentulism had a negative impact on fruit and vegetable consumption.

Contrary to some previous studies [24, 32–34], this study did not find an association between having edentulism and heart problems, stroke, asthma, arthritis, diabetes and depression. In a study in Indonesia the prevalence and severity of periodontitis (and consequently tooth loss) was not associated with arthritis [60] and among elderly in Indonesia, tooth loss was not associated with diabetes and heart diseases [10]. The diet and dietary habits of edentulous individuals in Indonesia may not be putting them at increased risk of heart diseases and diabetes [2]. It is also possible, since in this study arthritis, asthma, diabetes, and heart diseases were assessed by self-reported diagnosed conditions; they were underreported and thus contributing to these findings [2]. Sudiono [10] proposes that among elderly in Indonesia the loss of teeth may have been influenced by "a low demand for dental hygiene" and that "improvement of dental awareness and education in oral hygiene measures in such populations might reduce both diseases (dental caries and periodontitis) responsible for tooth loss and could improve quality of life in Indonesia."

Study limitations

Edentulism was only measured with one question. Oral examinations should be conducted in future investigations. The data analysed were based on a cross-sectional survey, so no causative conclusions be drawn between independent study variables and the prevalence of edentulism. Finally, the analysis was limited to the variables included in IFLS-5, and other factors such as inadequate oral hygiene and dental attendance found significant in previous investigations should be included in future research.

Conclusions

Almost one in ten older adults (50 years and above) Indonesians were edentate. Results suggest that overall and/or among men or women that older age, living in five major island groups, having functional disability, tobacco quitters and users and those with low social capital was associated with edentulism. The identified associated factors of edentulism may be utilized in oral health programmes targeting older adults in Indonesia.

Abbreviations
BMI: Body Mass Index; CES-D: Centres for Epidemiologic Studies Depression Scale; DBP: Diastolic Blood Pressure; EA: Enumeration Area; IFLS: Indonesian Family Life Survey; SBP: Systolic Blood pressure

Acknowledgments
The research was conducted based on the IFLS-5 conducted by RAND (http://www.rand.org/labor/FLS/IFLS.html). We thank RAND for providing the access to the survey data and the study participants who provided the survey data.

Funding
The authors received no specific funding for this work.

Authors' contributions
KP and SP conceived and designed the analysis. KP drafted the manuscript and SP made critical revision of the manuscript for key intellectual content. Both authors read and approved the final version of the manuscript.

Competing interests
The authors declare that they have no competing interests.

Author details
[1]ASEAN Institute for Health Development, Mahidol University, Salaya, Thailand. [2]Department of Research & Innovation, University of Limpopo, Turfloop, South Africa. [3]HIV/AIDS/STIs and TB (HAST) Research Programme, Human Sciences Research Council, Private Bag X41, Pretoria 0001, South Africa.

References
1. Tyrovolas S, Koyanagi A, Panagiotakos DB, Haro JM, Kassebaum NJ, Chrepa V, Kotsakis GA. Population prevalence of edentulism and its association with depression and self-rated health. Sci Rep. 2016;6:37083. https://doi.org/10.1038/srep37083.
2. Peltzer K, Hewlett S, Yawson AE, Moynihan P, Preet R, Wu F, Guo G, Arokiasamy P, Snodgrass JJ, Chatterji S, Engelstad ME, Kowal P. Prevalence of loss of all teeth (edentulism) and associated factors in older adults in China, Ghana, India, Mexico, Russia and South Africa. Int J Environ Res Public Health. 2014;11(11):11308–24. https://doi.org/10.3390/ijerph111111308.
3. Kassebaum NJ, Smith AGC, Bernabé E, Fleming TD, Reynolds AE, Vos T, Murray CJL, Marcenes W, GBD 2015 Oral Health Collaborators. Global, regional, and national prevalence, incidence, and disability-adjusted life years for oral conditions for 195 countries, 1990-2015: a systematic analysis for the global burden of diseases, injuries, and risk factors. J Dent Res. 2017; 96(4):380–7. https://doi.org/10.1177/0022034517693566.
4. GBD 2015 DALYs and HALE Collaborators. Global, regional, and national disability-adjusted life-years (DALYs) for 315 diseases and injuriesand healthy life expectancy (HALE), 1990-2015: a systematic analysis for the global burden of disease study 2015. Lancet. 2016;388(10053):1603–58. https://doi.org/10.1016/S0140-6736(16)31460-X.
5. Sussex PV. Edentulism from a New Zealand perspective -a review of the literature. NZ Dental J. 2008;104:84–96.
6. Thomson WM. Monitoring edentulism in older New Zealand adults over two decades: a review and commentary. Int J Dent. 2012;2012 https://doi.org/10.1155/2012/375407.
7. Kossioni AE. Current status and trends in oral health in community dwelling older adults: a global perspective. Oral Health Prev Dent. 2013;11:331–40.
8. Hewlett SA, Yawson AE, Calys-Tagoe BN, Naidoo N, Martey P, Chatterji S, Kowal P, Mensah G, Minicuci N, Biritwum RB. Edentulism and quality of life among older Ghanaian adults. BMC Oral Health. 2015;15:48. https://doi.org/10.1186/s12903-015-0034-6.
9. Ministry of Health Republic of Indonesia. Report on Result of National Basic Health Research (RISKESDAS). Indonesia: the National Institute of Health Research and Development, 2007.
10. Sudiono J. The features of degenerative diseases and their association with the loss of teeth in the elderly of East Jakarta (Indonesia). Southeast Asian J Trop Med Public Health. 2008;39(1):184–9.
11. Ren C, McGrath C, Yang Y. Edentulism and associated factors among community-dwelling middle-aged and elderly adults in China. Gerodontology. 2017;34(2):195–207. https://doi.org/10.1111/ger.12249.
12. Olofsson H, Ulander EL, Gustafson Y, Hörnsten C. Association between socioeconomic and health factors and edentulism in people aged 65 and older - a population-based survey. Scand J Public Health. 2017; https://doi.org/10.1177/1403494817717406.
13. Starr JM, Hall RJ, Macintyre S, Deary IJ, Whalley LJ. Predictors and correlates of edentulism in the healthy old people in Edinburgh (HOPE) study. Gerodontology. 2008;25(4):199–204. https://doi.org/10.1111/j.1741-2358.2008.00227.x.

14. Arora M, Schwarz E, Sivaneswaran S, Banks E. Cigarette smoking and tooth loss in a cohort of older Australians: the 45 and up study. J Am Dent Assoc. 2010;141:1242–9.

15. Kailembo A, Preet R, Stewart Williams J. Common risk factors and edentulism in adults, aged 50 years and over, in China, Ghana, India and South Africa: results from the WHO Study on global AGEing and adult health (SAGE). BMC Oral Health. 2016;17(1):29. https://doi.org/10.1186/s12903-016-0256-2.

16. Musacchio E, Perissinotto E, Binotto P, Sartori L, Silva-Netto F, Zambon S, Manzato E, Corti MC, Baggio G, Crepaldi G. Tooth loss in the elderly and its association with nutritional status, socio-economic and lifestyle factors. Acta Odontol Scand. 2007;65(2):78–86.

17. Saman DM, Lemieux A, Arevalo O, Lutfiyya MN. A population-based study of edentulism in the US: does depression and rural residency matter after controlling for potential confounders? BMC Public Health. 2014;14:65. https://doi.org/10.1186/1471-2458-14-65.

18. Islas-Granillo H, Borges-Yañez SA, Lucas-Rincón SE, Medina-Solís CE, Casanova-Rosado AJ, Márquez-Corona ML, Maupomé G. Edentulism risk indicators among Mexican elders 60-year-old and older. Arch Gerontol Geriatr. 2011;53:258–62.

19. de Pablo P, Dietrich T, McAlindon TE. Association of periodontal disease and tooth loss with rheumatoid arthritis in the US population. J Rheumatol. 2008;35(1):70–6.

20. Kim EK, Jung YS, Kim KH, Kim KR, Kwon GH, Choi YH, Lee HK. Social capital and oral health: the association of social capital with edentulism and chewingability in the rural elderly. Arch Gerontol Geriatr. 2018;74:100–5. https://doi.org/10.1016/j.archger.2017.10.002.

21. Tsakos G, Sabbah W, Chandola T, Newton T, Kawachi I, Aida J, Sheiham A, Marmot MG, Watt RG. Social relationships and oral health among adults aged 60 years or older. Psychosom Med. 2013;75:178–86.

22. Medina-Solís CE, Pontigo-Loyola AP, Pérez-Campos E, Hernández-Cruz P, Avila-Burgos L, Mendoza-Rodríguez M, Maupomé G. Edentulism and other variables associated with self-reported health status in Mexican adults. Med Sci Monit. 2014;20:843–52. https://doi.org/10.12659/MSM.890100.

23. De Marchi RJ, Hugo FN, Padilha DM, Hilgert JB, Machado DB, Durante PC, Antunes MT. Edentulism, use of dentures and consumption of fruit and vegetables in south Brazilian community-dwelling elderly. J Oral Rehabil. 2011;38(7):533–40. https://doi.org/10.1111/j.1365-2842.2010.02189.x.

24. Tsakos G, Herrick K, Sheiham A, Watt RG. Edentulism and fruit and vegetable intake in low-income adults. J Dent Res. 2010;89(5):462–7. https://doi.org/10.1177/0022034510363247.

25. Felton DA. Complete edentulism and comorbid diseases: an update. J Prosthodont. 2016;25(1):5–20. https://doi.org/10.1111/jopr.12350.

26. Toniazzo MP, Amorim PS, Muniz FW, Weidlich P. Relationship of nutritional status and oral health in elderly: Systematic review with meta-analysis. Clin Nutr. 2017; https://doi.org/10.1016/j.clnu.2017.03.014.

27. Tôrres LH, da Silva DD, Neri AL, Hilgert JB, Hugo FN, Sousa ML. Association between underweight and overweight/obesity with oral health among independently living Brazilian elderly. Nutrition. 2013;29(1):152–7. https://doi.org/10.1016/j.nut.2012.05.011.

28. Österberg T, Dey DK, Sundh V, Carlsson GE, Jansson JO, Mellström D. Edentulism associated with obesity: a study of four national surveys of 16,416 swedes aged 55–84 years. Acta Odontol Scand. 2010;68:360–7.

29. Nascimento GG, Leite FR, Conceição DA, Ferrúa CP, Singh A, Demarco FF. Is there a relationship between obesity and tooth loss and edentulism? A systematic review and meta-analysis. Obes Rev. 2016;17(7):587–98. https://doi.org/10.1111/obr.12418.

30. Ayo-Yusuf OA, Ayo-Yusuf IJ. Association of tooth loss with hypertension. S Afr Med J. 2008;98:381–5.

31. Peres MA, Tsakos G, Barbato PR, Silva DA, Peres KG. Tooth loss is associated with increased blood pressure in adults–a multidisciplinary population-based study. J Clin Periodontol. 2012;39(9):824–33. https://doi.org/10.1111/j.1600-051X.2012.01916.x.

32. Medina-Solís CE, Pontigo-Loyola AP, Pérez-Campos E, Hernández-Cruz P, Ávila-Burgos L, Kowolik MJ, Maupomé G. Association between edentulism and angina pectoris in Mexican adults 35 years of age and older: a multivariate analysis of a population-based survey. J Periodontol. 2014;85:406–16.

33. Del Brutto OH, Mera RM, Zambrano M, Del Brutto VJ. Severe edentulism is a major risk factor influencing stroke incidence in rural Ecuador (The Atahualpa Project). Int J Stroke. 2017;12(2):201–4. https://doi.org/10.1177/1747493016676621.

34. Emami E, de Souza RF, Kabawat M, Feine JS. The impact of edentulism on oral and general health. Int J Dent. 2013;2013:498305. https://doi.org/10.1155/2013/498305.

35. Starr JM, Hall R. Predictors and correlates of edentulism in healthy older people. Curr Opin Clin Nutr Metab Care. 2010;13(1):19–23. https://doi.org/10.1097/MCO.0b013e328333aa37.

36. Yu YH, Lai YL, Cheung WS, Kuo HK. Oral health status and self-reported functional dependence in community-dwelling older adults. J Am Geriatr Soc. 2011;59(3):519–23. https://doi.org/10.1111/j.1532-5415.2010.03311.x.

37. Asia A, Kusdhany L, Rahardjo A, Bachtiar A. Association between tooth loss and the development of dementia on the Indonesian elders. JSM Dent. 2015;3(1):1050.

38. Adiatman M, Ueno M, Ohnuki M, Hakuta C, Shinada K, Kawaguchi Y. Functional tooth units and nutritional status of older people in care homes in Indonesia. Gerodontology. 2013;30(4):262–9. https://doi.org/10.1111/j.1741-2358.2012.00673.x.

39. Strauss J, Witoelar F, Sikoki B. The Fifth Wave of the Indonesia Family Life Survey (IFLS5): Overview and Field Report. 2016. WR-1143/1-NIA/NICHD, 2016.

40. Peltzer K, Pengpid S. High prevalence of depressive symptoms in a national sample of adults in Indonesia: childhood adversity, sociodemographic factors and health risk behaviour. Asian J Psychiatr. 2018;33:52–9. https://doi.org/10.1016/j.ajp.2018.03.017.

41. Wen CP, David Cheng TY, Tsai SP, Chan HT, Hsu HL, Hsu CC, Eriksen MP. Are Asians at greater mortality risks for being overweight than Caucasians? Redefining obesity for Asians. Public Health Nutr. 2009;12:497–506.

42. Katz S, Ford AB, Moskowitz RW, Jackson BA, Jaffe MW. Studies of illness in the aged. JAMA. 1963;185(12):914–9.

43. Lawton MP, Brody EM. Assessment of older people: self-maintaining and instrumental activities of daily living. The Gerontologist. 1969;9(3-Part-1):179–86.

44. Chobanian AV, Bakris GL, Black HR, Cushman WC, Green LA, Izzo JL, et al. Seventh report of the Joint National Committee of Prevention, Detection, Evaluation, and Treatment of High Blood Pressure. Hypertension. 2003;42:1206–52.

45. Andresen EM, Malmgren JA, Carter WB, Patrick DL. Screening for depression in well older adults: evaluation of a short form of the CES-D (Center for Epidemiologic Studies Depression Scale). Am J Prev Med. 1994;10(2):77–84.

46. van der Velden U, Amaliya A, Loos BG, Timmerman MF, van der Weijden FA, Winkel EG, Abbas F. Java project on periodontal diseases: causes of tooth loss in a cohort of untreated individuals. J Clin Periodontol. 2015;42(9):824–31. https://doi.org/10.1111/jcpe.12446.

47. Doğan BG, Gökalp S. Tooth loss and edentulism in the Turkish elderly. Arch Gerontol Geriatr. 2012;54:e162–e166.

48. Gaio EJ, Haas AN, Carrard VC, Oppermann RV, Albandar J, Susin C. Oral health status in elders from South Brazil: a population-based study. Gerodontology. 2012;29:214–23.

49. Hugo FN, Hilgert JB, de Sousa Mda L, da Silva DD, Pucca GA Jr. Correlates of partial tooth loss and edentulism in the Brazilian elderly. Community Dent Oral Epidemiol. 2007;35:224–32.

50. Mendes DC, Poswar Fde O, de Oliveira MV, Haikal DS, da Silveira MF, Martins AM, De Paula AM. Analysis of socio-demographic and systemic health factors and the normative conditions of oral health care in a population of the Brazilian elderly. Gerodontology. 2012;29:e206–14.

51. Moreira Rda S, Nico LS, Tomita NE. Spatial risk and factors associated with edentulism among elderly persons in Southeast Brazil. Cad Saude Publica. 2011;27:2041–54.

52. Hanson BS, Liedberg B, Owall B. Social network, social support and dental status in elderly Swedish men. Community Dent Oral Epidemiol. 1994;22:331–7.

53. Wennström A, Ahlqwist M, Stenman U, Björkelund C, Hakeberg M. Trends in tooth loss in relation to socio-economic status among Swedish women, aged 38 and 50 years: repeated cross-sectional surveys 1968–2004. BMC Oral Health. 2013;13 https://doi.org/10.1186/1472–6831–13–63.

54. Takeuchi K, Aida J, Kondo K, Osaka K. Social participation and dental health status among older Japanese adults: a population-based cross-sectional study. PLoS One. 2013;8(4):e61741.

55. Rodrigues SM, Oliveira AC, Vargas AM, Moreira AN, E Ferreira EF. Implications of edentulism on quality of life among elderly. Int J Environ Res Public Health. 2012;9(1):100–9. https://doi.org/10.3390/ijerph9010100.

56. Northridge ME, Ue FV, Borrell LN, De La Cruz LD, Chakraborty B, Bodnar S, Marshall S, Lamster IB. Tooth loss and dental caries in community-dwelling older adults in northern Manhattan. Gerodontology. 2012;29:e464–e473.

57.   Leite FRM, Nascimento GG, Scheutz F, López R. Effect of smoking on periodontitis: a systematic review and meta-regression. Am J Prev Med. 2018; https://doi.org/10.1016/j.amepre.2018.02.014.

58.   Rauen MS, Moreira EA, Calvo MC, Lobo AS. Oral condition and its relationship to nutritional status in the institutionalized elderly population. J Am Diet Assoc. 2006;106:1112–4.

59.   Lee JS, Weyant RJ, Corby P, Kritchevsky SB, Harris TB, Rooks R, Rubin SM, Newman AB. Edentulism and nutritional status in a biracial sample of well-functioning, community-dwelling elderly: the health, aging, and body composition study. Am J Clin Nutr. 2004;79:295–302.

60.   Susanto H, Nesse W, Kertia N, Soeroso J, Huijser van Reenen Y, Hoedemaker E, Agustina D, Vissink A, Abbas F, Dijkstra PU. Prevalence and severity of periodontitis in Indonesian patients with rheumatoid arthritis. J Periodontol. 2013;84(8):1067–74. https://doi.org/10.1902/jop.2012.110321.

13

Dental health between self-perception, clinical evaluation and body image dissatisfaction

Ancuta Banu[1], Costela Şerban[2*] (iD), Marius Pricop[2], Horatiu Urechescu[2] and Brigitha Vlaicu[3]

Abstract

Background: Self-perception of oral health status is a multidimensional construct that includes psychological, psychosocial and functional aspects of oral health. Contemporary concepts suggest that the evaluation of health needs should focus on clinical standards and socio-dental indicators that measure the impact of health/disease on the individual quality of life. Oral health cannot be dissociated from general health. This study evaluates a possible association between oral health status, body size, self-perception of oral health, self-perception of body size and dissatisfaction with body image in prepubertal children with mixed dentition, targeting the completion of children's health status assessment which will further allow the identification of individuals at risk and could be further used as an evaluation of the need for specific interventions.

Methods: The present study is cross-sectional in design and uses data from 710 pre-pubertal children with mixed dentition. The outcome variables comprised one item self-perception of oral health: dmft/DMFT Index and Dental Aesthetic Index, body size, self-assessed body size and desired body size. Multiple logistic regression analyses were performed. The level of significance was set at 5%.

Results: More than a half (53.1%) of the participants with mixed dentition reported that their oral health was excellent or very good. In the unadjusted model, untreated decayed teeth, dmft score and body dissatisfaction levels had a significant contribution to poor self-perception of oral health, but after adjustment for gender, BMI status, dmft score, DMFT score and DAI score, only untreated decayed teeth OR = 1.293, 95%CI (1.120–1.492) and higher body dissatisfaction levels had a significant contribution.

Conclusion: It was concluded that the need for dental treatment influenced self-perception of oral health in prepubertal children with mixed dentition, especially with relation to untreated decayed teeth. Since only body dissatisfaction levels, but not BMI, were related to poor self-perception of oral health, which involves a psychological component, further studies should evaluate the risk factors of body dissatisfaction, in order to plan health care directed to this age group, and with the purpose to positive parenting strategies.

Keywords: Self-perception of oral health, Mixed dentition, Decayed teeth, Body dissatisfaction

* Correspondence: costela.serban@umft.ro
[2]Department 3 Functional Sciences, "Victor Babes" University of Medicine and Pharmacy Timişoara, 14 Spl. Tudor Vladimirescu, 300172 Timişoara, Romania
Full list of author information is available at the end of the article

Background

Self-perception of oral health status is a multidimensional construct that includes oral disease, tissue damage, modified functional capacity, pain, and aesthetics - psychological and psychosocial components. Self-reported oral health status is a relatively simple and easy method of assessment, which can be routinely collected and has several uses, such as the assessment of perceived treatment needs, and as a monitoring tool for health promotion intervention. Although most studies on contributors to oral health perception targeted adult populations, there have been some studies performed on children and adolescents which have shown good consistency over time of one item self-rated oral health, and its importance in taking preventive measures [1, 2]. It has been concluded that self-reported oral health has an impact on both well-being and quality of life [3]. In children and adolescents, oral health-related quality of life has been proved to be impacted by several oral conditions such as dental caries or malocclusion, but also by psychological components such as self-esteem and positive self-image [4–8].

With the rise in prevalence of childhood obesity, several studies have attempted to explore the links between dental decay and obesity, concluding that they share common etiological, social and behavioural factors [9].

The association of weight status with the body image is formed through the subjective judgment of body size by children and has been demonstrated in numerous studies that have focused on satisfaction with body shape. Dissatisfaction with body image was judged to increase with age among the groups of children and adolescents studied [10]. A negative body image was correlated with depression, anxiety, low self-esteem, obsessive-compulsive behaviours [11], and inadaptive behaviours in adolescence [12].

Objectives

Since it is demonstrated that effective prevention strategies improve the oral health status and considering the before-demonstrated link between the oral health perception and the previously mentioned items (body image, self-esteem and self-image) we might hypothesize that by identifying a cluster of target patients in which screening and pro-active prevention strategies will have an increased impact leading to an increased quality of life with all the associated benefits. Thus, to be able to improve the screening strategies and identification of most vulnerable patients, this study aimed to evaluate a possible association between oral health status, body size, self-perception of oral health, self-perception of body size and dissatisfaction with body image in pre-pubertal children with mixed dentition.

Method

Sample

Data was taken from the program for monitoring and control of oral health status of the population of Timişoara, Romania undertaken in the Maxillo-Facial Surgery Clinic of City Hospital Timişoara with the support of the City Hall in Timişoara and the Timiş County School Inspectorate. The program was promoted in all 40 Primary and Middle Schools from Timisoara, Romania, and all attending students were invited to participate. In Romania the school is compulsory until the age of 16, representing 11 grades: from the preparatory school year to the tenth grade. The sample was obtained by availability.

The sample size was considered as being representative of the city of Timişoara, which, at the last referendum had 319,279 inhabitants with a proportion of children attending school with age range 7–18 years of 9.4% [13]. Taking into account our actual sample size of 710 participants, the calculated margin of error for the sample is 3.6%.

Selection criteria for participants:

- inclusion criteria: children in the selected age group (8–11 years), with mixed dentition, of normal weight and overweight by WHO (World Health Organization) 2007 criteria, children without a serious general illness, cooperative children, children whose parents have given informed consent.
- exclusion criteria: underweight children (as defined by WHO 2007 criteria), children with exclusive temporary or definitive dentition, children with genetic or post-traumatic malformations, children with a serious general illness, children with rare conditions.

Out of the total of 945 children examined, a sample of 710 primary school children was obtained which had no missing data on outcome variables. The group had a mean age of 114 (+/− 11.3) months. 52.8% (375) of the sample were boys.

Data collection started in May 2015 and continued for 8 weeks. The children were evaluated clinically and with a questionnaire-based interview, performed on the same day. The children responded voluntarily to the personalized interview, which was adapted to their age, with questions covering the self-assessment of their oral health status, their perception of body image and their desired body shape. The following information was recorded: gender, date of birth, date of consultation. Evaluation was conducted by examiners licensed both in medicine and dentistry. The dental clinical examiner is maxillo-facial surgery specialist and has competence in Pedodontics and Orthopedic dentistry.

Weight was measured by a single examiner, in minimal clothing, without shoes, to the nearest 0.1 kg, with a calibrated mechanical step scale; height was measured to the nearest 0.5 cm under the same conditions using a standard stadiometer from the medical office.

Body mass index (BMI) was calculated from weight and height measurements, based on the following formula: BMI = weight (kg)/height (m)^2. WHO AnthroPlus macros were used for assessing growth and adiposity status (BMI-z score). Furthermore, children were classified according to WHO recommendations of normal weight category, overweight and obesity [14].

Perceived body image and **desired body image** were measured using the Pictorial Body Image Instrument [15], a well-established method for assessing body image dissatisfaction, which facilitated the children's choices and their communication with the examiner. The boys and girls were presented with a set of seven drawings of children, matched to the respondent's gender, ranging in size from very thin to obese, and numbered from one (very thin) to seven (obese).

Body image dissatisfaction was calculated as the discrepancy between the perceived and the desired body images assessed as part of the questionnaire. A score of zero indicated that the child was satisfied with his/her size, a positive score indicated that the child wanted to be thinner, and a negative score indicated that the child wanted to be larger.

The endo-oral clinical examination was performed by a single examiner, in a dental chair, with the help of a mouth mirror, probe, and William's probe which was used to determine the overjet and overbite. The following were recorded:

- number of teeth that are decayed (d for primary teeth, D for permanent teeth), missing (m for primary teeth, M for permanent teeth), or filled (f for primary teeth, F for permanent teeth) and were computed the dmft/DMFT index for mixed dentition, according to WHO recommendations [16]. dmft/DMFT index is established as the measure of caries experience in dental epidemiology.
- parameters Dental Aesthetic Index (DAI): overjet, underjet, missing teeth, diastema, anterior open bite, anterior crowding, anterior spacing, largest anterior irregularity (mandible and maxilla), anterior-posterior molar relationship.

The Dental Aesthetic Index were computed according to WHO recommendations [16]. It has two components: a clinical component and an aesthetic component and it links the clinical and aesthetic components mathematically to produce a single score that combines the physical and the esthetic aspects of occlusion. DAI was adopted as a cross-cultural index by the World Health Organization for the assessment of orthodontic treatment needs.

Perceived oral health status was measured on a 7 item Likert scale that comprised the following possible answers: excellent, very good, good, average, poor, very poor and I do not know option. The question was: "How would you rate your overall oral health?". Since self-perceived oral health status is a latent construct, the best approach in registering the participants' subjective opinion on this topic is a Likert-type ordinal scale answer.

Data analysis

Data analysis was performed using the Statistical Program for Social Sciences for Windows (IBM-SPSS, Version 18). Perceived oral health status was the main outcome of the study. The main explanatory variables were clinical oral status (dmft score, DMFT score, number of untreated decayed teeth), BMI categories and body image dissatisfaction. Other variables included in the analysis were the participant's gender and age. For numerical variables, descriptive summary measures of central tendency were computed. For ordinal or nominal variables, frequency (%/N) were computed. For comparisons between genders of continuous variables under the presumption of normality t-tests were used and for continuous variables which failed in the assumption of normality and homogeneity of variance, and categorical variables Man-Whitney test was used.

Using the clinical indicators (dmft score, DMFT score, DAI score and number of untreated decayed teeth) as dependent variables, four general linear models were used to test differences between gender (M/F) and age groups (8–9 years / 10–11 years) and their interaction, using Estimated Marginal Means, and comparing their main effects using Sidak correction for multiple comparisons. Using body dissatisfaction as a dependent variable, and gender, BMI categories and their interaction as predictors, another general linear model was constructed, applying Sidak correction for multiple comparisons.

Logistic regression was applied for the prediction of poor self-perception of oral health, which, after recoding self-perception of oral health, resulted in: excellent and very good as high self-perception of oral health and the rest of answers as poor self-perception of oral health. As independent predictors we have used gender, clinical oral indicators (dmft score, DMFT score, DAI score, total number of untreated decayed teeth), BMI categories and body dissatisfaction levels in absolute discrepancy. Univariate OR were computed separately for all independent variables. In the following step a model was constructed.

All statistical tests performed were 2-tailed and statistical significance was defined by a p value < 0.05.

Results

Self-perception of oral health

Descriptive statistics of self-perception of oral health status are presented in Table 1. No respondents rated their oral health status as bad, or very bad, and those categories were collapsed. More than half (53.1%) of the group rated their oral health status as excellent or very good. Almost 10% of the group could not rate their oral health status.

No significant differences were found between "I do not know" responders and lower class self-raters (collapsed good and average raters) ($p > 0.05$), therefore in further analysis for the prediction of lower class of self-perception of oral health, they were considered together with lower self-raters.

Oral health

For the sample, dmft and DMFT scores and Dental Aesthetic Index (DAI) score were calculated and descriptive statistics are presented in Table 1.

Using the general linear model with gender (male vs female) and age groups (8–9 years vs 10–11 years) as factors, four different models were constructed for dmft score, DMFT score and DAI score and the total number of untreated decayed teeth. Only models constructed for dmft score ($p = 0.017$), DMFT score ($p = 0.005$) and for

the total number of decayed teeth ($p = 0.036$) reached statistical significance (Table 2).

For dmft score, significant differences were observed between genders, females having a higher dmft score, compared to males ($p = 0.016$, partial eta squared = 0.008) with the 8–9 year old age group having a significantly higher score than the 10–11 year old age group ($p = 0.035$, partial eta squared = 0.006), but their interaction was not statistically significant, $p = 0.877$. For DMFT score, significant differences were found between age groups, with the 10–11 year old group having a higher DMFT score, compared to 8–9 year old group ($p = 0.001$, partial eta squared = 0.017) but not between genders ($p = 0.587$), or the interaction between gender and age group ($p = 0.272$).

For the total number of untreated decayed teeth, significant differences were only observed between genders, females having a higher number, compared to males ($p = 0.007$, partial eta squared = 0.010) but the differences between age groups ($p = 0.306$) and their interaction ($p = 0.877$) were not statistically significant.

The general linear model for DAI score did not reach significance, $p = 0.080$ (Table 2).

BMI status

Prevalence of overweight is 14.4% (54) for boys and 19.1% (64) for girls and the prevalence of overweight

Table 1 Descriptive statistics for outcome variables ($N = 710$ participants)

			Gender		Statistical test / significance level	Total
			M	F		
Age (months)		Mean +/− SD	113.81 +/− 11.4	114.24 +/− 11.3	* / 0.615	114.01 +/− 11.3
Perception of oral health	Excellent	% (n)	27.5% (103)	32.2% (108)	** / 0.521	29.7 (211)
	Very good	% (n)	25.6% (96)	20.9% (70)		23.4 (166)
	good	% (n)	19.5% (73)	18.5% (62)		19.0 (135)
	average	% (n)	17.1% (64)	19.7% (66)		18.3 (130)
	I do not know	% (n)	10.4% (39)	8.7% (29)		9.6 (68)
BMI categories	normal weight	% (n)	76.3% (286)	78.2% (262)	** / 0.293	77.2 (548)
	overweight	% (n)	14.4% (54)	19.1% (64)		16.6 (118)
	obese	% (n)	9.3% (35)	2.7% (9)		6.2 (44)
BMI Z-score		Mean +/− SD	0.97 +/− 1.38	0.78 +/− 1.34	* / 0.068	0.88 +/− 1.36
dmft score		Mean +/− SD	1.71 +/− 1.97	2.08 +/− 2.13	* / 0.017	1.89 +/− 2.06
DMFT score		Mean +/− SD	0.85 +/− 1.09	0.88 +/− 1.11	* / 0.720	0.86 +/− 1.10
DAI score		Mean +/− SD	23.70 +/− 7.74	23.26 +/− 6.48	* / 0.406	23.49 +/− 7.17
Orthodontic treatment need		% (n)	36.3 (136)	36.7 (123)	** / 0.901	36.5 (259)
Total no of untreated decayed teeth		Mean +/− SD	1.74 +/− 1.83	2.14 +/− 2.09	* / 0.006	1.93 +/− 1.97

Note: * t-test ** Mann-Whitney
SD standard deviation

Table 2 General linear models (GLM) for oral health indicators as dependent variables by gender and age group (N = 710 participants)

	Variables	Categories		Mean +/– SD	Significance	Partial Eta Squared
dmft	Gender	male (375)		1.71 +/– 1.971	0.016	0.008
		female (335)		2.08 +/– 2.132		
	Age groups	8–9 years (449)		2.01 +/– 2.124	0.035	0.006
		10–11 years (261)		1.68 +/– 1.916		
	Gender * Age Group (Interaction)	male	8–9 years (242)	1.84 +/– 2.087	0.877	0.000
			10–11 years (133)	1.48 +/– 1.722		
		female	8–9 years (207)	2.20 +/– 2.156		
			10–11 years (128)	1.89 +/– 2.086		
DMFT	Gender	male (375)		0.85 +/– 1.095	0.587	0.000
		female (335)		0.88 +/– 1.105		
	Age groups	8–9 years (449)		0.76 +/– 0.960	0.001	0.017
		10–11 years (261)		1.05 +/– 1.285		
	Gender * Age Group (Interaction)	male	8–9 years (242)	0.78 +/– 1.010	0.272	0.002
			10–11 years (133)	0.98 +/– 1.228		
		female	8–9 years (207)	0.73 +/– 0.900		
			10–11 years (128)	1.12 +/– 1.344		
DAI	Gender	male (375)		23.70 +/– 7.744	0.328	0.001
		female (335)		23.26 +/– 6.478		
	Age groups	8–9 years (449)		23.97 +/– 7.550	0.021	0.008
		10–11 years (261)		22.68 +/– 6.406		
	Gender * Age Group (Interaction)	male	8–9 years (242)	23.98 +/– 8.015	0.349	0.001
			10–11 years (133)	23.21 +/– 7.227		
		female	8–9 years (207)	23.95 +/– 6.986		
			10–11 years (128)	22.14 +/– 5.397		
Decayed teeth	Gender	male (375)		1.74 +/– 1.835	0.007	0.010
		female (335)		2.14 +/– 2.091		
	Age groups	8–9 years (449)		1.98 +/– 1.944	0.306	0.001
		10–11 years (261)		1.84 +/– 2.011		
	Gender * Age Group (Interaction)	male	8–9 years (242)	1.79 +/– 1.849	0.972	0.000
			10–11 years (133)	1.63 +/– 1.811		
		female	8–9 years (207)	2.20 +/– 2.032		
			10–11 years (128)	2.05 +/– 2.188		

GLM dependent variable dmft, F(3) = 3431, p = 0.017, partial eta squared = 0.014, adjusted R squared = 0.010
GLM dependent variable DMFT, F(3) = 4337, p = 0.005, partial eta squared = 0.018, adjusted R squared = 0.014
GLM dependent variable DAI, F(3) = 2257, p = 0.080, partial eta squared = 0.010, adjusted R squared = 0.005
GLM dependent variable Decayed teeth, F(3) = 2858, p = 0.036, partial eta squared = 0.012, adjusted R squared = 0.008

and obesity is 23.7% (89) for boys and (73) 21.8% for girls. For this sample, no statistical differences were found between genders related to BMI z-score (p = 0.068), nor between the proportion of BMI categories, between genders (p = 0.293) (Table 1).

Body image dissatisfaction
Of all the students included in our study, 43.8% (311) are satisfied with their body image. 45.6% (324) reported they would like to be thinner (35.2% by 1 level, 8.6% by 2 levels and 1.8% by 3 levels) and 35.2% (250) that they wanted to be heavier (10.1% by 1 level and 0.4% by 2 levels).

General linear model was applied in order to quantify the influence of gender, BMI categories or their interaction on satisfaction levels. Gender (p = 0.549) and the interaction of gender and BMI categories (p = 0.578) did not contribute significantly to the model (Table 3).

BMI categories significantly influenced the outcome, F(2) = 11.37, $p < 0.001$. The result was further explored

Table 3 General linear model (GLM) for dependent variable body dissatisfaction level by gender, BMI categories and interaction of gender and BMI categories (N = 710 participants)

Variables	Categories		Mean body dissatisfaction level +/− SD	Significance	Partial Eta Squared
Gender	male (375)		0.49 +/− 0.889	0.548	0.001
	female (335)		0.44 +/− 0.852		
BMI categories	normal weight (548)		0.39 +/− 0.853	< 0.001	0.031
	overweight (118)		0.68 +/− 0.856*		
	obese (44)		0.93 +/− 0.925*		
Gender* BMI categories	male	normal weight (286)	0.42 +/− 0.870	0.578	0.002
		overweight (54)	0.65 +/− 0.894		
		obese (35)	0.89 +/− 0.932		
	female	normal weight (262)	0.35 +/− 0.835		
		overweight (64)	0.70 +/− 0.830		
		obese (9)	1.11 +/− 0.928		

Note: *GLM* dependent variable Body dissatisfaction levels, $F(5) = 5.213$, $p < 0.001$, partial eta squared = 0.036
*mean body dissatisfaction significantly higher in overweight ($p = 0.003$) and obese ($p = 0.001$) compared with normal weight children, results adjusted by Sidak method for multiple comparisons

with post-hoc tests with Sidak correction for multiple comparisons. Normal weight children had a significant higher level of satisfaction when compared with overweight children (mean difference = 0.29, p = 0.003) and with obese children (mean difference = 0.613, p = 0.001). The differences between levels of satisfaction in overweight and obese children were not statistically significant (mean difference = 0.323, p = 0.201).

For the body image dissatisfaction measure, the absolute discrepancy was also calculated to remove the direction and the extent of dissatisfaction.

Predictors of poor self-perception of oral health status
In univariate unadjusted logistic regression, gender, BMI categories, DMFT and DAI score did not significantly contribute to the prediction of poor self-rated oral health. Untreated decayed teeth, dmft score and body dissatisfaction levels had significant contributions in univariate analysis (Table 4).

In the model, when controlling for gender, BMI categories, dmft score, DMFT score and DAI score, the unique contributors were the number of untreated decayed teeth and the levels of dissatisfaction with the body (Table 4).

Table 4 Logistic regression results for the predictors of poor self-evaluation of oral health status (N = 710 participants)

	Unadjusted OR*	95% C.I. for OR	Model OR**	95% C.I. for OR
Gender (Male)	1.003	(0.746–1.347)	1.055	(0.776–1.435)
BMI categories	$p = 0.745$			$p = 0.969$
Overweight vs Normal weight	1.045	(0.702–1.557)	1.029	(0.682–1.552)
Obese vs Normal weight	1.268	(0.685–2.345)	1.076	(0.567–2.040)
dmft score	1.075	(1.000– 1.156)	.911	(0.806–1.030)
DMFT score	1.083	(0.947– 1.238)	.899	(0.763–1.058)
DAI	1.006	(0.985– 1.027)	1.004	(0.983–1.025)
Untreated decayed teeth	1.154	(1.068– 1.246)	1.293	(1.120–1.492)
Body image dissatisfaction	$p = 0.006$			$p = 0.003$
1 level vs no dissatisfaction	1.585	(1.157– 2.172)	1.605	(1.164–2.211)
2 levels vs no dissatisfaction	1.820	(1.059– 3.129)	2.040	(1.168–3.564)
3 levels vs no dissatisfaction	3.393	(1.023– 11.260)	3.617	(1.057–12.373)

Dependent variable: poor self-evaluation of oral health
Independent variables: Gender, BMI categories, dmft score, DMFT score, DAI score, total number of decayed teeth
*Unadjusted OR were calculated separately for each individual variable
**Model adjusted for gender, BMI categories, dmft score, DMFT score, DAI score; log likelihood chi-square: 31.364, Prob > chi-square: 0.001, Pseudo R-square: 0.043

Body image dissatisfaction has a unique contribution in the prediction of poor self-rated health: the higher the level of dissatisfaction, the higher probability of a poor evaluation class: when compared with the students who did not exhibit dissatisfaction with their body image, those who had one level of dissatisfaction had an OR = 1.61, those with 2 levels of dissatisfaction had an OR = 2.04 and those with 3 levels of dissatisfaction had an OR = 3.61. Body image dissatisfaction had similar OR and 95% confidence intervals in adjusted and unadjusted models, showing that the relation is not confounded.

In the adjusted model, when controlling for dmf and DMF scores, for each extra untreated decayed tooth there is a 29% higher probability of poor self-rated oral evaluation. In the unadjusted model, when dmft and DMFT scores were not controlled for, the probability was lower, for each extra untreated decayed tooth there was a 15% higher probability of poor evaluation. In the correlation matrix, the mean total number of decayed teeth was correlated with the dmft score (tau = 0.688, $p < 0.001$) and the DMFT score (tau = 0.408, $p < 0.001$), therefore dmft score and DMFT score are confounders and have to be controlled for, in the prediction of poor self-rated oral health.

Discussion

According to the literature [17], from the end of the first period of mixed dentition and the beginning of the second period of mixed dentition children with mixed dentition present an optimal morpho-functional and aesthetic balance, dento-alveolar harmony, balanced occlusal relations in the three planes, the dental upper arch circumscribing the dental lower arch with a vestibular cusp, the upper incisors covering the lower one with a contact point or incisal step of 1–2 mm, permanent molars in the cusp-groove or cusp-cusp relationship, fraenums labiis on the maxillary midline and skull base, and absence of diastema. The caries of the deciduous teeth disrupt the development of the dento-maxillary apparatus, this balance being lost.

For this age group, as far as it is known, self-rated oral health status has never been evaluated regarding its oral clinical indicators (carious experience and malocclusion) and body shape and body image dissatisfaction as contributing risk factors.

In this study, self-perception of oral health was not related to clinical epidemiological oral health indicators or dento-occlusal aesthetic indicators, with the exception of untreated decayed teeth. Although dmft Index, DMFT Index, dmft/DMFT Index have been used intensively in clinical settings in order to assess dental caries prevalence, as well as dental treatment needs among populations [18], for this age group, only the cumulated "decayed" component of both scores is associated with

self-perceived oral health with an OR = 1.293, 95%CI (1.120, 1.492), as has been previously reported [19]. Since the proximal consequence of dental decay is pain [20], it is likely that the contribution of decayed untreated teeth to self-reported oral health is viewed by children through their subjective measure. Untreated cavitated dentine lesions and their consequences negatively influence the quality of life in children [21].

The presence of malocclusion did not relate to self-perception of oral health, although, in older adolescents and adults, malocclusion has physical, social, and psychological effects on oral conditions as well as on the quality of life [22]. It might be that at this age self-consciousness regarding facial aesthetics is not well established. The need for orthodontic treatment for this mixed dentition population is high (36,5%), possibly related to the fact that, orthodontic treatment is rarely applied in deciduous dentition and is more often recommended to be applied at phase I in early mixed dentition, as soon as the upper lateral incisors are erupted [23], so it is likely that our population is not well informed about orthodontic treatment. A recent governmental report [24] showed that only 10% of children with malocclusion and dental malposition benefited of orthodontic treatment in Romania. Children and adolescents mainly seek orthodontic treatment due to dissatisfaction with their dento-facial appearance, orthodontic counselling, and the influence of peers who wear braces [22].

Dissatisfaction with the body image is a complex indicator. During pre-pubertal and pubertal years, children's bodies are in transition regarding shape, weight status and appearance. Children have a unique vision of reality. Body image is influenced by media, parents, peers, romantic peers, all of whom shape beliefs about the ideal body. Internalization and perceived pressure to align oneself to social norms can be used to explain the links between measured and perceived body weight [25, 26]. In this study, dissatisfaction with body image was associated with poor self-perception of oral health status. This relation can be explained through psychological traits such as self-esteem, life satisfaction, quality of life, sense of coherence, anxiety and depression [27–33]. Several Delphi consensus studies have agreed that the prevention of the onset of body dissatisfaction [34] and childhood depression and anxiety disorders [35] can be achieved through a variety of positive parenting strategies that include healthy eating patterns discussions, establishing and maintaining a good relationship, being involved and supporting increasing autonomy, establishing family rules and consequences, and encouraging habits of good health.

Our study had several limitations. First, it is a cross sectional study. Then, a selection bias has to be considered, since our participants were self-selected from pupils attending primary school. Since our results are based on participants from urban area, which have higher access to healthcare services, it will be important to have a broader image of the impact of a diversified environment. The lack of data on parents' education level, on indicators of socio-economic status, socio-cultural status, oral health-related behaviours, are other limitations. However, the analysis was adjusted by gender, weight categories and oral clinical indicators.

Conclusions

Oral health perception is a good and cheap indicator of the tooth decay treatment need in pre-adolescents with mixed dentition, which can impact oral health outcomes and reduces risks of morbidity. Oral health surveillance in mixed dentition population should include information on self-perceived oral health. The association of self-perception of oral health with dissatisfaction with body image, but not BMI, underlines that even at this age, oral health is included in the general perception of body status. Given that body image dissatisfaction may exacerbate emotional distress, and because in adolescence there is an increased risk of developing a negative body image and an increased vulnerability to social-cultural influences, this should be a primary goal for clinical interventions. Planning for medical intervention should include therapeutic interventions appropriate to needs and motivational particularities of preadolescents.

Abbreviations

BMI: Body mass index; CI: Confidence interval; d/D: Decayed teeth (for deciduous dentition in lower case and for permanent teeth in uppercase); DAI: Dental aesthetic index; dmft/DMFT: Decayed, missing, filled teeth (for deciduous dentition in lower case and for permanent teeth in uppercase); f/F: filled teeth (for deciduous dentition in lower case and for permanent teeth in uppercase); GLM: General linear model; m/M: missing teeth (for deciduous dentition in lower case and for permanent teeth in uppercase); OR: Odds ratio; SD: Standard deviation; WHO: World Health Organization

Authors' contributions

AB, MP and BV designed the study; AB and HU were involved in clinical evaluation of participants, AB and CS analysed and interpreted the data, AB, HU and CS drafted the manuscript, MP and BV reviewed and completed the manuscript. All authors approved the final version of the manuscript.

Competing interests

The authors declare that they have no competing interests.

Author details

¹Department 2, Discipline of Maxillofacial Surgery, Faculty of Dentistry, "Victor Babeş" University of Medicine and Pharmacy Timişoara, 5 Take Ionescu Bvd, 300062 Timisoara, Romania. ²Department 3 Functional Sciences, "Victor Babeş" University of Medicine and Pharmacy Timişoara, 14 Spl. Tudor Vladimirescu, 300172 Timişoara, Romania. ³Department 14 Microbiology, "Victor Babeş" University of Medicine and Pharmacy Timişoara, 16 Victor Babeş Bvd, 300226 Timişoara, Romania.

References

1. Gururatana O, Baker SR, Robinson PG. Determinants of children's oral-health-related quality of life over time. Community Dent Oral Epidemiol. 2014;42(3):206–15. https://doi.org/10.1111/cdoe.12080.
2. Astrom AN, Mashoto K. Determinants of self-rated oral health status among school children in northern Tanzania. Int J Paediatr Dent. 2002;12:90–100. https://doi.org/10.1046/j.1365-263X.2002.00341.x.
3. Chalmers NI, Wislar JS, Boynes SG, Doherty M, Nový BB. Improving health in the United States: oral health is key to overall health. J Am Dent Assoc. 2017;148(7):477–80. https://doi.org/10.1016/j.adaj.2017.04.031.
4. Paula JS, Sarracini KLM, Meneghim MC, Pereira AC, Ortega EMM, Martins NS, Mialhe FL. Longitudinal evaluation of the impact of dental caries treatment on oral health-related quality of life among schoolchildren. Eur J Oral Sci. 2015;123:173–8.
5. Liu Z, McGrath C, Hägg U. The impact of malocclusion/orthodontic treatment need on the quality of life. A systematic review. Angle Orthod. 2009 May;79(3):585–91. https://doi.org/10.2319/042108-224.1.
6. da Rosa GN, Del Fabro JP, Tomazoni F, Tuchtenhagen S, Alves LS, Ardenghi TM. Association of malocclusion, happiness, and oral health–related quality of life (OHRQoL) in schoolchildren. J Public Health Dent. 2016;76:85–90. https://doi.org/10.1111/jphd.12111.
7. Foster Page LA, Thomson MW, Ukra A, Farella M. Factors influencing adolescents' oral health-related quality of life (OHRQoL). Int J Paediatr Dent. 2013;23:415–23.
8. Maida CA, Marcus M, Hays RD, et al. Qual Life Res. 2015;24:2739. https://doi.org/10.1007/s11136-015-1015-6.
9. Kantovitz KR, Pascon FM, Rontani RMP, Gavião MB, Pascon FM. Obesity and dental caries–a systematic review. Oral Health Prev Dent. 2006;4(2):137–44.
10. Mulasi-Pokhriyal U, Smith C. Assessing body image issues and body satisfaction/dissatisfaction among American children 9–18 years of age using mixed methodology. Body Image. 2010;7:341–8. https://doi.org/10.1016/j.bodyim.2010.08.002.
11. Paxton SJ, Franko DL. Body image and eating disorders. In: Cucciare MA, Weingardt KR, editors. Using technology to support evidence-based behavioral health practices: a Clinician's guide. 1st ed: Routledge; 2010.
12. Mellor D, McCabe M. Ricciardelli et al. sociocultural influences on body dissatisfaction and body change behaviors among Malaysian adolescents. Body Image. 2009;6:121–8. https://doi.org/10.1016/j.bodyim.2008.11.003.
13. National Institute of Statistics. Population Census 2011. Table 8. Stable population by ethnicity – counties, municipalities, cities, communes. 2013. [cited 2017 Apr 16] Available from: http://www.recensamantromania.ro/rezultate-2/. (Romanian).
14. WHO. WHO Anthro (version 3.2.2, January 2011) and macros. [cited 2017 Apr 16] Available from: http://www.who.int/childgrowth/software/en/.
15. Collins ME. Body figure perceptions and preferences among preadolescent children. Int J Eat Disord. 1991;10:199–208. https://doi.org/10.1002/1098-108X(199103)10:2<199::AID-EAT2260100209>3.0.CO;2-D.
16. WHO. Oral health surveys: basic methods. 5th ed. Geneva: ORH/EPID; 2013.
17. Dorobat V, Stanciu D. [Orthodontics and dento-facial orthopedics]. Editura Medicală Bucureşti, 2009. (Romanian).
18. Broadbent JM, Thomson WM. For debate: problems with the DMF index pertinent to dental caries data analysis. Community Dent Oral Epidemiol. 2005;33(6):400–9. https://doi.org/10.1111/j.1600-0528.2005.00259.x.
19. Pattussi MP, Anselmo Olinto MT, Hardy R, Sheiham A. Clinical, social and psychosocial factors associated with self-rated oral health in Brazilian adolescents. Community Dent Oral Epidemiol. 2007;35(5):377–86. https://doi.org/10.1111/j.1600-0528.2006.00339.x.
20. Ferraz NK, Nogueira LC, Pinheiro ML, Marques LS, Ramos-Jorge ML, Ramos-Jorge J. Clinical consequences of untreated dental caries and toothache in preschool children. Pediatr Dent. 2014;36(5):389–92.
21. Leal SC, Bronkhorst EM, Fan M, Frencken JE. Untreated Cavitated dentine lesions: impact on Children's quality of life. Caries Res. 2012;46:102–6. https://doi.org/10.1159/000336387.
22. Gonçalves Vieira-Andrade R, Martins de Paiva S, Silva Marques L. Impact of Malocclusions on Quality of Life from Childhood to Adulthood, Issues in Contemporary Orthodontics, Prof. Farid Bourzgui (Ed.), 2015. InTech, DOI: https://doi.org/10.5772/59485. Available from: https://www.intechopen.com/books/issues-in-contemporary-orthodontics/impact-of-malocclusions-on-quality-of-life-from-childhood-to-adulthood.
23. Suresh M, Ratnaditya A, Kattimani VS, Karpe S. One phase versus two phase treatment in mixed dentition: a critical review. J Int Oral Health. 2015;7(8):144–7.

24. National Institute of Public Health Bucharest. National Report of Oral Health status in children and young people. 2012. [cited 2017 Iun 18] Available from: http://insp.gov.ro/sites/cnepss/wp-content/uploads/2014/12/Raport-national-de-sanatate-orala-la-copii-si-tineri-2012.pdf. (Romanian).

25. Tatangelo G, McCabe M, Mellor D, Mealey A. A systematic review of body dissatisfaction and sociocultural messages related to the body among preschool children. Body image. 2016;18:86–95. https://doi.org/10.1016/j.bodyim.2016.06.003.

26. Voelker DK, Reel JJ, Greenleaf C. Weight status and body image perceptions in adolescents: current perspectives. Adolesc Health Med Ther. 2015;6:149–58. https://doi.org/10.2147/AHMT.S68344.

27. Benyamini Y, Leventhal H, Leventhal EA. Self-rated oral health as an independent predictor of self-rated general health, self-esteem and life satisfaction. Soc Sci Med. 2004;59(5):1109–16. https://doi.org/10.1016/j.socscimed.2003.12.021.

28. Biby EL. The relationship between body dysmorphic disorder and depression, self-esteem, somatization, and obsessive–compulsive disorder. J Clin Psychol. 1998;54(4):489–99.

29. Locker D. Self-esteem and socioeconomic disparities in self-perceived oral health. J Public Health Dent. 2009;69(1):1–8. https://doi.org/10.1111/j.1752-7325.2008.00087.x.

30. Lindmark U, Hakeberg M, Hugoson A. Sense of coherence and its relationship with oral health–related behaviour and knowledge of and attitudes towards oral health. Comm Dent Oral Epidemiol. 2011;39(6):542–53. https://doi.org/10.1111/j.1600-0528.2011.00627.x.

31. Sischo L, Broder HL. Oral health-related quality of life: what, why, how, and future implications. J Dent Res. 2011;90(11):1264–70. https://doi.org/10.1177/0022034511399918.

32. Anttila S, Knuuttila M, Ylöstalo P, Joukamaa M. Symptoms of depression and anxiety in relation to dental health behavior and self-perceived dental treatment need. Eur J Oral Sci. 2006;114(2):109–14. https://doi.org/10.1111/j.1600-0722.2006.00334.x.

33. Stevens SD, Herbozo S, Morrell HE, Schaefer LM, Thompson JK. Adult and childhood weight influence body image and depression through weight stigmatization. J Health Psychol. 2016;22(8):1084–93. https://doi.org/10.1177/1359105315624749.

34. Hart LM, Damiano SR, Chittleborough P, Paxton SJ, Jorm AF. Parenting to prevent body dissatisfaction and unhealthy eating patterns in preschool children: a Delphi consensus study. Body Image. 2014;11(4):418–25. https://doi.org/10.1016/j.bodyim.2014.06.010.

35. Yap MB, Fowler M, Reavley N, Jorm AF. Parenting strategies for reducing the risk of childhood depression and anxiety disorders: a Delphi consensus study. J Affect Disord. 2015;183:330–8. https://doi.org/10.1016/j.jad.2015.05.031.

14

An observation on the severity of periodontal disease in past cigarette smokers suffering from rheumatoid arthritis- evidence for a long-term effect of cigarette smoke exposure?

Márk Antal[1*], Emese Battancs[1], Márta Bocskai[2], Gábor Braunitzer[3] and László Kovács[2]

Abstract

Background: Rheumatoid arthritis (RA) and cigarette smoking are both risk factors for periodontal disease (PD). Previous research suggests that systemic inflammatory conditions and cigarette smoking may act in synergy, and their co-occurrence leads to a much higher risk of developing severe stage PD than what the combination of their individual risks would suggest. We originally sought to test this in the case of RA, but it turned out that the majority of our patients were former smokers, who smoked for prolonged periods in the past. For that reason, we decided to shift our focus toward the possible effects of past chronic cigarette smoke exposure.

Methods: The data of 73 RA patients and 77 healthy controls were analyzed. The participants received a full-mouth periodontal examination to determine their periodontal status. Rheumatological indices and data on past tobacco use were also recorded. Both the patient and the control groups were divided into former smoker and non-smoker subgroups for the analyses. Non-smoker controls were used as the reference group.

Results: In the control group, smoking in history increased the odds of developing both the moderate and the severe stages of PD, but the change was not statistically significant. RA significantly, increased the odds of developing both stages in itself, but the highest odds were seen in the former smoker RA group.

Conclusion: Based on this surprising observation of ours, we hypothesize that chronic cigarette smoke might bring about permanent changes in the periodontal tissues, leading to their hypersensitivity to inflammatory challenges.

Keywords: Rheumatoid arthritis, Periodontal disease, Chronic inflammation, Late sequelae, Tobacco smoking

Background

The connection between periodontal disease (PD) and various systemic conditions of an autoimmune/dysimmune background is well documented [1–5]. Rheumatoid arthritis (RA) is an immune mediated disease with a particularly well established link to PD [6–9]. While the exact immunological mechanisms have not been clarified, there is evidence to suggest that the presence of citrullinated proteins (and antibodies against them) is the link [10–12].

In this respect, the role of the periodontal pathogen, *Porphyromonas gingivalis* is emphasized, the only periodontal pathogen that expresses the citrullinating enzyme peptidyl-arginine deiminase (PPAD) [9, 13, 14]. Compared to the general population, subjects with PD are at an increased risk of developing RA, and vice versa [9, 15], which suggests that once they are established, they mutually aggravate each other.

Cigarette smoking is a known risk factor for both PD [16–18] and RA [19–21]. Cigarette smoking promotes oral bacterial colonization [22] and smoking itself has been shown to promote citrullination [23], evidenced by the fact that an association was found between tobacco

---

* Correspondence: antal.mark@stoma.szote.u-szeged.hu
[1]Faculty of Dentistry, Department of Aesthetic and Operative Dentistry, University of Szeged, 6720 Tisza Lajos körút, Szeged 64, Hungary
Full list of author information is available at the end of the article

exposure and anti-cyclic citrullinated peptide (anti-CCP) titers in RA patients [24]. It follows that cigarette smoking may be an additional aggravating factor in both PD and RA, especially when the two conditions are comorbid.

In 2014, we published a study about the effects of cigarette smoking on the severity of PD in psoriasis [25]. In that study, we found that while both psoriasis and smoking significantly elevated the odds that the individual will develop advanced PD, when both risk factors were present, the odds multiplied, well beyond the combined odds. We concluded that cigarette smoking probably acted as a permissive factor, and we articulated a hypothesis about the possible role of toll-like receptor 4 (TLR-4). The hypothesis was that smoking exerts this effect through the upregulation of TLR-4.

In their review [26], Baka and co-workers point out that as cigarette smoking promotes bacterial colonization, it may well be that smokers are exposed to an increased burden of *P. gingivalis*, whereby they are constantly exposed to a potent antigen.

Based on these premises, we wished to find out about if smoking acts as a booster of periodontal deterioration also in the context of RA. This is an important question with practical bearings. For instance, severe PD was reported to hamper the efficacy of anti-TNF (tumor necrosis factor) therapy [27].

To answer the question, we collected data on 82 RA patients and 100 controls who met all the inclusion and exclusion criteria and also gave their informed consent. At this point, though, we were faced with a difficulty: most of our patients turned out to be non-smokers (NS). Only eight of them smoked at the time of the study, and the rest had either quit or never ever smoked in their lives. The majority of our patient sample, therefore, consisted of non-smokers and former smokers (FS) who had quit smoking long before.

While we have a wealth of information about the immunological consequences of current smoking [28–31], we know almost nothing about the permanent immunological changes that chronic exposure to cigarette smoke may bring about - and that may remain even if the smoker quits. Considering that the majority of our formerly smoking patients had smoked for at least a decade before they quit, and that chronic exposure to cigarette smoke was proven to induce genome level changes [32–34], we decided to shift our focus and concentrate on the effects of past smoking. We hypothesized that the periodontal status of patients with no smoking history would be significantly poorer than that of healthy controls (the effect of RA), and we wished to know if past smoking would be associated with poorer periodontal status to any extent. We were also interested in the relationship between the rheumatological factors and the periodontal status.

Methods

Both RA patients and healthy controls were recruited on a voluntary basis.

Patients were eligible for the study if they met the 2010 European League against Rheumatism and American College of Rheumatology (EULAR/ACR) criteria for rheumatoid arthritis [35]. Exclusion criteria for both groups were determined based on the literature of the subject and included obesity (body mass index - BMI≥30), excessive alcohol consumption, drug abuse, diabetes mellitus, diseases causing neutropenia and local or systemic inflammatory conditions (other than RA) [36]. Poor oral hygiene, defined as Simplified Oral Health Index (OHI-S)- > 3 [37] was also an exclusion criterion.

Required sample size was calculated with G*Power 3.1. 5. (University of Kiel, Germany), a software designed especially for statistical power and sample size computation [38]. The software allows the computation of achieved statistical power (post-hoc) and required sample size (a priori). As mostly categorical variables were to be analyzed, a priori sample size estimation was performed for crosstabs/chi square/contingency tables, with the following input parameters: effect size (w): 0.3; α: 0. 05;power (1-β): 0.9; df: 3. Required sample size turned out to be $n = 158$ (for four groups: RA smoker/former smoker; control smoker/former smoker).

RA Patients ($n = 82$) were recruited from among the patients of the Department of Rheumatology, University of Szeged. The control group ($n = 100$) was recruited from among people attending mandatory lung screening in the same city and the same period. After removing the actual smokers from the sample, we were left with 150 participants (73 patients and 77 controls), yielding a statistical power of 0.88.

The study was approved by the Institutional and Regional Ethics Committee for Medical Biological Research at the University of Szeged (approval No.144/2014), and the study design conformed to the Declaration of Helsinki in all respects. Written informed consent was obtained from all participants.

Demographic and tobacco use data were collected by a questionnaire. Participants were divided into FS and non-smoker groups, based on their self-reported tobacco use in the past. In both the patient and the control groups, a subject was considered a FS if they smoked for at least one year in the past as a habit and without interruption. Sixty-four percent of the FS controls and 74 % of the FS RA patients provided tobacco use information that could be used for the analyses.

The clinical disease severity of PD is still a matter of debate, and several methods are available in the literature [39]. We decided to use the staging proposed by Fernandes and colleagues [40]. The reason for using this

Table 1 The applied clinical staging and the corresponding pathological/pathophysiological changes [40, 41]

CLINICAL STAGING (Fernandes et al., 2009)	PATHOLOGY/PATHOPHYSIOLOGY (Ohlrich et al., 2009)
1.NO CLINICAL SIGNS- no clinical attachment loss (CAL) or bleeding on probing (BOP)	(NO LESION- NOT CLASSIFIED EXPLICITLY IN OHLRICH ET AL.)
(GINGIVITIS-NOT CLASSIFIED EXPLICITLY IN FERNANDES ET AL.)	1. INITIAL LESION – up to 4 days following plaque accumulation. Polymorphonuclear leukocytes (PMN), complement activation, loss of connective tissue. Mast cells release tumor necrosis factor alpha, PMNs migrate into the gingival sulcus, but as the bacteria are protected by the biofilm, abortive phagocytosis occurs. PMNs release lysosomal contents, which leads to further tissue destruction.
2.EARLY PERIODONTITIS- CAL $\geq$1 mm in $\geq$2 teeth	2. EARLY/STABLE LESION- 7-21 days after plaque accumulation, clinically evident approximately from day 12. Dominantly macrophages and lymphocytes (CD4$^+$:CD8$^+$ 2:1). Perivascular inflammatory infiltrate. Intercellular spaces between epithelial cells widen, bacterial products infiltrate the gingival tissues at a higher rate. Escalation of response. If plaque removed, tissue remodeling can take place.
3.MODERATE PERIODONTITIS- 3 sites with CAL $\geq$4 mm and at least 2 sites with probing depth (PRD) $\geq$3 mm	3. ESTABLISHED OR PROGRESSIVE LESION- dominantly a B cell/plasma cell response. High levels of IL-1 and IL-6: connective tissue loss, breakdown of bone.
4. SEVERE PERIODONTITIS- CAL $\geq$6 mm in $\geq$2 teeth and PRD $\geq$5 mm in $\geq$1 site	4. ADVANCED LESION- Overt loss of attachment. High levels of IL-1, TNF α and PGE$_2$ stimulate fibroblasts and macrophages to produce matrix metalloproteases. The junctional epithelium progresses in apical direction (deepening periodontal pocket). Oligoclonal Th$_2$ (CD4$^+$) dominance.

classification was that its clinical staging matches the pathological/pathophysiological changes in PD very well [41], and that we had had previous experience with it [25]. The staging requires the following parameters to be recorded: bleeding on probing (BOP; the presence or absence of bleeding within 15 s after probing), probing depth (PRD; in millimeters), and clinical attachment level (CAL; to describe the position of the soft tissue in relation to the cemento-enamel junction). All subjects received a full-mouth examination and their periodontal status was classified into one of the four categories of the staging: healthy(0); early (1); moderate (2); severe (3). For the examination, Williams probes (Hu-Friedy Manufacturing Co., Chicago, USA) were used. Table 1 shows the categories of the applied staging and the corresponding pathological/pathophysiological status. Although there is some lack of overlap in the first stage of the PD, it may not influence any of the results as nor the initial lesion, nor the gingivitis is having real influence on the immune sytem and the gingival health. Gingivitis itself is a reversible form of the disease.

To characterize the patient population from a rheumatological point of view, the following indices and laboratory values were recorded: IgM rheumatoid factor seropositivity and levels (RF) measured with nephelometry, anti-citrullinated peptide antibody (ACPA) seropositivity and levels with antigenic specificity to mutated citrullinated vimentin (aMCV) measured with ELISA, disease activity score (DAS28-ESR) at the latest visit and its average of the past 12 months, and the HAQ-DI disability index. Data on the conventional and biological disease modifying antirheumatic drug (DMARD) and corticosteroid therapy of the patients were also recorded. Laboratory values were determined as part of the routine examinations (i.e. not especially for this study).

We divided the subjects into four groups based on the presence/absence of RA and smoking in the past. To express the odds that a member of a given group develops a given clinical degree of periodontal disease, multinomial logistic regression analysis was conducted and the odds ratios were calculated. In the multinomial

Table 2 Demographic and tobacco use characteristics of the studied groups

Group	Sex ratio F(%):M(%)	Smoke-free for (mean years, SD)	Smoked for (mean years, SD)	Cigarettes smoked per day (rounded average, SD)	Age in years (mean, SD)
CNS (n = 55)	44(80):11(20)	NA	NA	NA	55.7 (13.3)
CS (n = 22)	12(54):10 (45)	11.3(12.5)	13.8(10.2)	11 (7.9)	58.1 (13.5)
PNS (n = 42)	33(79): 9 (21)	NA	NA	NA	56.5 (12.7)
PS (n = 31)	24(77):7 (23)	16.4(12.2)	18.3(11.4)	14 (10.2)	59.3 (13.6)

CNS control, never smoked, *CS* control, used to smoke, *PNS* patient, never smoked, *PS* patient, used to smoke

Table 3 A brief rheumatological characterization of the patient population by smoking in patient history

Rheumatoid factor positivity [> 30 U/ml] n (%)	FS	20 (64.5)
	NS	24 (57.1)
Anti-citrullinated peptide antibody positivity [> 20 U/ml] n(%)	FS	20 (64.5)
	NS	25 (59.5)
Patients on conventional DMARD therapy n (%)	FS	25 (80.6)
	NS	36 (85.7)
Patients on biological DMARD therapy (%)	FS	17 (54.8)
	NS	18 (42.8)
DAS28 at visit mean (SD; range)	FS	(n = 21) 3.10 (1.42; 0.97–6.52)
	NS	(n = 35) 2.94 (1.30; 0.79–6.33)
Average DAS28 in the previous 12 months mean (SD; range)	FS	(n = 10) 3.20 (1.68; 1.38–5.22)
	NS	(n = 8) 2.41 (1.30; 1.20–5.30)
HAQ mean (SD)	FS	(n = 15) 0.98 (0.84)
	NS	(n = 7) 2.21 (0.70)

FS former smoker, *NS* never smoked, *DMARD* disease-modifying antirheumatic drug, *DAS28* disease activity score, *HAQ* score on the health assessment questionnaire for rheumatoid arthritis. Where data from not all patients were available, the actual number of patients is given in parentheses

model, disease severity (healthy, early, moderate, severe) was defined as the outcome variable, group was the factor, and age and sex were covariates. Within-group analyses (Mann-Whitney U tests) were also performed in the patient group, according to the smoking status, to see if past smoking had any effect on the rheumatological indices. For the analyses, SPSS 21.0 (IBM, USA) was used.

Results

The demographic and tobacco use characteristics of the four studied groups are given in Table 2. It can be seen that the vast majority of the participants were females. This is because RA affects predominantly women and the control group was selected to match the patient group age- and gender-wise as closely as possible.

The within-group comparisons in the patient group did not indicate significant difference in any of the rheumatological indices between FS and non-smokers (data not shown). To test the effect of RF/aMCV positivity on periodontal status, a separate multinomial regression analysis was conducted. While no statistically significant effects were found, seropositivity for RF increased the odds of the moderate stage to 1.65, and that of the severe stage to 2.51. The rheumatological indices of the patient group are summarized in Table 3.

The periodontal status and CAL data of each group is shown in Table 4. It is noteworthy that while the majority of the cases in both control groups falls into the healthy and early stages, in the patient groups the situation is just the opposite. This tendency is the most remarkable among the patients who used to smoke. 81% of them were classified as having moderate or severe PD. Note also that in the patient groups nobody was found who could be classified as periodontally healthy.

The results of the multinomial regression analysis are given in Table 5. The analysis indicated no significant influence of either age or sex on periodontal status. Male

Table 4 Periodontal status in the examined groups according to Fernandes et al. (38). Data are given as n (%, rounded percentages). CAL values are also shown (mm, mean ± SD). The conventions are the same as in Table 1

	RA				Control			
	n		CAL		n		CAL	
Total	73		3.55 (±1.62)		77		2.03 (±1.17)	
	PNS		PS		CNS		CS	
	n	CAL	n	CAL	n	CAL	n	CAL
Total	42	3.18 (±1.39)	31	4.06 (±1.79)	55	2.08 (±1.26)	22	1.91 (±0.89)
Healthy	0	NA	0	NA	8 (15)	0.67 (±0.30)	4 (18)	0.76 (±0.40)
Early	12 (29)	1.81 (±0.21)	6 (19)	1.89 (±0.31)	30 (55)	1.52 (±0.39)	12 (55)	1.76 (±0.37)
Modrate	22 (52)	3.07 (±0.32)	12 (39)	3.50 (±0.89)	13 (24)	3.35 (±0.21)	5 (23)	3.19 (±0.25)
Severe	8 (19)	5.52 (±1.21)	13 (42)	5.57 (±1.46)	4 (7)	4.99 (±0.14)	1 (5)	4.72 (±NA)

Table 5 Results of the multinomial regression analysis. The odds ratios (Exp(B)) express the odds that a member of the given group develops the given stage of periodontal disease. Controls who never smoked and early stage periodontal disease served as reference (as no periodontally healthy individuals were found in the patient group, healthy could not be used as reference). B: correlation coefficient; df: degrees of freedom

Periodontal status (reference: early)		B	df	Sig.	Exp(B)	95% CI for Exp(B)
moderate	RA- used to smoke	1.529	1	0.011	4.615	1.423–14.966
	RA- never smoked	1.442	1	0.003	4.231	1.623–11.030
	Control- used to smoke	0.932	1	0.090	2.538	0.866–7.442
	Control-never smoked	–	–	–	–	–
	Male sex	0.223	1	0.643	1.250	0.487–3.212
	Age	0.002	1	0.896	1.002	
severe	RA- used to smoke	2.788	1	0.000	16.250	3.917–67.412
	RA- never smoked	1.609	1	0.022	5.000	1.265–19.762
	Control- used to smoke	0.405	1	0.666	1.500	0.238–9.465
	Control-never smoked	–	–	–	–	–
	Male sex	0.839	1	0.867	2.315	0.703–7.619
	Age	0.028	1	0.176	1.029	0.972–1.033

sex appears to be associated with an increased risk for both the moderate and the severe stages, but given the under-representation of the male sex in this study, we would not draw conclusions from this. As for the odds of developing the moderate or severe stages, these were significantly higher in both patient groups for both stages as compared to controls who never smoked. Controls who used to smoke did not have significantly higher odds to develop any of these stages than controls who never smoked, while an increment was definitely seen. The highest significant odds ratio for the severe stage (16.25) was found in the RA group of FS.

Discussion

A part of these findings is merely the corroboration of known facts. RA has been known as a risk factor for PD for some time [6–8], and our results demonstrate the same: the presence of RA in itself is enough to significantly increase the odds that the patient will develop a more severe stage of PD.

We also found that past smoking did not have a significant effect on any of the rheumatological indices and that there was no association between these indices and periodontal status. The lack of the effect of past smoking on the rheumatological status as expressed by these indices might be best explained by the time passed since the patient stopped smoking. While cigarette smoke must have been an extra immunological stimulus while the patient was still smoking, and it might as well have boosted the immunological memory against citrullinated proteins [42], these effects are unlikely to be reflected in indices characterizing a much narrower time window.

How come that no association was found between the specific RA indices and the periodontal status, while, as pointed out before, being in the RA group in itself significantly increased the odds of the more severe PD stages? Given that other studies describing larger populations found significant association with rheumatoid factor positivity and anti-citrullinated peptide antibody production [43, 44], we think that our sample size was probably too small to allow reliable assessment at the level of the individual indices, considering their greater variability.

The main finding of this study, however, is also the most difficult to explain. The finding that the FS RA patients had the highest and significant odds ratio for the severe stage of PD is really an unexpected one. From the results it appears that the effect is not mediated by the actual rheumatological status, the presence of RA with a longer period of cigarette smoke exposure in the past is enough. This suggests that long-term cigarette smoking might permanently sensitize the periodontium, but at this point we could only speculate about the possible mechanisms, and it is because of that reason that we put this up for debate.

Conclusions

While this study definitely has its limitations, we think that our quasi-accidental finding about the effect of past smoking on periodontal health in RA deserves attention. This finding implies that long-term exposure to cigarette smoke might have a permanent sensitizing effect on the human periodontal tissues, which is not reversible by quitting smoking.

Abbreviations
ACP: Anti-citrullinated peptide antibody; aMCV: Mutated citrullinated vimentin; anti-CCP: Anti-cyclic citrullinated peptide; anti-TNF: Anti-tumor necrosis factor; BMI: Body mass index; BOP: Bleeding on probing;

CAL: Clinical attachment level; CNS: Control, never smoked; CS: Control, used to smoke; DAS28-ESR: Disease activity score; FS: Former smokers; NS: Non-smokers; OHI-S: Simplified Oral Health Index; PD: Periodontal disease; PNS: Patient, never smoked; PPAD: Peptidyl-arginine deiminase; PRD: Probing depth; PS: Patient, used to smoke; RA: Rheumatoid arthritis; RF: Rheumatoid factor; TLR-4: Toll-like receptor 4

Authors' contributions
MA organized the study; MA and EB performed the periodontal examinations and recorded patient data; MB and LK performed the rheumatological examinations and recorded patient data; GB performed the data analysis; EB, MB, LK, MA and GB prepared the manuscript. All authors have read and approved the final version of the manuscript.

Competing interests
The authors declare that they have no competing interests.

Author details
[1]Faculty of Dentistry, Department of Aesthetic and Operative Dentistry, University of Szeged, 6720 Tisza Lajos körút, Szeged 64, Hungary. [2]Faculty of Medicine, Department of Rheumatology and Immunology, University of Szeged, 6725 Kálvária sugárút, Szeged 57, Hungary. [3]Laboratory for Perception & Cognition and Clinical Neuroscience, Nyírő Gyula Hospital, 1135 Lehel utca, Budapest 59, Hungary.

References
1. Kim J, Amar S. Periodontal disease and systemic conditions: a bidirectional relationship. Odontology. 2006;94(1):10–21.
2. Grossi SG, Genco RJ. Periodontal disease and diabetes mellitus: a two-way relationship. Ann Periodontol. 1998;3(1):51–61.
3. Shlossman M. Diabetes mellitus and periodontal disease–a current perspective. Compend. 1994;15(8):1018. 1020–1014 passim; quiz 1032
4. Preus HR, Khanifam P, Kolltveit K, Mork C, Gjermo P. Periodontitis in psoriasis patients: a blinded, case-controlled study. Acta Odontol Scand. 2010;68(3):165–70.
5. Shlossman M, Knowler WC, Pettitt DJ, Genco RJ. Type 2 diabetes mellitus and periodontal disease. J Am Dent Assoc. 1990;121(4):532–6.
6. Mercado F, Marshall RI, Klestov AC, Bartold PM. Is there a relationship between rheumatoid arthritis and periodontal disease? J Clin Periodontol. 2000;27(4):267–72.
7. Mercado FB, Marshall RI, Bartold PM. Inter-relationships between rheumatoid arthritis and periodontal disease. A review. J Clin Periodontol. 2003;30(9):761–72.
8. Mercado FB, Marshall RI, Klestov AC, Bartold PM. Relationship between rheumatoid arthritis and periodontitis. J Periodontol. 2001;72(6):779–87.
9. Koziel J, Mydel P, Potempa J. The link between periodontal disease and rheumatoid arthritis: an updated review. Curr Rheumatol Rep. 2014; 16(3):408.
10. Nesse W, Westra J, van der Wal JE, Abbas F, Nicholas AP, Vissink A, Brouwer E. The periodontium of periodontitis patients contains citrullinated proteins which may play a role in ACPA (anti-citrullinated protein antibody) formation. J Clin Periodontol. 2012;39(7):599–607.
11. Detert J, Pischon N, Burmester GR, Buttgereit F. The association between rheumatoid arthritis and periodontal disease. Arthritis Res Ther. 2010;12(5):218.
12. Lundberg K, Wegner N, Yucel-Lindberg T, Venables PJ. Periodontitis in RA- the citrullinated enolase connection. Nat Rev Rheumatol. 2010;6(12):727–30.
13. Hendler A, Mulli TK, Hughes FJ, Perrett D, Bombardieri M, Houri-Haddad Y, Weiss EI, Nissim A. Involvement of autoimmunity in the pathogenesis of aggressive periodontitis. J Dent Res. 2010;89(12):1389–94.
14. Wegner N, Wait R, Sroka A, Eick S, Nguyen KA, Lundberg K, Kinloch A, Culshaw S, Potempa J, Venables PJ. Peptidylarginine deiminase from Porphyromonas gingivalis citrullinates human fibrinogen and alpha-enolase: implications for autoimmunity in rheumatoid arthritis. Arthritis Rheum. 2010; 62(9):2662–72.
15. Pons-Fuster A, Rodriguez Agudo C, Galvez Munoz P, Saiz Cuenca E, Pina Perez FM, Lopez-Jornet P. Clinical evaluation of periodontal disease in patients with rheumatoid arthritis: a cross-sectional study. Quintessence Int. 2015;46(9):817–22.
16. Bergstrom J. Cigarette smoking as risk factor in chronic periodontal disease. Community Dent Oral Epidemiol. 1989;17(5):245–7.
17. Tonetti MS. Cigarette smoking and periodontal diseases: etiology and management of disease. Ann Periodontol. 1998;3(1):88–101.
18. Martinez-Canut P, Lorca A, Magan R. Smoking and periodontal disease severity. J Clin Periodontol. 1995;22(10):743–9.
19. Heliovaara M, Aho K, Aromaa A, Knekt P, Reunanen A. Smoking and risk of rheumatoid arthritis. J Rheumatol. 1993;20(11):1830–5.
20. Hazes JM, Dijkmans BA, Vandenbroucke JP, de Vries RR, Cats A. Lifestyle and the risk of rheumatoid arthritis: cigarette smoking and alcohol consumption. Ann Rheum Dis. 1990;49(12):980–2.
21. Costenbader KH, Karlson EW. Cigarette smoking and autoimmune disease: what can we learn from epidemiology? Lupus. 2006;15(11):737–45.
22. Kumar PS, Matthews CR, Joshi V, de Jager M, Aspiras M. Tobacco smoking affects bacterial acquisition and colonization in oral biofilms. Infect Immun. 2011;79(11):4730–8.
23. Makrygiannakis D, Hermansson M, Ulfgren AK, Nicholas AP, Zendman AJ, Eklund A, Grunewald J, Skold CM, Klareskog L, Catrina AI. Smoking increases peptidylarginine deiminase 2 enzyme expression in human lungs and increases citrullination in BAL cells. Ann Rheum Dis. 2008;67(10):1488–92.
24. Lee DM, Phillips R, Hagan EM, Chibnik LB, Costenbader KH, Schur PH. Quantifying anti-cyclic citrullinated peptide titres: clinical utility and association with tobacco exposure in patients with rheumatoid arthritis. Ann Rheum Dis. 2009;68(2):201–8.
25. Antal M, Braunitzer G, Mattheos N, Gyulai R, Nagy K. Smoking as a permissive factor of periodontal disease in psoriasis. PLoS One. 2014;9(3):e92333.
26. Baka Z, Buzas E, Nagy G. Rheumatoid arthritis and smoking: putting the pieces together. Arthritis Res Ther. 2009;11(4):238.
27. Savioli C, Ribeiro AC, Fabri GM, Calich AL, Carvalho J, Silva CA, Viana VS, Bonfa E, Siqueira JT. Persistent periodontal disease hampers anti-tumor necrosis factor treatment response in rheumatoid arthritis. J Clin Rheumatol. 2012;18(4):180–4.
28. O'Leary SM, Coleman MM, Chew WM, Morrow C, McLaughlin AM, Gleeson LE, O'Sullivan MP, Keane J. Cigarette smoking impairs human pulmonary immunity to Mycobacterium tuberculosis. Am J Respir Crit Care Med. 2014; 190(12):1430–6.
29. Lee J, Taneja V, Vassallo R. Cigarette smoking and inflammation: cellular and molecular mechanisms. J Dent Res. 2012;91(2):142–9.
30. Arnson Y, Shoenfeld Y, Amital H. Effects of tobacco smoke on immunity, inflammation and autoimmunity. J Autoimmun. 2010;34(3):J258–65.
31. Morris GF, Danchuk S, Wang Y, Xu B, Rando RJ, Brody AR, Shan B, Sullivan DE. Cigarette smoke represses the innate immune response to asbestos. Physiol Rep. 2015;3(12). https://doi.org/10.14814/phy2.12652.
32. Lee KW, Pausova Z. Cigarette smoking and DNA methylation. Front Genet. 2013;4:132.
33. Dogan MV, Shields B, Cutrona C, Gao L, Gibbons FX, Simons R, Monick M, Brody GH, Tan K, Beach SR, et al. The effect of smoking on DNA methylation of peripheral blood mononuclear cells from African American women. BMC Genomics. 2014;15:151.
34. Zeilinger S, Kuhnel B, Klopp N, Baurecht H, Kleinschmidt A, Gieger C, Weidinger S, Lattka E, Adamski J, Peters A, et al. Tobacco smoking leads to extensive genome-wide changes in DNA methylation. PLoS One. 2013;8(5):e63812.
35. Aletaha D, Neogi T, Silman AJ, Funovits J, Felson DT, Bingham CO 3rd, Birnbaum NS, Burmester GR, Bykerk VP, Cohen MD, et al. Rheumatoid arthritis classification criteria: an American College of Rheumatology/ European league against rheumatism collaborative initiative. Arthritis Rheum. 2010;62(9):2569–81.
36. Genco RJ, Borgnakke WS. Risk factors for periodontal disease. Periodontology 2000. 2013;62(1):59–94.

37. Greene JC, Vermillion JR. The simplified oral hygiene index. J Am Dent Assoc. 1964;68:7–13.

38. Faul F, Erdfelder E, Lang AG, Buchner A. G*power 3: a flexible statistical power analysis program for the social, behavioral, and biomedical sciences. Behav Res Methods. 2007;39(2):175–91.

39. Leroy R, Eaton KA, Savage A. Methodological issues in epidemiological studies of periodontitis–how can it be improved? BMC Oral Health. 2010;10:8.

40. Fernandes JK, Wiegand RE, Salinas CF, Grossi SG, Sanders JJ, Lopes-Virella MF, Slate EH. Periodontal disease status in gullah african americans with type 2 diabetes living in South Carolina. J Periodontol. 2009;80(7):1062–8.

41. Ohlrich EJ, Cullinan MP, Seymour GJ. The immunopathogenesis of periodontal disease. Aust Dent J. 2009;54(Suppl 1):S2–10.

42. James EA, Rieck M, Pieper J, Gebe JA, Yue BB, Tatum M, Peda M, Sandin C, Klareskog L, Malmstrom V, et al. Citrulline-specific Th1 cells are increased in rheumatoid arthritis and their frequency is influenced by disease duration and therapy. Arthritis Rheumatol. 2014;66(7):1712–22.

43. The J, Ebersole JL. Rheumatoid factor (RF) distribution in periodontal disease. J Clin Immunol. 1991;11(3):132–42.

44. Terao C, Asai K, Hashimoto M, Yamazaki T, Ohmura K, Yamaguchi A, Takahashi K, Takei N, Ishii T, Kawaguchi T, et al. Significant association of periodontal disease with anti-citrullinated peptide antibody in a Japanese healthy population - the Nagahama study. J Autoimmun. 2015;59:85–90.

15

Root form and canal morphology of maxillary first premolars of a Yemeni population

Elham M. Senan[1*], Hatem A. Alhadainy[2,5], Thuraia M. Genaid[3] and Ahmed A. Madfa[1,4]

Abstract

Background: The purpose of this study was to investigate variations in the root canal systems of permanent maxillary first premolars in a Yemeni population using a clearing technique.

Methods: Two hundred fifty permanent maxillary first premolar teeth extracted from Yemeni individuals were collected. A small hole in the center of the occlusal surface of each tooth was prepared and pulp tissue was removed by immersion in 5.25% sodium hypochlorite. Teeth were stored in 5–10% nitric acid solution for 5–6 days. Next, teeth were rinsed, dried, and dehydrated using ascending concentrations of ethanol (70, 95, and 100%) successively for 12 h each. Waterproof black ink was injected into the dried dehydrated teeth. Stained teeth were then rendered clear by immersion in methyl salicylate solution (98%) until evaluation. Root canal morphology of each tooth was then examined.

Results: 54.8% of teeth were single-rooted, while 44.4% were double-rooted and only 0.8% had three separated roots. The most common canal system configuration was Vertucci type IV (55.6%). Eight specimens of the single-rooted premolars (3.2%) had new canal configurations that have not been recognized in previous published studies. Accessory canals and inter-canal communications were detected in a total of 52.8 and 34.4% of the specimens, respectively. The apical foramen was located centrally to the apex in 84.9% and apical deltas were found in 13.2% of the studied sample.

Conclusions: Yemeni permanent maxillary first premolars are mainly single-rooted and predominantly present Vertucci type IV canal morphology. The finding of additional canal configurations in this study is low but should be kept in mind when performing endodontic therapy for these teeth.

Keywords: Maxillary first premolar, Root canal morphology, Yemeni population, Clearing technique

Background

Root canal treatment is an essential part of comprehensive, quality dental care [1]. Successful endodontic treatment depends on complete root canal cleansing and shaping, three-dimensional hermetic root canal system obturation, and well-fitting coronal restorations with no leakage [2]. However, lack of thorough knowledge about teeth internal anatomy is one of the main reasons for treatment failure in endodontics. Thus, dental practitioners must be familiar with root canal morphology of

teeth to be treated. Such knowledge can aid in localization and negotiation of canals, as well as their subsequent management [3]. Unfortunately, root canal morphology varies greatly among different populations and even in different individuals within the same population. Therefore, an accurate knowledge of root canal morphology and its anatomical variations is essential for a successful root canal treatment [4].

Maxillary first premolar represents one of the most difficult teeth to be treated endodontically. A number of studies exhibited great variations in root anatomy and root canal morphology [5–13]. These variations in number and type of root canals are probably some of the most widely described anomalies in the literature. The presence of two canals must be considered normal [14, 15], but racial

* Correspondence: elhamdent06@yahoo.com
[1]Restorative and Prosthodontic Department, College of Dentistry, University of Science and Technology, Sana'a, Yemen
Full list of author information is available at the end of the article

differences in the root canal morphology of maxillary first premolar have been established [14–17].

Numerous studies have dealt with the evaluation of root canal morphology among different populations using various techniques, such as radiographs, decalcification, sectioning, replication and computerized-aided techniques [11–13, 18–21]. Of all these techniques, teeth clearing technique has considerable value in studying the morphology of root canal system. This is because clearing technique provides a three-dimensional view of the pulp cavity in relation to the exterior of teeth and allows a comprehensive examination of the pulp chamber and root canal system [4].

Clinically, it is important to identify the root and canal morphology prevalent in a population to reduce errors during root canal treatment. However, no study in Yemen has yet investigated the incidence of root canal configurations in any tooth. Therefore, the purpose of this study was to evaluate root and canal morphology of permanent maxillary first premolar teeth in a Yemeni population using a clearing technique.

Methods

The present study was approved by the Medical Ethics Committee (MEC) of Faculty of Medicine and Health Sciences at University of Science and Technology, Sana'a, Yemen (MECA NO.: 2016/13). Two hundred fifty recently extracted maxillary first premolars were collected from Yemeni patients attending various orthodontic clinics in Sana'a city. All teeth were identified at the time of extraction as maxillary first premolars from Yemeni patients attending orthodontic clinics. All patients signed consents acknowledging that their teeth will be used in the study. Teeth sample was collected in one and a half year.

Gender of the patient was not recorded and the age range was 20–45 years. The extracted teeth were thoroughly washed and cleaned to remove blood, saliva, or debris. They were then placed in 5.25% sodium hypochlorite solution for 30 min to remove organic debris from the surface. If there was calculus, it was removed using scaler (miniPiezon®, Electro Medical Systems EMS, Nyon, Switzerland). The cleaned specimens were then saved in 10% formalin solution (Oxford Laboratory, Mumbai, India) until further investigation was carried out [13].

External root morphology was determined visually and the findings were recorded. The specimens were classified into three groups based on the forms and number of roots as follows: single-rooted, double-rooted and three-rooted premolars. After recording the external root morphology of the specimens, a small hole in the center of the occlusal surface of each tooth was prepared as access to the pulp cavity. The specimens were then immersed in 5.25% sodium hypochlorite for 4 h to remove pulpal tissues. They were then rinsed under running tap water for 2 h and dried overnight. Afterwards, the specimens were decalcified with 10% nitric acid (Gainlad Chemical Co., Clwyd, UK) for 3 days followed by 5% nitric acid for 2–3 days at room temperature. The nitric acid solution was changed daily and agitated once a day to speed the process of decalcification. Then, the specimens were tested for softness by inserting a needle into the coronal region [13]. Decalcified specimens were then rinsed thoroughly and stored in water overnight and were bench-dried for 3 h. They were dehydrated in successive solutions of 70, 95 and 100% ethanol (Scharlau Co., European Union); each for 12 h. Once the dehydration process was completed, teeth were allowed to bench-dry for 2 h.

To clearly view the root canal system, waterproof black ink (Sanford rotring GmbH, Hamburg, Germany) was coronally injected into the pulp chambers using an endodontic irrigation syringe with a 27 gauge needle (BU Kwang Medical Inc., Seoul, Korea) until the ink was seen out through the apical foramen. Excess ink was then removed from the surface of the specimens with gauze soaked in ethanol. The stained specimens were then bench-dried for 4 h. Finally, transparency was achieved by placing the specimens in 98% methyl salicylate (ACROS Organics, New Jersey, USA).

Standardized pictures of the transparent cleared teeth were obtained by digital photographing both mesio-distally and bucco-lingually with a fixed distance (10 cm) and zoom (× 2.5). Photographs were taken with a light-illuminated white paper wet with methyl salicylate solution as a background. Evaluation of cleared teeth images was performed independently by two endodontists, each with an experience of more than five years. This was done after calibration to Vertucci canal types' classification. Inter-examiner agreement was evaluated using Kappa test on SPSS. The following observations were recorded: (i) number and type of root canals; (ii) presence and location of both accessory canals and inter-canal communications (ICCs); (iii) location and number of apical foramina and (iv) presence of apical deltas.

Results

Morphology and number of roots

Of the 250 maxillary first premolars studied, 137 teeth had one root (54.8%), whilst 36.4% were single-tipped root apex and the rest (18.4%) had double-tipped root apex. Of the 111 (44.4%) double-rooted premolars, 29.2% had two separated roots and 15.2% had two fused roots (they exhibited bifurcation in the apical third). Two premolars of the study sample (0.8%) had three separated roots (Fig. 1).

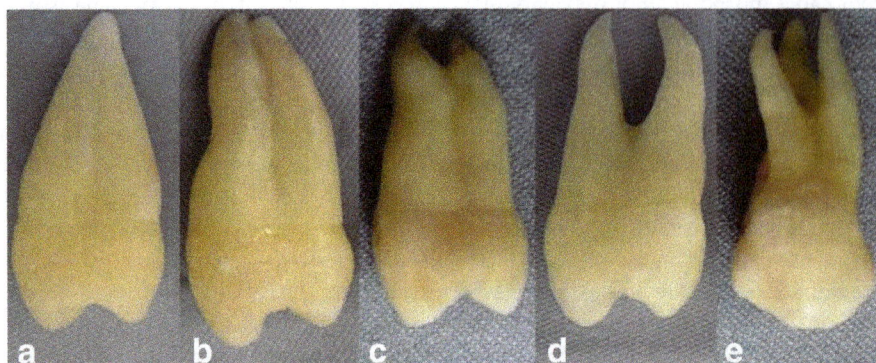

Fig. 1 Clinical photographs showing variations in number of root and morphology in permanent maxillary first premolars.**a** One root with single tip, (**b**) one root with double tips, (**c**) fused two roots, (**d**) separated two roots and (**e**) separated three roots

Number and type of root canals

The data for number and type of root canal system were revealed in Table 1. Single-rooted premolars demonstrated a wide variation of canal configurations (Figs. 2, 3,4). Seventy-four of the single-rooted specimens had one canal (54.1%) of either Vertucci type I (24.1%), III (14.6%), V (8.8%) or VII (6.6%) configuration, while 35.7% (*n* = 49) of the specimens had two canals of either type II (8.0%), IV (24.8%) or VI (2.9%) configuration. In addition, four cases of the single-rooted premolars had two canals (2.9%) of either Gulabivala type III (2.2%), or IV (0.7%) configuration. Furthermore, two cases of the single-rooted premolars had three canals (1.5%) of either Gulabivala type I (0.7%), or (3–2–1) Sert & Bayirli (0.7%) configuration (Table 1). Moreover, eight specimens of the single-rooted premolars had one canal (3.2%) with new canal configurations that have not been recognized in previous studies (Table 1, Fig. 4).

On the other hand, the double-rooted specimens exhibited Vertucci types IV and V in 105 (94.6%) and 2 (1.8%), respectively (Table 1, Figs. 2 and 3). In addition, both Gulabivala type III (1.8%) and (2–3-2) Sert & Bayirli (1.8%) configurations were found in two specimens. Of the three-rooted specimens, both cases exhibited three canals (Table 1, Fig. 2).

Accessory canals, inter-canal communications, apical foramina and deltas

Accessory canals were detected in a total of 132 (52.8%) of the specimens (Table 1). They were more frequently observed in the apical third as compared to cervical and middle thirds of the roots. Inter-canal communications (ICCs) were present in 86 (34.4%) of the specimens. ICCs were more prevalent in the single-rooted group (25.2%) compared to the double-rooted (9.2%) premolars (Table 1). The apical foramen was located centrally to the apex in 84.9% of the studied sample. Out of all the canals; canals exiting in single foramina were 77.5%; whereas, 19.7%

exited in two separate foramina. Only in 2.8% of the specimens, three apical foramina were present (Table 2). Apical deltas were found in 33 specimens (13.2%), of which 29 (11.6%) were in single-rooted group and 4 (1.6%) were in double-rooted premolars. However, apical deltas were not detected in the three-rooted premolars (Table 2).

Discussion

This is the first study in Yemen that evaluated root and canal morphology of permanent maxillary first premolar teeth. Several methods are used to investigate root canal morphology, including root sectioning, modeling, radiographic examination, tooth-clearing technique, cone-beam computed tomography (CBCT) and micro-computed tomography (micro-CT) imaging. Neelakantan et al. [22] compared the efficacy of four tomography methods with digital radiography and a tooth-clearing technique and concluded that only two tomography methods, CBCT and peripheral quantitative computed tomography, were as accurate as canal staining and tooth-clearing technique in identifying root canal systems. On the other hand, clearing technique was replaced with micro-CT technology which was proven to be the current reference method for the ex vivo study of the root canal anatomy. Micro-CT is preferred upon teeth clearing method due to the significant low detection of Vertucci type I canal in cleared teeth and fine anatomical details when compared to micro-CT method [23]. This limitation of teeth clearing method can be explained by incomplete diffusion of ink dye leading to distorted internal anatomy of cleared teeth and resulting in a different root canal type [23–25]. Although micro-CT has gained popularity because it provides accuracy, high resolution, and can be applied for detailed quantitative and qualitative measurements of the root canal anatomy, micro-CT is not available in all parts of the world, especially underdeveloped and developing countries. Moreover, the cost and radiation dose of micro-CT are other factors. In this study,

Table 1 The different anatomical features of Yemeni permanent maxillary first premolars

Features	Single-rooted n (%)	Double-rooted n (%)	Three-rooted n (%)	Total n (%)
Vertucci classification				
Type I (1)	33 (24.1%)	0 (0.0%)	0 (0.0%)	33 (13.2%)
Type II (2–1)	11 (8.0%)	0 (0.0%)	0 (0.0%)	11 (4.4%)
Type III (1–2-1)	20 (14.6%)	0 (0.0%)	0 (0.0%)	20 (8.0%)
Type IV (2)	34 (24.8%)	105 (94.6%)	0 (0.0%)	139 (55.6%)
Type V (1–2)	12 (8.8%)	2 (1.8%)	0 (0.0%)	14 (5.6%)
Type VI (2–1-2)	4 (2.9%)	0 (0.0%)	0 (0.0%)	4 (1.6%)
Type VII (1–2–1-2)	9 (6.6%)	0 (0.0%)	0 (0.0%)	9 (3.6%)
Type VIII (3)	0 (0.0%)	0 (0.0%)	2 (100%)	2 (0.8%)
Gulabivala classification				
Type I (3–1)	1 (0.7%)	0 (0.0%)	0 (0.0%)	1 (0.4%)
Type III (2–3)	3 (2.2%)	2 (1.8%)	0 (0.0%)	5 (2.0%)
Type IV (2–1–2-1)	1 (0.7%)	0 (0.0%)	0 (0.0%)	1 (0.4%)
Additional types				
Type (3–2-1) Sert & Bayirli	1 (0.7%)	0 (0.0%)	0 (0.0%)	1 (0.4%)
Type (2–3-2) Sert & Bayirli	0 (0.0%)	2 (1.8%)	0 (0.0%)	2 (0.8%)
New types				
Type (1–2-3)	2 (1.5%)	0 (0.0%)	0 (0.0%)	2 (0.8%)
Type (1–2–1–2-1)	2 (1.5%)	0 (0.0%)	0 (0.0%)	2 (0.8%)
Type (1–2–1-3-2)	1 (0.7%)	0 (0.0%)	0 (0.0%)	1 (0.4%)
Type (1–2–1–2-3-2)	1 (0.7%)	0 (0.0%)	0 (0.0%)	1 (0.4%)
Type (1–3-4)	1 (0.7%)	0 (0.0%)	0 (0.0%)	1 (0.4%)
Type (1–2–1-3-2)	1 (0.7%)	0 (0.0%)	0 (0.0%)	1 (0.4%)
No. accessory canals				
Accessory canals present	65 (47.4%)	66 (59.5%)	1 (50%)	132 (52.8%)
Accessory canals absent	72 (52.6%)	45 (40.5%)	1 (50%)	118 (47.2%)
Accessory canals in				
Cervical third	4 (5.4%)	9 (11.7%)	0 (0.0%)	13 (8.5%)
Middle third	16 (21.6%)	29 (37.7%)	1 (50%)	46 (30.1%)
Apical third	54 (73.0%)	39 (50.6%)	1 (50%)	94 (61.4%)
No. ICCs				
ICCs present	63 (46.0%)	23 (20.7%)	0 (0.0%)	86 (34.4%)
ICCs absent	74 (54.0%)	88 (79.3%)	2 (100%)	164 (65.6%)
ICCs in				
Cervical third	30 (33.0%)	13 (46.5%)	0 (0.0%)	43 (36.2%)
Middle third	39 (42.9%)	9 (32.1%)	0 (0.0%)	48 (40.3%)
Apical third	22 (24.1%)	6 (21.4%)	0 (0.0%)	28 (23.5%)

canal staining and teeth clearing technique was used as suggested by Peiris [13], to determine the root canal morphology. Apart from being inexpensive and easy to conduct, other important advantages of clearing technique include retaining the original form of the canal, enabling the assessment of canal form and morphology with maintenance of the samples for long time [22].

Root canal morphology has been classified in different ways by several investigators in the literature [4, 26–30]. Weine et al. [26] classification includes four types depending on the pattern of division of the main root canal of a tooth along its course from the floor of the pulp chamber to the root apex. Meanwhile, Vertucci [4] categorized the root canal morphology in a more descriptive manner into

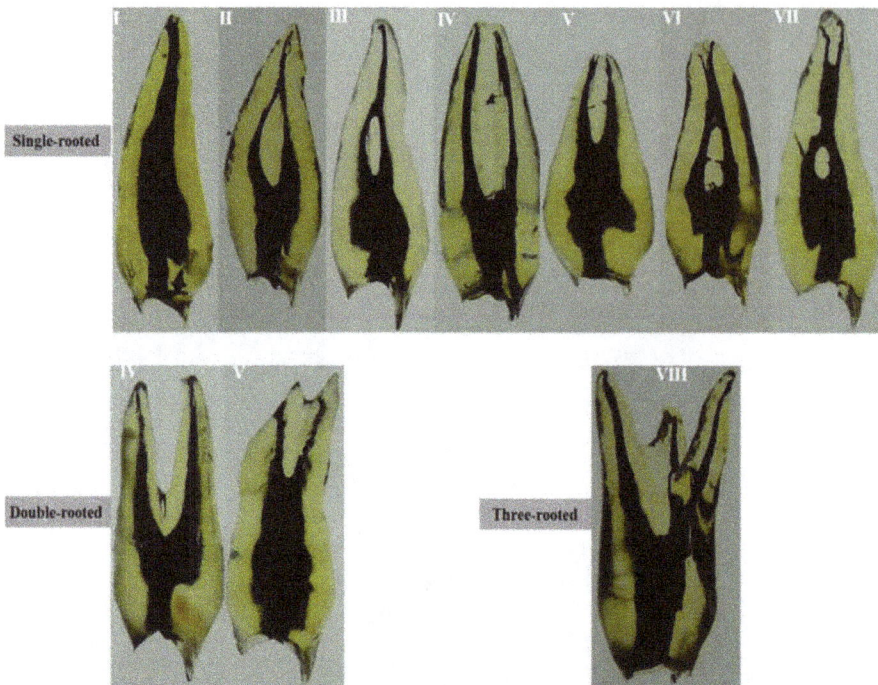

Fig. 2 Cleared teeth demonstrating Vertucci's canal configurations of Yemeni permanent maxillary first premolars

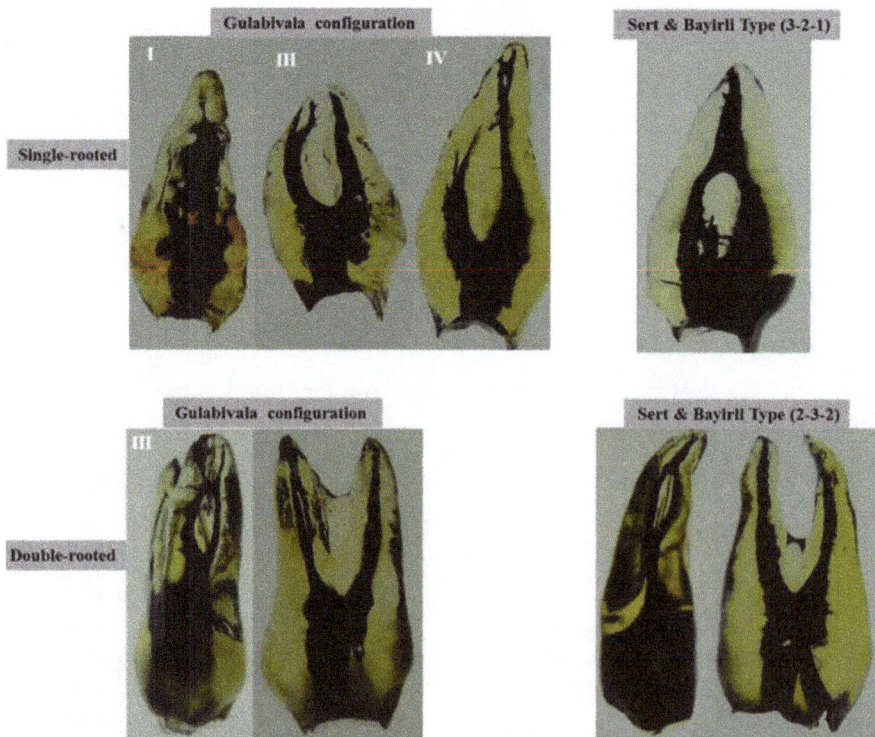

Fig. 3 Cleared teeth demonstrating supplemental canal configurations of Yemeni permanent maxillary first premolars

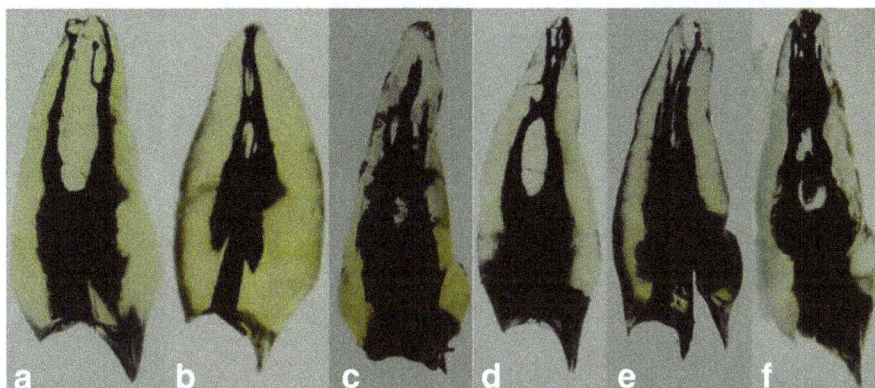

Fig. 4 Cleared teeth showing new canal types of Yemeni permanent maxillary first premolars. **a** Type (1–2-3), (**b**) Type (1–2-1-2-1), (**c**) Type (1–2-1-3-2), (**d**) Type (1–2-1-2-3-2), (**e**) Type (1–3-4), and (**f**) Type (1–2-1-3-2)

eight types within three main groups. The first group includes three canal types (types I, II, and III), all with one apical foramen. The second one includes four canal types (types IV, V, VI, and VII), all exiting with two apical foramina. The third one includes the last canal type in this classification (type VIII) with three apical foramina. Gulabivala et al. [27, 28] developed two root canal classification systems that were based on observations of root canal configurations within mandibular molars in a sample of Burmese and Thai individuals, respectively. Additional types not present in Vertucci et al. classification were found. A different approach to root canal classification has been offered by Sert and Bayirli [29], who proposed a classification system

differentiated by sex on the mandibular and maxillary permanent teeth among Turkish individuals. Fourteen new root canal configurations not included in other previous classification systems were described. Ordinola-Zapata et al. [31] used micro-CT imaging to evaluate of C-shaped mandibular first premolars in a Brazilian subpopulation. They reported several new anatomical variations and complexities of the root canal anatomy that were not included in previous classifications. Ahmed et al. [30, 32, 33] proposed new coding system for classifying root main and accessory canal morphology as well as teeth with anomalies to provide detailed information of the tooth and its root and canal anatomical features. In the present study, Vertucci classification [4] was used as

Table 2 Distribution of apical foramina and deltas of Yemeni permanent maxillary first premolars

Features	Single-rooted n (%)	Double-rooted n (%)		Three-rooted n (%)			Total n (%)
		B	P	MB	DB	P	
Apical foramen location							
Centrally in the apex	104 (75.9%)	101 (91.0%)	99 (89.2%)	2 (100%)	2 (100%)	2 (100%)	310 (84.9%)
Laterally	17 (12.4%)	10 (9.0%)	12 (10.8%)	0 (0.0%)	0 (0.0%)	0 (0.0%)	39 (10.7%)
Both	16 (11.7%)	0 (0.0%)	0 (0.0%)	0 (0.0%)	0 (0.0%)	0 (0.0%)	16 (4.4%)
No. of apical foramina							
One	61 (44.5%)	106 (95.5%)	110 (99.1%)	2 (100%)	2 (100%)	2 (100%)	283 (77.5%)
Two	66 (48.2%)	5 (4.5%)	1 (0.9%)	0 (0.0%)	0 (0.0%)	0 (0.0%)	72 (19.7%)
Three	10 (7.3%)	0 (0.0%)	0 (0.0%)	0 (0.0%)	0 (0.0%)	0 (0.0%)	10 (2.8%)
Apical deltas							
Apical delta present	29 (21.2%)	3 (2.7%)	1 (0.9%)	0 (0.0%)	0 (0.0%)	0 (0.0%)	33 (13.2%)
Apical delta absent	108 (78.8%)	108 (97.3%)	110 (99.1%)	2 (100%)	2 (100%)	2 (100%)	332 (86.8%)

Table 3 In vitro studies on root morphology of the permanent first maxillary premolar

Author	Year	Population	Sample (n)	Single-rooted (%)	Double-rooted (%)	Three-rooted (%)
Vertucci & Gegauff	1979	North America	400	39.5	56.5	4
Walker	1987	China	100	60	40	0
Pecora et al.	1991	Brazil	240	55.8	41.7	2.5
Loh	1998	Singapore	957	49.4	50.6	0
Kartal et al.	1998	Turkey	300	37.3	61.3	1.3
Chaparro et al.	1999	Andalusia	150	40	56.7	3.3
Lipski et al.	2005	Poland	142	15.5	74	9
Atieh	2008	Saudia Arabia	246	17.9	80.9	1.2
Awawdeh et al.	2008	Jordan	600	30.8	68.4	0.8
Present study	–	Yemen	250	54.8	44.4	0.8

reference because it is the most widely used classification in the literature and is still used in newly published papers [23, 34, 35]. Therefore, for the previous reasons, and also for easier results comparison, it was used in this study. However, additional root canal configurations [27–29] along with Vertucci classification were taken into consideration in this study.

Previous studies of the number of roots in maxillary first premolars showed various results. The prevalence of single-rooted maxillary first premolars (54.8%) in Yemeni population was in agreement with the findings of Pecora et al. [7], who reported that 55.8% of their specimens had one root. Walton & Torabinejad [36] referred to the existence of 50% of maxillary first premolars with two roots. In the present study, the prevalence of double-rooted premolars was in 44.4% of the specimens. The prevalence of three-rooted maxillary first premolars (0.8%) in this study was consistent with other studies performed in Turkish, Saudi, and Jordanian

populations [8, 11, 12]. The number of roots of the maxillary first premolars as reported in previously mentioned studies and studies elsewhere [37–39] is summarized in Table 3 alongside the results of this study.

Vertucci & Gegauff [5] reported that maxillary first premolar was the only tooth which showed all eight types of Vertucci canal configurations. This was in accordance with this study in which all eight types of Vertucci canal configurations were found. In addition, in the current study, 2.8% of premolars showed types I, III, and IV of Gulabivala [27, 28] canal configurations, and 1.2% of Sert & Bayirli [29] additional canal types. More interesting findings of this study were the new root canal configurations found in eight premolars (3.2%). Although these canal types represent a low percentage but their treatment is challenging. Table 4 summarizes the percentage of root canal configurations in maxillary first premolars reported in previous studies [8, 10–13, 37–39] along with the results of the present study.

Table 4 In vitro studies on root canal configuration of the permanent first maxillary premolar

Author	Year	Population	Sample (n)	Vertucci's root canal configuration (%)								Additional types (%)
				I	II	III	IV	V	VI	VII	VIII	
Vertucci & Gegauff	1979	North America	400	8	18	–	62	7	–	–	5	–
Caliskan et al.	1995	Turkey	100	3.9	5.9	–	78.4	5.9	5.9	–	–	–
Kartal et al.	1998	Turkey	300	8.7	1	–	71.3	14.7	2.3	0.3	1.3	–
Chaparro et al.	1999	Andalusia	150	1.3	37.3	–	58	–	–	–	3.3	–
Sert & Bayirli	2004	Turkey	200	10.5	12.5	5.5	61.5	3.5	1	–	3	–
Lipski et al.	2005	Poland	142	2.1	6.3	–	82.4	–	–	–	9.2	–
Peiris[a]	2008	Sri Lanka	153	1.3	16.3	2	64	5.9	5.9	0.7	–	3.9
	2008	Japan	81	4.9	29.6	2.5	45.7	2.5	8.6	–	–	6.2
Atieh	2008	Saudia Arabia	246	8.9	26.8	–	63	–	–	–	1.2	–
Awawdeh et al.	2008	Jordan	600	3.3	10.2	0.3	79.7	2	2.3	–	1.5	0.7
Weng et al.	2009	China	95	6.3	22.1	3.2	64.2	3.2	1	–	–	–
Present study	–	Yemen	250	13.2	4.4	8.0	55.6	5.6	1.6	3.6	0.8	7.2

[a]This study was performed in a Sri Lankan and Japanese populations

Table 5 In vitro studies on root canal morphology (accessory canals, inter-canal communications, apical foramina, deltas) of the permanent first maxillary premolar

Author	Year	Population	Sample (n)	Accessory Canals (%)	ICCs (%)	Apical Foramina		Deltas (%)
						Central (%)	Lateral (%)	
Vertucci & Gegauff	1979	North America	400	49.5[a]	34.2	12	88 [a]	3.2
Caliskan et al.	1995	Turkey	100	33.3	17.7	33.3	66.7	21.6
Kartal et al.	1998	Turkey	300	26	7	15.3	84.7	7.7
Sert & Bayirli	2004	Turkey	200	33	12	34	76	30.7
Awawdeh et al.	2008	Jordan	600	19.3	7	60	40	4.3
Weng et al.	2009	China	95	51.7	–	–	–	–
Present study	–	Yemen	250	52.8	34.4	84.9	15.1	13.2

[a] Percentage is from canals number (788) not teeth number

The occurrence of accessory canals in this study was 52.8% with maximum number noticed in the apical third (37.6%) of the roots. This was in accordance with text book of endodontics, where the highest incidence of accessory canals was found in the apical third of the root [40]. Different investigators [5, 8, 12, 29, 38, 39] have reported variations in the prevalence of accessory canals in maxillary first premolars (Table 5).

Inter-canal communications (ICCs) or transverse anastomoses/isthmuses were present in 34.4% of the specimens with highest percentage being in the middle third of the root (19.2%). This was in agreement with textbook of endodontics, where highest incidence of ICCs was found in the middle third of the root [40]. An isthmus is a narrow, ribbon-shaped communication between two root canals that contains pulp or pulpally derived tissue. It functions as a bacterial reservoir. This communication is of clinical significance as it may be difficult to debride and fill adequately [41, 42]. The prevalence of ICCs in maxillary first premolars as reported in studies elsewhere [5, 8, 12, 29, 38] is summarized in Table 5 alongside the results of this study.

The location of apical foramen is of clinical significance during working length determination, which often depends on the average position of the apical constriction relative to the root apex [41, 42]. In the present study, the apical foramen was found to be central in 84.9% of the studied specimens. This is much higher than previous studies that showed that the apical foramen was centrally-located in 12 to 60% of their specimens (Table 5). The low percentage of laterally-located apical foramina in this study in comparison to other studies may be due to ethnicity. In addition, teeth used in the present study were collected from young patients attending orthodontic clinics. Obviously, age would mostly affect apical foramina location due to deposition of secondary dentine within the root canal that moves the

site of the apical constriction away from the apex. These may explain why in this study the apical foramina were centrally-located in most studied specimens compared to previous studies [5, 8, 12, 29, 38] (Table 5). Apical deltas were observed in 13.2% of the collected Yemeni maxillary first premolars. The incidence of apical deltas in the maxillary first premolar as reported in previous studies [5, 8, 12, 29, 38] is summarized in Table 5 alongside the findings of this study.

Conclusion

Yemeni permanent maxillary first premolars are mainly single-rooted and predominantly present type IV Vertucci canal morphology. The finding of additional canal configurations in this study is low but should be kept in mind when performing endodontic therapy for these teeth. The results of the present study further confirm the importance of a thorough knowledge of root canal morphology for each population and the need of a careful exploration and radiographic examination of these teeth prior to endodontic therapy.

Abbreviations
CBCT: cone-beam computed tomography; ICCs: Inter-canal communications; MEC: Medical Ethics Committee; micro-CT: micro-computed tomography

Acknowledgements
The authors would like to acknowledge the co-operation received from the staff of the orthodontic clinics from where the teeth sample for this study was collected.

Funding
This study was entirely funded by University of Science and Technology, Sana'a, Yemen.

Authors' contributions
ES contributed with research concept, sample collection, technical steps, data collection, statistical analysis, writing the original draft and reviewing

and editing the final manuscript. HA contributed with research concept, supervision, sample evaluation, statistical analysis, writing the original draft and critical reviewing and editing of the final manuscript. TG contributed with supervision and writing the original draft. AM contributed with statistical analysis, writing the original draft and reviewing and editing the final manuscript. All authors read and approved the final manuscript

Authors' information

ES is a Lecturer of Endodontics at the Restorative and Prosthodontic Department, College of Dentistry, University of Science and Technology, Sana'a, Yemen.
HA is a Professor of Endodontics and a visiting professor at University of Alberta, Canada, on leave from the Department of Endodontics, Faculty of Dentistry, Tanta University, Tanta, Egypt.
TG is a Professor of Conservative Dentistry at the Department of Conservative Dentistry, Faculty of Dentistry, Tanta University, Tanta, Egypt.
AM is an Associate Professor of Endodontics at the Department of Conservative Dentistry, Faculty of Dentistry, Thamar University, Dhamar, Yemen, and at the Restorative and Prosthodontic Department, College of Dentistry, University of Science and Technology, Sana'a, Yemen.

Competing interests

The authors declare that they have no competing interests.

Author details

[1]Restorative and Prosthodontic Department, College of Dentistry, University of Science and Technology, Sana'a, Yemen. [2]Department of Dentistry, University of Alberta, Edmonton, Canada. [3]Department of Conservative Dentistry, Faculty of Dentistry, Tanta University, Tanta, Egypt. [4]Department of Conservative Dentistry, Faculty of Dentistry, Thamar University, Dhamar, Yemen. [5]Department of Endodontics, Faculty of Dentistry, Tanta University, Tanta, Egypt.

References

1. Lai W-H, Ho S-C, Weng T-Y, Huang S-T. Profile of nonsurgical root canal treatment under the National Health Insurance in Taiwan in 2006. J Dent Sci. 2009;4:187–90.
2. Chen G, Chang Y-C. Effects of liquid- and paste-type EDTA on smear-layer removal during rotary root-canal instrumentation. J Dent Sci. 2011;6:41–7.
3. Awawdeh LA, Al-Qudah AA. Root form and canal morphology of mandibular premolars in a Jordanian population. Int Endod J. 2008;41:240–8.
4. Vertucci FJ. Root canal anatomy of the human permanent teeth. Oral Surg Oral Med Oral Pathol. 1984;58:589–99.
5. Vertucci FJ, Gegauff A. Root canal morphology of the maxillary first premolar. J Am Dent Assoc. 1979;99:194–8.
6. Walker RT. Root form and canal anatomy of maxillary first premolars in a southern Chinese population. Dent Traumatol. 1987;3:130–4.
7. Pecora JD, Saquy PC, SousaNeto MD, Woelfel JB. Root form and canal anatomy of maxillary first premolars. Braz Dent J. 1991;2:87–94.
8. Kartal N, Ozcelik B, Cimilli H. Root canal morphology of maxillary premolars. J Endod. 1998;24:417–9.
9. Loh HS. Root morphology of the maxillary first premolar in Singaporeans. Aust Dent J. 1998;43:399–402.
10. Lipski M, Woźniak K, Łagocka R, Tomasik M. Root and canal morphology of the human maxillary first premolar. Durham Anthropol J. 2005;12:2–3.
11. Atieh MA. Root and canal morphology of maxillary first premolars in a Saudi population. J Contemp Dent Pract. 2008;9:46–53.
12. Awawdeh LA, Abdullah H, Al-Qudah AA. Root form and canal morphology of Jordanian maxillary first premolars. J Endod. 2008;34:956–61.
13. Peiris R. Root and canal morphology of human permanent teeth in a Sri Lankan and Japanese population. Anthropol Sci. 2008;116:123–33.
14. Neelakantan P, Subbarao C, Ahuja R, Subbarao CV. Root and canal morphology of Indian maxillary premolars by a modified root canal staining technique. Odontology. 2011;99:18–21.
15. Koçani F, Kamberi B, Dragusha E, Kelmendi T, Sejfija Z. Correlation between anatomy and root canal topography of first maxillary premolar on kosovar population. Open J Stomatol. 2014;4:332–9.
16. Trope M, Elfenbein L, Tronstad L. Mandibular premolars with more than one root canal in different race groups. J Endod. 1986;12:343–5.
17. Sieraski SM, Taylor GN, Kohn RA. Identification and endodontic management of three-canaled maxillary premolars. J Endod. 1989;5:29–32.
18. Mayo CV, Montgomery S, Rio C. A computerized method for evaluating root canal morphology. J Endod. 1986;12:2–7.
19. Baurmann M. A new approach to demonstration of root canal anatomy. J Dent Educ. 1994;28:704–8.
20. Blaskovic-Subat V, Smojver I, Maricic D, Sutaalo J. A computerized method for the evaluation of root canal morphology. Int Endod J. 1995;28:290–6.
21. Omer OE, Ai Shalabi RM, Jennings M, Glennon J, Claffey NM. A comparison between clearing and radiographic techniques in the study of the root-canal anatomy of maxillary first and second molars. Int Endod J. 2004;37:291–7.
22. Neelakantan P, Subbarao C, Subbarao CV. Comparative evaluation of modified canal staining and clearing technique, cone-beam computed tomography, peripheral quantitative computed tomography, spiral computed tomography and plain and contrast medium-enhanced digital radiography in studying root canal morphology. J Endod. 2010;36:1547–51.
23. Ordinola-Zapata R, Bramante CM, Versiani MA, Moldauer BI, Topham G, Gutmann JL, Nuñez A, Duarte MA, Abella F. Comparative accuracy of the clearing technique, CBCT and micro-CT methods in studying the mesial root canal configuration of mandibular first molars. Int Endod J. 2017;50:90–6.
24. Kim Y, Perinpanayagam H, Lee JK, Yoo YJ, Oh S, Gu Y, Lee SP, Chang SW, Lee W, Baek SH, Zhu Q. Comparison of mandibular first molar mesial root canal morphology using micro-computed tomography and clearing technique. Acta Odonto Scandi. 2015;73:427–32.
25. Lee KW, Kim Y, Perinpanayagam H, Lee JK, Yoo YJ, Lim SM, Chang SW, Ha BH, Zhu Q, Kum KY. Comparison of alternative image reformatting techniques in micro–computed tomography and tooth clearing for detailed canal morphology. J Endod. 2014;40:417–22.
26. Weine FS, Healey HJ, Gerstein H, Evanson L. Canal configuration in the mesiobuccal root of the maxillary first molar and its endodontic significance. Oral Surg Oral Med Oral Pathol. 1969;28:419–25.
27. Gulabivala K, Aung TH, Alavi A, Ng YL. Root and canal morphology of Burmese mandibular molars. Int Endod J. 2001;34:359–70.
28. Gulabivala K, Opasanon A, Ng YL, Alavi A. Root and canal morphology of Thai mandibular molars. Int Endod J. 2002;35:56–62.
29. Sert S, Bayirli GS. Evaluation of the root canal configurations of the mandibular and maxillary permanent teeth by gender in the Turkish population. J Endod. 2004;30:391–8.
30. Ahmed HM, Versiani MA, De-Deus G, Dummer PM. A new system for classifying root and root canal morphology. Int Endodo J. 2017;50:761–70.
31. Ordinola-Zapata R, Monteiro Bramante C, Gagliardi Minotti P, Cavalini Cavenago B, Gutmann JL, Moldauer BI, Versiani MA, Duarte H. Micro-CT evaluation of C-shaped mandibular first premolars in a Brazilian subpopulation. Int Endod J. 2015;48:807–13.
32. Ahmed HM, Neelakantan P, Dummer PM. A new system for classifying accessory canal morphology. Int Endod J. 2018;51:164–76.
33. Ahmed HM, Dummer PM. A new system for classifying tooth, root and canal anomaly. Int Endod J. 2017;12 In Press
34. Mokhtari H, Niknami M, Zonouzi HR, Sohrabi A, Ghasemi N, Golzar AA. Accuracy of cone-beam computed tomography in determining the root canal morphology of mandibular first molars. Iran Endod J. 2016;11:101–5.
35. Akhlaghi NM, Khalilak Z, Vatanpour M, Mohammadi S, Pirmoradi S, Fazlyab M, Safavi K. Root canal anatomy and morphology of mandibular first molars in a selected Iranian population: an in vitro study. Iran Endod J. 2017;12:87–91.
36. Walton R, Torabinenjad M. Principles and Practice of Endodontics. 2nd ed. Philadelphia: W.B. Saunders Co; 1996. p. 177–8.
37. Chaparro AJ, Segura JJ, Guerrero E, Jiménez-Rubio A, Murillo C, Fetio JJ. Number of roots and canals in maxillary first premolars: study of an Andalusian population. Dent Traumatol. 1999;15:65–7.
38. Caliskan MK, Pehlivan Y, Sepetcioglu F, Turkun M, Tuncer SS. Root canal morphology of human permanent teeth in a Turkish population. J Endod. 1995;21:200–4.

39. Weng XL, Yu SB, Zhao SL, Wang HG, Mu T, Tang RY, Zhou XD. Root canal morphology of permanent maxillary teeth in the Han nationality in Chinese Guanzhong area: a new modified root canal staining technique. J Endod. 2009;35:651–6.
40. Hargreaves KM, Cohen S. Pathways of the pulp, vol. 139. 10th ed. Louis Missouri: CV Mosby; 2011.
41. Weine FS. The enigma of the lateral canal. Dent Clin N Am. 1984;28:833–52.
42. Vertucci FJ. Root canal morphology and its relationship to endodontic procedures. Endod Topics. 2005;10:3–29.

16

Assessment of oral health and cost of care for a group of refugees in Germany

Katja Goetz[*] , Wiebke Winkelmann and Jost Steinhäuser

Abstract

Background: There is a research gap concerning the evaluation of the oral healthcare of refugees. Therefore, the aim of this study was to evaluate the oral health of refugees and to estimate the costs of oral care.

Methods: The study was conceptualized as a pilot study. The study participants were refugees who lived either in collective living quarters or at a reception center in a region of the federal state of Schleswig-Holstein, Germany. The cross-sectional design was complemented by dental screening. Data were collected from August 2016 until July 2017. The basic condition of the teeth was evaluated using a convenience sample by a single dentist. The assessment of caries was carried out visually in accordance with the International Caries Detection and Assessment System from code 3 and higher. The DMF-T (decayed, (D), missing, (M), filled (F), teeth (T)) index was calculated. The costs of oral care were analyzed for conservative treatment (filling or extraction) and for prosthetic treatment (missing teeth) in the form of a bridge or crown.

Results: The dental screening was attended by 102 refugees, with a mean age of 28 years. A total of 49% of the study sample suffered from toothache, and the DMF-T index had a mean of 6.89. For 92% of the study sample, treatment was indicated, and a cost estimate of the treatment could be calculated. The average cost of conservative treatment was estimated to be 205.86 EUR, and the average cost of prosthetic treatment was estimated to be 588.0 EUR. The oral healthcare costs of the different treatment procedures were higher for refugees that presented with toothache than for those without toothache, with the exception of prosthetic treatment procedures.

Conclusions: There is a lack of population-based data that survey the oral health status of refugees. Therefore, the current study presents an initial overview regarding the oral health status and the potential costs of oral healthcare of refugees.

Keywords: Cost of care, Dental screening, Oral health, Refugees

Background

Oral health is essential for well-being and is a quality-of-life determinant [1]. There is a strong relationship between oral health and general health. For example, severe periodontal disease is associated with type 2 diabetes [2]. Moreover, periodontal disease and dental caries are the two most prevalent oral afflictions worldwide [2]. Effective prevention of these diseases is related to access to oral healthcare, periodic assessment of oral health and individual oral health behavior [2]. Therefore, it may be assumed that refugees are a high-risk group for developing oral disease because of their limited access to dental care. Various factors, such as limited access to oral healthcare, oral care products and to nutritious food and clean water could lead to poor oral health status, including the development of periodontal disease or dental caries. Moreover, factors such as access to and organization of healthcare in the country of origin could contribute to the poor oral health of refugees, which is shown in the oral health database provided by the World Health Organization (WHO) [3].

* Correspondence: katja.goetz@uni-luebeck.de
Institute of Family Medicine, University Hospital Schleswig-Holstein, Campus Luebeck, Ratzeburger Allee 160, 23538 Luebeck, Germany

By the end of 2016, there were approximately 22.5 million refugees and 2.8 million asylum seekers worldwide [4, 5]. Over 55% of these refugees originate from South Sudan, Afghanistan, and Syria countries with human rights violations [4, 5]. In Europe, there were approximately 5.2 million refugees, and 669,500 refugees had entered Germany by the end of 2016 [5]. In Germany, the asylum policy has no limit regarding the entry of refugees. The entitlements to medical care by refugees in Germany are detailed in the Asylum-Seekers' Benefits Act (AsylbLG), and §4, 6 AsylBLG specifically regulates the access to health care, which is limited [6, 7]. These laws detail what types of health problems allow for access to healthcare. According to §4 AsylBLG, these constitute acute diseases and pain that requires medical or dental treatment [6].

Different systematic reviews show a research gap concerning the evaluation of the oral healthcare of refugees [8, 9]. Therefore, the aim of this study was to evaluate the oral health of refugees in one region in Germany and to estimate the costs of oral care on the basis of regular and restricted access.

Methods

The currents study was conceptualized as a pilot study with a cross-sectional design.

Design and participants

This study complies with the Strengthening the Reporting of Observational Studies in Epidemiology (STROBE) guidelines [10]. The study participants were refugees who lived in either collective living quarters or at a reception center in one region of the federal state of Schleswig-Holstein, Germany. The participants were recruited to the project "Mobile Medical Practice" (Rollende Arztpraxis). The "Rollende Arztpraxis" was financed by the Damp-Stiftung and provided general practice care for refugees in rural regions of Schleswig-Holstein [11]. In connection with this project, dental screening was offered in the "Rollende Arztpraxis" in a non-dental setting. This was a small bus that was furnished with equipment such as a treatment table, a chair, an emergency electrocardiogram, a spirometer, a defibrillator and a pocket Doppler. The dentist used the treatment table for dental screenings, enabling the refugees to lie down so that a more effective evaluation of the oral health status could be obtained. The dentist used magnifying glasses with light, a plane mouth mirror and a dental probe for the screening.

The examination of oral health was performed by a dentist supported by interpreters who provided translation in different languages. The following languages could be translated by the interpreters: Arabic, Farsi, Persian and Russian. Three interpreters were available, which was in agreement with the facility manager of the collective living quarters and reception center. The dental screening service was announced in advance so that the interpreters could be arranged.

A calibration of the dentist was not addressed because it is not part of the recommendations included in the STROBE guidelines [10].

A dentist in the region was recommended if a participant suffered from pain or the screening showed the need for dental treatment. The data were collected from August 2016 until July 2017.

After verbal and written information was given by the interpreter, written informed consent was obtained from each participant. Participation in the study was completely voluntary.

Measurements

The measurement process consisted of a two-step procedure. First, sociodemographic data were collected, and then the dental screening was carried out.

Sociodemographic data

The sociodemographic data included gender, age, country of origin, number of months residing in Germany and the location where they were currently living. This questionnaire was in the German language and was translated by the interpreter. The questionnaire was a separate step, decoupled from the oral health screening.

Evaluation of oral health

Information regarding oral health was obtained from different questions, such as the date of the last visit to a dentist, daily dental hygiene, access to dental hygiene products and the presence or absence of toothache. All questions were in German and were translated by the interpreter for the refugee. The toothache pain level was determined by a visual analogue scale ranging from 0 (no pain) to 10 (extremely strong pain). The condition of the teeth was evaluated by a dentist. Dental caries were assessed visually in accordance with the International Caries Detection and Assessment System from code 3 and higher [12]. The tools used for the oral health screening were as follows: magnifying glasses with light, a plane mouth mirror and a dental probe. The results were entered into a paper-based schematic that depicted all 32 teeth, including five areas in the posterior region (mesial, occlusal, distal, buccal and oral), five areas in the front tooth region (mesial, distal, incisal, labial and oral), and the root and tooth necks. The questionnaire of the evaluation of the oral health was added as Additional file 1.

Data analysis

Data analysis was performed using SPSS 24.0 (SPSS Inc., IBM). Continuous data were summarized using the mean and standard deviation. Categorical data were presented as frequency counts and percentages. Student's t-test with case exclusion was used for the comparison between toothache (yes/no) and healthcare costs (conservative, prosthetic and overall costs). Additionally, refugees who were in need of a removable denture were considered as a fixed denture within the analysis because this is covered by standard care.

Calculation of the DMF-T index

The DMF-T (decayed, (D), missing, (M), filled (F), teeth (T)) index was calculated. With this index, it is possible to assess the patient's individual risk of caries. All teeth, excepting the wisdom teeth, were included in the calculation to obtain the sum score, which ranged from 0 to 28. A score of 0 indicates that all teeth are without decay, and no teeth are missing, filled or destroyed. Furthermore, the DMF-T index can be divided into four categories: less than 5.0 indicates a very low risk of caries, 5.0 to 8.9 indicates a low risk of caries, 9.0 to 13.9 indicates a moderate risk of caries, and greater than 13.9 indicates a high risk of caries [13].

Methodology of healthcare cost estimation

The estimation of costs was based on destroyed and decayed teeth that required conservative treatment in the form of tooth filling or extraction and on missing teeth that required a prosthetic treatment in the form of a bridge or crown. The costs of oral healthcare were estimated using two different German statutory health insurance plans and were averaged. The calculated costs included payments that would be reimbursed in a regular care setting, material costs and treatment costs. An overview of the estimated costs for the different treatment procedures is provided in Table 1.

Ethical approval

Ethical approval for this research study was obtained from the University of Luebeck in June 2016 (Approval No. 16–123). Participation in the study was voluntary. No additional data were evaluated.

Results

One hundred and two refugees and asylum seekers participated in the pilot study and attended a dental screening. The total number of refugees residing in the participating collective living quarters and reception center is unknown. Therefore, no response rate can be calculated. Table 2 presents the sociodemographic characteristics of the participants. More than 80% of the responding refugees were male. The mean age

Table 1 Methodology to estimate oral healthcare costs (in EUR)

	Procedure	Mean of costs (in EUR)
Conservative treatment: Destroyed teeth		
Lower jaw (one root)	Block anesthesia	11.62
	Extraction	9.68
	Overall cost	21.30
Lower jaw (≥ two roots)	Block anesthesia	11.62
	Extraction	14.52
	Overall cost	26.14
Upper jaw (one root)	Infiltration anesthesia	7.75
	Extraction	9.68
	Overall cost	17.43
Upper jaw (≥ two roots)	Infiltration anesthesia	7.75
	Extraction	14.52
	Overall cost	22.27
Conservative treatment: Decayed teeth		
Parts of lower jaw	Block anesthesia	11.62
	Indirect pulp capping	5.81
	Areas of filling (min)	31.00
	Areas of filling (max)	56.14
	Overall cost (min/max)	48.43 / 73.57
Upper jaw	Infiltration anesthesia	7.75
	Indirect pulp capping	5.81
	Areas of filling (min)	31.00
	Areas of filling (max)	56.14
	Overall cost (min/max)	44.56 / 69.70
Prosthetic treatment: Crown	Full cast	143.27
	Unveneered	152.94
	Overall cost	296.21
Prosthetic treatment: Bridge	Full cast	114.23
	Vestibular veneer	124.00
	Pontic	60.00
	Overall cost	298.23

was 28.6 years (SD = 10.3). Participants were from nine different countries; over 24% migrated from Afghanistan, 18% migrated from Iraq, and 14% migrated from Syria.

Oral health of refugees

The evaluation of oral health is presented in Table 3. Over 84% of the study participants did not visit a dentist regularly during their childhood. Nearly 50% of the participants practiced dental hygiene twice per day. The presence of toothache afflicted 49% of the participants, with a mean of 4.51 (SD = 1.9) on the pain scale. The

Table 2 Sociodemographic data of the study sample ($n = 102$)

Characteristic		Number
Months residing in Germany, mean (SD);range		13.9 (5.6) 3–24
Age, mean (SD);range		28.6 (10.3) 16–64
Gender, n (%)	Female	18 (17.6%)
	Male	84 (82.4%)
Residence, n (%)	Reception center	21 (20.6%)
	Collective living quarters	81 (79.4%)
Country of origin, n (%)	Afghanistan	25 (24.5)
	Iraq	19 (18.6)
	Syria	15 (14.7)
	Eritrea	14 (13.7)
	Yemen	11 (10.8)
	Armenia	7 (6.9)
	Somalia	5 (4.9)
	Iran	4 (3.9)
	Chechnya	2 (2.0)

SD standard deviation

DMF-T index had a mean of 6.89 (SD = 5.5). Healthy dentition was present in 13.7% of the participants. A moderately high DMF-T index (> 9.0) was observed in 25.5% of the refugees.

The following means and standard deviations were observed for the individual DMF-T components: for decayed teeth (DT), a mean of 2.90 (SD = 2.04); for missing teeth (MT), a mean of 3.88 (SD = 2.95); and for filled teeth (FT), a mean of 3.76 (SD = 2.94).

Estimation of oral healthcare costs

For 92% ($n = 94$) of the study population, some form of treatment was indicated. The estimated healthcare costs of the study population were divided into conservative treatment and prosthetic treatment and are presented in Table 4. Conservative treatment in cases requiring the extraction of destroyed teeth was indicated for 77 participants, and the mean cost was calculated to be 82.64 EUR (SD = 62.65). The healthcare costs for conservative treatment were calculated on the basis of 93 participants with a minimum mean of 157.47 EUR (SD = 106.0) and a maximum mean of 205.86 EUR (SD = 153.20). Prosthetic treatment was indicated for 44 participants, and the mean cost was calculated to be 588.0 EUR (SD = 395.77).

Table 3 Oral health and DMF-T index of refugees

Variable		Number (%)
Year of last dental visit	2017	31(30.4%)
	2016	29 (28.5%)
	2015	4 (3.9%)
	2014	9 (8.8%)
	< 2014	26 (25.5%)
Regular visits to a dentist during childhood	No	86 (84.3%)
	Once per year	11 (10.8%)
	Twice per year	5 (4.9%)
Daily dental hygiene	Once per day	45 (44.1%)
	Twice per day	50 (49.0%)
	More than twice per day	7 (6.9%)
Was there a time without access to dental hygiene products?	No	47 (46.1%)
	Yes	55 (53.9%)
Do you currently have a toothache?	No	52 (51.0%)
	Yes	50 (49.0%)
Toothache on the pain scale[a], mean (SD); range		4.51 (1.9); 2–10
DMF-T index, mean (SD)		6.89 (5.5)
Categorization of DMF-T Index, n (%)	No index (0.0)	14 (13.7%)
	Very low Index (< 5.0)	38 (37.3%)
	Low Index (5.0–8.9)	24 (23.5%)
	Moderate Index (9.0–13.9)	14 (13.7%)
	High Index (> 13.9)	12 (11.8%)

[a]ranged from 0 (no pain) to 10 (extremely strong pain), SD standard deviation

Table 4 Conservative and prosthetic treatment – estimation of oral healthcare costs (in EUR)

Conservative treatment		Mean (SD), range (in EUR)
Destroyed teeth (n = 77)		82.64 (62.65), 17.43–359.21
Decayed teeth (n = 61)	Minimum	135.77 (93.57), 44.56–412.65
	Maximum	209.54 (144.84), 69.70–638.91
Overall costs for conservative treatment (n = 93)	Minimum	157.47 (106.0), 17.43–508.50
	Maximum	205.86 (153.20), 17.43–734.76
Prosthetic treatment		Mean (SD), range
Crown (n = 4)		183.90 (81.3), 143.27–305.88
Bridge (n = 43)		587.90 (390.88), 228.46–1680.92
Overall costs for prosthetic treatment (n = 44)		588.0 (395.8), 143.27–1680.92
Overall oral healthcare costs (n = 94)	Minimum	431.03 (445.94), 22.27–1747.65
	Maximum	487.91 (463.54), 22.27–1973.91

SD standard deviation, n number of refugees who require treatment

Table 5 shows the comparison of toothache (yes/no) and healthcare costs. The healthcare costs for the different treatment procedures were greater for refugees with toothache than for those without toothache, with the exception of prosthetic treatment procedures. A significant difference was found for conservative treatment procedures, with an average difference of 46.9 EUR (minimum) and 74.6 EUR (maximum). For the overall oral healthcare, an average difference of 102.5 EUR (minimum) and 129.0 EUR (maximum) was found.

Discussion

Our results present an initial overview of oral health status and the potential costs of oral healthcare of refugees in one region in the federal state of Schleswig-Holstein, Germany. The study was conceptualized as a pilot study to obtain preliminary data on the oral health status and costs of oral healthcare of refugees. The sociodemographic data obtained in the study concerning the origin of the refugees were comparable to the official statistics of

Schleswig-Holstein, which show that Afghanistan, Iraq and Syria are the primary countries from which people immigrate [14]. Moreover, our results concerning the distribution of gender show a high proportion of male refugees, which coincides with another study on the oral healthcare of refugees [15]. There are multiple reasons for the gender imbalance. The official statistics from the Federal Agency of Migration and Refugees show that more men than women are refugees [16]. It can also be assumed that social values and standards, such as traditional gender roles and culture in the country of origin could influence the utilization of healthcare [17]. However, more information is needed to explain why men are more likely than women to utilize oral healthcare services, and this question should be investigated in further studies.

The evaluation of oral health revealed a low level of preventive behavior during childhood. Over 84% of the participants did not visit a dentist during their childhood. The professional recommendation is to visit a dentist at least once per year [18]. When accounting for

Table 5 Comparison of oral healthcare costs for refugees with and without toothache (in EUR, using Student's t-test with case exclusion)

Treatment procedures		Toothache	Mean (SD) (in EUR)	Average difference	p-value
Cost for conservative treatment	Minimum	Yes (n = 48)	180.2 (106.3)	46.9	0.03
	Minimum	No (n = 45)	133.3 (101.2)		
	Maximum	Yes (n = 48)	242.0 (155.6)	74.6	0.02
	Maximum	No (n = 45)	167.3 (142.3)		
Cost for prosthetic treatment		Yes (n = 26)	572.2 (380.5)	−38.6	0.75
		No (n = 16)	610.8 (427.1)		
Overall oral healthcare costs	Minimum	Yes (n = 49)	480.1 (440.8)	102.5	0.27
	Minimum	No (n = 45)	377.6 (450.2)		
	Maximum	Yes (n = 49)	540.7 (453.6)	129.0	0.18
	Maximum	No (n = 45)	411.7 (469.9)		

SD standard deviation

the global health workforce statistics, the low number of dentists in countries such as Afghanistan, Iraq and Syria is likely to be an important barrier to oral healthcare access and therefore to adequate prevention [19]. However, it is well known that preventive dental visits in childhood influence one's oral health in adulthood [20]. Our study sample presented a DMF-T index of 6.9, which is lower than that of the general population in Germany (11.2 for young adults) [21]. However, a comparison of the individual DMF-T components between the refugees and the general population showed similar results, with a lower proportion of DT and a higher proportion of MT and FT for the refugee population [21]. Similar results were also obtained in a different study on the oral healthcare of refugees in Germany [15]. Furthermore, our findings are comparable to a study from Australia that revealed that the oral health status of refugees is poorer than that of the general population [22]. Oral health status depends not only on access to care but also on the social status of an individual [21]. One possible explanation for the data could be that our study participants have a relatively high to moderate social status. Additional research would be helpful to clarify how the social status of refugees affects their oral health.

A dental care report by one statutory health insurance organization indicated that 8.9% of the insured adult population has had an extraction [23]. This is in contrast to our sample, where an extraction was recommended for 75.5% of the refugees. However, if the refugees were not experiencing pain, then no treatment was offered, according to the definition of restricted access in §4 AsylBLG [6]. This restricted access for refugees could have an impact on healthcare costs. The reimbursed costs for health insurance will be lower due to the restricted access, as not all refugees need treatment, and therefore, they will not incur any cost. However, the direct and indirect costs cannot be estimated. In our sample, 50 refugees stated that they currently suffered from toothache. In these cases, §4 AsylBLG would grant them treatment, and it would be more expensive than if there was no access limitation regarding toothache. Postponing treatment until there is pain is not preventive action. Therefore, it can be assumed that restricted access may lead to discrimination of refugee's healthcare, and it may also lead to higher costs [24]. Moreover, it is possible that persons who have poor oral health, such as missing teeth, might have problems obtaining employment, which is an important part of the integration process for refugees in a foreign society [25].

Limitations

The number of participants was rather small. Participation in the dental screening was voluntary; therefore, there may have been a potential selection bias. Moreover, the number of how many refugees were asked for participation was unknown. It is possible that refugees who did not have any oral health problems were less likely to seek oral healthcare, and this should be considered when interpreting our results. Furthermore, it is not possible to link the sociodemographic data and the oral health status of the refugees. Therefore, a regression analysis with adjustments to evaluate the potential effects of age, gender and country of origin on oral health status was not possible and should be confirmed in further studies. The questionnaire that was used to evaluate oral health was not based on the questionnaire used in the German oral healthcare study [21]. Moreover, potential bias may have been present in the dental screening process because only one dentist screened the refugees, and no additional dentist was available for verification of the screening results. It was not possible to follow up with the refugees regarding whether or not they contacted the recommended dentists in the region and what type of treatment they received. Additionally, no assessment of the periodontium or oral mucosa was performed because of a lack of resources, such as limited time, finances and personal equipment with which to carry out the dental screening process. However, such an assessment should be performed in further studies.

Calculating a cost estimate for the different treatment procedures is quite difficult because all of the existing statutory health insurances ($n = 113$) in Germany vary in their level of reimbursed costs [26]. The healthcare costs presented in this study are hypothetical because of the restricted healthcare access of the refugees. The true costs cannot be calculated. Finally, this was a cross-sectional study; therefore, we cannot draw causal links from these findings.

Conclusions

There is a lack of population-based data that survey the oral health status of refugees. It should be considered whether an oral health screening could be part of an initial medical examination. Standardized tools for oral health assessments are available from the WHO that could be used by advanced-stage dental students. These assessments would aid in the prevention of oral disease.

Abbreviations

AsylbLG: Asylum-seekers' benefits act; DMF-T index: Decayed, missing, filled-teeth index; DT: Decayed teeth; EUR: Euro; FT: Filled teeth; MT: Missing teeth; SD: Standard deviation; STROBE: Strengthening the reporting of observational studies in epidemiology; WHO: World Health Organization

Acknowledgments

The authors would like to thank the refugees who participated in the study.

Funding
This study did not receive funding.

Authors' contributions
All authors contributed to this study. KG, WW and JS participated in the conception and design of the study. WW performed the dental screenings. KG performed the statistical analyses and drafted the manuscript. WW and JS critically revised the manuscript draft and approved its final version. All authors have read and approved the final version of this manuscript.

Competing interests
The authors declare that they have no competing interests.

References
1. Hescot P. The new definition of oral health and relationship between oral health and quality of life. Chin J Dent Res. 2017;20:189–92.
2. Linden GJ, Lyons A, Scannapieco FA. Periodontal systemic associations: review of the evidence. J Clin Periodontol. 2013;40(Suppl14):8–19.
3. Oral Health Databases. 2017. https://www.mah.se/CAPP/Country-Oral-Health-Profiles/According-to-Alphabetical/?id=41424&id=41424. Accessed 15 Dec 2017.
4. UNHCR Statistics for Germany. 2017. http://www.unhcr.org/dach/de/services/statistiken. Accessed 15 Dec 2017.
5. UNHCR Global trends. Forced displacement in 2016. 2017. http://www.unhcr.org/statistics/unhcrstats/5943e8a34/global-trends-forced-displacement-2016.html. Accessed 15 Dec 2017.
6. Asylum-Seekers' Benefits Act, Paragraph 4. https://www.gesetze-im-internet.de/asylblg/__4.html. Accessed 15 Dec 2017.
7. Asylum-Seekers' Benefits Act, Paragraph 6. https://www.gesetze-im-internet.de/asylblg/__6.html. Accessed 15 Dec 2017.
8. Bozorgmehr K, Mohsenpour A, Saure D, Stock C, Loerbroks A, Joos S, Schneider C. Systematic review and evidence mapping of empirical studies on health status and medical care among refugees and asylum seekers in Germany (1990-2014). Bundesgesundheitsblatt Gesundheitsforschung Gesundheitsschutz. 2016;59:599–620.
9. Keboa MT, Hiles N, Macdonald ME. The oral health of refugees and asylum seekers: a scoping review. Glob Health. 2016;12:59.
10. Von Elm E, Altman DG, Egger M, Pocock SJ, Gotzsche PC, Vandenbroucke JP. The strengthening the reporting of observational studies in epidemiology (STROBE) statement: guidelines for reporting observational studies. Int J Surg. 2014;12:1495–9.
11. Damp-Stiftung. http://www.damp-stiftung.de/index.php?id=projekte_gesundheitswesen. Accessed 15 Dec 2017.
12. Dikmen B. Icdas II criteria (international caries detection and assessment system). J Istanb Univ Fac Dent 2015;49:63–72.
13. Word Health Organization. Oral health survey: basic methods, 5th edition. Geneva: World Health Organization; 2013. http://apps.who.int/iris/bitstream/10665/97035/1/9789241548649_eng.pdf?ua=1. Accessed 15 Dec 2017
14. Immigration to the federal state of Schleswig-Holstein, Germany. 2017. http://www.schleswig-holstein.de/DE/Fachinhalte/F/fluechtlingeSH/Downloads/zuwanderungsbericht/2017_Oktober_Zuwanderungsbericht.pdf?__blob=publicationFile&v=4. Accessed 15 Dec 2017.
15. Splieth CH, Takriti M, Alani A. Flüchtlinge in Deutschland – Mundgesundheit, Versorgungsbedarfe und deren Kosten. Abschlussbericht. https://www.bzaek.de/fileadmin/PDFs/b/Studie_Mundgesundheit_Fluechtlinge.pdf. Accessed 14 March 2017
16. Federal Ministry of Migration and Refugees. Report on asylum, current statistics. http://www.bamf.de/SharedDocs/Anlagen/DE/Downloads/Infothek/Statistik/Asyl/aktuelle-zahlen-zu-asyl-februar-2018.html?nn=7952222. Accessed 14 March 2017.
17. Diehl C, Koenig M, Ruckdeschel K. Religiosity and gender equality: comparing natives and Muslim migrants in Germany. Ethn Racial Stud. 2009;32:278–301.
18. Bhaskar V, McGraw KA, Divaris K. The importance of preventive dental visits from a young age: systematic review and current perspective. Clin Cosmet Investig Dent. 2014;6:21–7.
19. Global health workforce statistics. https://rho.emro.who.int/rhodata/node.main.HWF?lang=en. Accessed 15 Dec 2017.
20. Nicolau B, Thomson WM, Steele JG, Allison PJ. Life-course epidemiology: concepts and theoretical models and is relevance to chronic oral conditions. Community Dent Oral Epidemiol. 2007;35:241–9.
21. Jordan AR, Micheelis W. Fünfte Deutsche Mundgesundheitsstudie. Deutscher Zahnärzte Verlag: Köln; 2016.
22. Davidson N, Skull S, Calache H, Murray S, Chalmers J. Holes a plenty: oral health status a major issue for newly arrived refugees in Australia. Aust Dent J. 2006;51:306–11.
23. Rädel M, Bohm S, Priess HW, Walter M. BARMER GEK Zahnreport 2017. Wuppertal: BARMER. 2017. https://www.barmer.de/blob/105420/367ca3131074f4f956ac6b028ce83abe/data/dl-barmer-zahnreport-2017.pdf. Accessed 15 Dec 2017.
24. Bozorgmehr K, Razum O. Effect of restricting access to health care on health expenditures among asylum-seekers and refugees: a quasi-experimental study in Germany, 1994–2013. PLoS One. 2015;10:e0131483.
25. Hamermesh D, Biddle J. Beauty and the labor market. Am Econ Rev. 1994; 85:1174–94.
26. Busse R, Blümel M, Knieps F, Bärnighausen T. Statutory health insurance in Germany: a health system shaped by 135 years of solidarity, self-governance, and competition. Lancet. 2017;390:882–97.

17

Comparison of caries lesion detection methods in epidemiological surveys: CAST, ICDAS and DMF

Ana Luiza Sarno Castro[1]*[iD], Maria Isabel Pereira Vianna[2] and Carlos Maurício Cardeal Mendes[3]

Abstract

Background: Although dental caries is a globally widespread disease, there is no consensus regarding the method that should be used for their detection. In recent decades, a variety of new methods have been proposed for measuring caries in a population. Three caries detection methods, the decayed, missing and filled (DMF) index, the International Caries Detection and Assessment System (ICDAS) and the Caries Assessment Spectrum and Treatment (CAST), were compared to provide information to guide future method choices.

Methods: This was a descriptive, cross-sectional study in which three methods were used to measure caries in students, staff and their dependents at UNEB (State University of Bahia), Salvador, Brazil. We compared the mean application time of each method and the frequencies obtained by each method using the following indicators: the most severe caries lesion per individual; the mean number of missing, filled and decayed teeth; and the disease extent.

Results: The mean time taken to apply the DMF was 3.8 min; for ICDAS, it took 8.9 min, and for CAST, 4.7 min. When calculating the indicator the most severe caries lesion per individual, the prevalence rates were as follows: 28.1% for DMF, 84.0% for ICDAS and 75.0% for CAST. The mean numbers of decayed, missing and filled teeth were 6.0 according to the DMF, 6.2 according to ICDAS and 5.9 according to CAST. When the disease extension indicator was used, the following percentages of teeth were affected by caries: DMF 22.12%, ICDAS 49.11% and CAST 33.2%.

Conclusions: The DMF underestimated the occurrence of caries lesions in individuals but was the fastest method to apply. ICDAS obtained detailed information regarding lesion severity, but it was a time-consuming method and difficult to analyse. CAST described disease distributions very well and identified lesion severities and preventive and curative needs in the examined group, and the time required to apply CAST was similar to that of the DMF.

Keywords: Epidemiology, DMF index, ICDAS, CAST, Epidemiological surveys

Background

Caries is a disease that is present in all countries around the world. The signs and symptoms accumulate with increasing age, with a prevalence of 100% in most adult populations [1]. The occurrence of caries is a major cause of pain, tooth loss, aesthetic and functional problems and work absenteeism [2].

Although caries is an oral disease that occurs worldwide, according to Baelum and Fejerskov [3], there is no consensus regarding which criteria and methods should be used for its detection, and few studies compare different methods for measuring caries in epidemiological surveys involving adult populations [4, 5].

In recent decades, a wide variety of new methods have been developed to measure caries in a population [6–13]. These methods measure caries lesions based on different diagnostic thresholds. Some methods are able to measure early non-cavitated enamel lesions, which are observed only after drying the tooth surface, as indicated in the International Caries Detection and Assessment System (ICDAS) [11]. Others can detect early non-cavitated enamel lesions without the need to dry the tooth surface, as indicated in the Caries Assessment Spectrum and Treatment (CAST) [14]. The method used most frequently

* Correspondence: alscastro@yahoo.com.br
[1]Department of Health, State University of Feira de Santana, Transnordestina, s/n, Novo Horizonte, Feira de Santana, Bahia CEP 44036-900, Brazil
Full list of author information is available at the end of the article

since the 1940s is the decayed, missing and filled (DMF) index [15], which has generally been used to detect caries from dentin lesions. This change in diagnostic threshold affects the results of the prevalence rates calculated using each method.

The limitations of the DMF index have been noted in the literature, and therefore, new indexes were developed, among them the ICDAS and CAST have stood out, which were validated and used in several countries and therefore were chosen for comparison with the DMF [1, 8, 16–22].

This study aimed to compare the ICDAS, CAST and the DMF in terms of their operational aspects and their capacity to determine the extent and severity of dental caries in the same sample of individuals, thus informing future choices in regard to which caries detection method should be used in a community. To the best of our knowledge, this is the first study to compare the three methods at the same time in an adult population.

Methods

Study design and sample type

This was a descriptive cross-sectional study, in which three caries measurement methods were applied in the same group. The students, employees and their dependents, who were attending the Medical, Dental and Social Service (SMOS) at the State University of Bahia – UNEB, located in Salvador, Bahia, Brazil, during the period from September 6 to December 13, 2016, were examined. Because it was a convenience sample, no inferential statistics were calculated [23]. Only adults are provided care by this dental service, and the inclusion criterion was being in the care of the service during the aforementioned period; therefore, all examined individuals were adults, and 73% were between 18 and 31 years of age.

Ethical aspects

The individuals were examined after being properly informed about the procedures of the study and signing informed consent forms. The work was approved by the Research Ethics Committee of the Sciences Institute of the Federal University of Bahia under CAAE number 48500115.2.0000.5662.

Examiner calibration

Four examiners, with the aid of three note-takers, applied the three caries detection methods to the study population. Calibration of the four examiners was performed from August 8 to August 26, 2016. Each week, professors were asked to teach about a particular method and guide the examiner calibration. Eighteen hours of training were devoted to each method, and a total of 54 h of examiner calibration training was provided.

On the morning of the first day of training, there was a lecture on the CAST method, followed in the afternoon by training with projected photos and with in vitro teeth, in ceramic pots with modelling clay. On the morning of the next day, five patients were examined by the four study examiners, who were supervised by an experienced examiner, the method criteria were discussed, and the hits and errors of the four examiners were compared until a consensus was reached on the classification of the conditions diagnosed in the patients. In the afternoon, five more patients were examined to calculate the inter-examiner Kendall's Coefficient of Concordance (Kendall's W) [24]. These same patients were examined three days later to calculate the intra-examiner Kendall's Coefficient of Concordance. The following week, the same procedure was performed for ICDAS, adding the use of two e-learning programmes, one from the site ICDAS.org [25] and the other from a training programme developed by Port and Zaleski [26]. In the third week, the same procedure used in the calibration of CAST was followed for the DMF index training.

CAST was used according to the recommendations of the method's manual [27]. ICDAS was used as recommended on the ICDAS.org site at the time of the examination [25]. The DMF was applied according to the manual of the latest epidemiological survey of the Brazilian Ministry of Health [28], with the diagnostic threshold for the decayed tooth component in the DMF measured in non-cavitated dentine lesions (codes 4, 5 and 6 of ICDAS and 4, 5 and 6 of CAST). Descriptions of all the codes for the three methods are provided in the Additional file 1: Appendix.

Data collection procedure

The examinations were conducted in the period from September 6, 2016, to December 13, 2016. The selected exam period corresponded to the period of greatest frequency in the classroom by the university students in the second semester of the academic year. An exam schedule was drawn such that each examiner used a different method each week, the first to examine prophylaxis with brush and floss to remove plaque and allow a better clinical examination for him and the other examiners. Three dental offices were used. The patients, when they arrived, were provided with explanations about the research, signed the informed consent, and received prophylaxis from the first examiner. The fist examiner applied one method, the patient remained in the chair and another examiner examined him. The examiners then alternated, each one applying a different method. Dental equipment (dental light, dental chair) and dental instruments (WHO probe and plain dental mirror) were used. A compressed air syringe was used to dry the teeth during application of the ICDAS, which is the only method that requires the use of this resource.

During the examinations, each examiner applied a different method each week, and 780 forms were completed using the three methods (each of the 260 patients was examined three times in the same session by different examiners applying ICDAS, CAST and the DMF so that each patient produced three forms). Re-examinations were performed in 10% of the sample for each method to compare the intra-examiner and inter-examiner reproducibility using Kendall's W Coefficient of Concordance [24].

Analysis method

The proportions and absolute, percentage and standardised mean differences obtained with each method were compared. The data were entered into Microsoft Excel (2007) and analysed in R [29].

The tooth surface was the analysis unit used to calculate Kendall's W (i.e., Kendall's coefficient of concordance). For each individual, 128 surfaces (those of 28 permanent teeth) were examined. The third molars were not included in the examination. Surfaces with sealants were regarded as healthy.

Kendall's W Coefficient of Concordance is suitable for testing the reliability of ordinal data and thus was used to test the intra- and inter-examiner agreement. This coefficient has the advantage of not being affected by the prevalence of the studied object [24].

The most severe caries lesion per individual was used as an indicator to identify those in need of restorative and preventive treatment. This indicator shows the highest caries score in the carious component observed in an individual; therefore, it shows the greatest need for treatment at the moment of examination.

For example, an individual with restorations, extracted teeth and enamel caries will be included as an individual who needs preventive treatment to prevent this enamel lesion from developing into a dentine lesion, and another individual with enamel caries and a lesion that reached the pulp will be classified as an individual with caries that can produce an odontogenic abscess. Thus, a priority for the service would be to attend to this individual. This manner of classifying the individual's situation and not the mean number of teeth affected by caries facilitates communication between planning epidemiologists and other professionals in the health area. The most severe caries lesion per individual was determined based on the maximum score per subject used by the group of researchers who developed CAST [30].

This indicator was used in the same way that prevalence calculations were performed by CAST [27]; that is, per individual, without considering the calculation of sealants, fillings and teeth extracted due to caries. A modification was incorporated relative to CAST, which

was the inclusion of enamel caries lesions when calculating disease prevalence.

Initially, data were recorded for the tooth surface. The most severe caries lesion per tooth was then recorded, according to the worst conditions encountered when using each method, and finally, the worst lesion observed per individual was recorded.

When calculating the most severe caries lesion per individual, scores related to sealants, fillings, extractions and excluded surfaces were ignored. The order of severity adopted, from lowest to highest, was as follows: non-cavitated enamel lesions detected after drying the tooth; non-cavitated enamel lesions detected without drying the tooth; cavitated enamel lesions; non-cavitated dentine lesions; cavitated dentine lesions; filled surface with cavitated dentine lesions and extensive dentine lesions with pulp involvement.

Differences in the percentages of individuals classified as having caries lesions according to each method calculated with the indicator of the most severe caries lesion were compared.

The methods were also compared in terms of extension of disease, which, according to Maltz et al. [31], is the number of teeth or surfaces affected by the disease.

Three units of measure were used according to the different purposes: the surface unit to be further detailed and sensitive was used to calculate the concordance between the examinees, the tooth unit was used to compare the extent that the caries reached the group, and the individual unit used to differentiate people according to the worst condition found by calculations using the indicator the most severe caries lesion per individual.

When using the tooth as the measurement unit, lesions found by each method were classified as pre-morbidity (enamel lesions), morbidity (non-cavitated dentine and cavitated dentine lesions), severe morbidity (dentine lesions that had reached the pulp) and mortality (extracted teeth) according to the CAST Manual classification [27].

The means for decayed, missing and filled teeth obtained by each method were compared. The data obtained from CAST and ICDAS can be converted into the mean DMF if the same diagnostic threshold applied for the caries lesion is used for all three methods to classify the tooth.(In the study, the diagnostic threshold was established for all three methods from D3, i.e., non-cavitated dentine lesions and cavitated dentin lesions) [25]. Thus, we can add the following: teeth classified as carious; teeth identified as filled; and teeth lost due to caries. The total can then be divided by the number of examined persons to calculate a mean of decayed, filled and lost teeth using each method.

To facilitate comparisons between the methods and to simplify reporting of the results obtained by ICDAS, all the method codes relating to fillings were grouped together such that the codes distinguishing various types of fillings were reported simply as filled.

In the present study, ICDAS was used as recommended on the ICDAS.org site at the time the study was conducted, without incorporating Exposed Pulp, Ulceration, Fistula, Abscess (PUFA), International Caries Classification & Management System (ICCMS) or Lesion Activity (LA) measures.

To calculate the application time of each index, each examination was timed from the first annotated code to the last recorded code. The mean times spent performing examinations using each of the different methods were calculated and compared using the mean percentage difference, which is the difference between two values divided by the average of the two values shown as a percentage.

The standardised mean difference (SMD) was also utilised, which expresses the size of the intervention effect in each study relative to the variability observed in that study. To interpret the SMD data, Cohen's d was used. Cohen's d is a rather simple statistical expression: specifically, it reflects the difference between two group outcomes divided by the population standard deviation and is represented in the following formula: $d = (\mu1 - \mu2)/\sigma$ [32, 33].

$$SMD = \frac{\text{Difference in mean outcome between groups}}{\text{Standard deviation of outcome among participants}}$$

Results

Overall intra- and inter-examiner agreement and general sample characteristics

Most of the examined individuals were students (70.3%), female (74.2%) and aged 18 to 31 years (73.0%), with a mean age of 28 and a standard deviation (SD) of 10 years.

The Kendall's W values found in the intra- and inter-examiner tests demonstrated a very good level of agreement, as Kendall's W values above 0.90 were observed for the four examiners during application of the methods [34]. All values of Kendall's W for the different examiners are provided in the Additional file 1: Appendix.

Comparison of methods in regard to the application time

The coefficient of variation (CV) is a standardised measure of dispersion expressed as a percentage; it is the ratio of the standard deviation to the mean, shows the extent of variability in relation to the mean, and is used to compare the heterogeneity of the number of applications found with different methods. As shown in Table 1, the fastest method was the DMF, in which the mean application time was 3.8 min. However, the DMF also presented the most heterogeneous results (39.5% coefficient of variation). The results for CAST were similar to those of the DMF, with a mean application time of

Table 1 Mean application times, in minutes, of the ICDAS, CAST and DMF methods

Method	Mean (SD)	CV (%)	Min–Max
CAST	4.7 (1.4)	29.8	1.5–7.0
DMF	3.8 (1.5)	39.5	1.2–8.2
ICDAS	8.9 (2.8)	31.5	3.3–18.0

CV coefficient of variation, *SD* standard deviation, *Min* minimum, *Max* maximum

approximately one additional minute (4.7 min). This method presented the least heterogenous data (coefficient of variation 29.8%). ICDAS took longer than both the DMF and CAST, with a mean of 8.9 min. Its coefficient of variation was similar to that of CAST (31.5%).

Table 2 reveals that the biggest differences observed were between the DMF and ICDAS (134.2% and 2.3) methods, while the smallest differences were found between the CAST and the DMF methods (23.7% and 0.6).

To interpret the magnitude of the standardised mean difference, Cohen [32] recommended thresholds based on standardised mean differences: 0.2 reflects a small effect; 0.5 reflects a medium effect; and greater than 0.8 reflects a large effect. Using these guidelines, the results indicate that the effect sizes show large differences between the ICDAS and both the DMF and CAST and a medium difference between CAST and the DMF.

Comparison between methods according to the most severe caries lesion per individual

The distribution of caries prevalence in the population was determined according to the indicator of the most severe caries lesion per individual. This prevalence includes individuals who had caries lesions according to the diagnostic threshold of each method. When this indicator was calculated using the DMF index, a caries prevalence of 28.1% was found among the individuals. However, when using ICDAS, a prevalence of 84.6% was found, and when CAST was applied, the prevalence was 75.0% (the prevalence corresponds to the complement of the absence of lesions shown in the first row of Table 3).

According to the CAST and ICDAS methods, the worst condition observed in approximately half of the

Table 2 Differences in the mean application times of the ICDAS, CAST and DMF methods

METHODS	Absolute mean difference (minutes)	Percentage mean difference (%)	Standardised mean difference
CAST X DMF	0.9	23.7	0.6
CAST X ICDAS	4.2	47.2	1.9
DMF X ICDAS	5.1	134.2	2.3

Table 3 Distribution of indicators of the most severe caries lesions per individual according to the ICDAS, CAST and DMF methods

MOST SEVERE CARIES LESION	ICDAS		CAST		DMF		STAGE
	N	Pr	N	Pr	N	Pr	
No lesions	40	15.4	65	25.0	187	71.9	Healthy
EL* after drying	25	9.6					Pre-morbidity
EL without drying	48	18.5					
Cavitated EL	74	28.4			-----		
EL without drying + cavitated EL			122	46.9			
Non-cavitated DL**	12	4.6	12	4.6			Morbidity
Cavitated DL			48	18.5			
Cavitated DL + extensive DL	61	23.5					
Extensive DL with pulp involvement			13	5.0			Severe morbidity
Non-cavitated DL + cavitated DL + extensive DL with or without pulp involvement					73	28.1	

*EL Enamel lesion ** DL Dentine lesion, Pr Prevalence

individuals was enamel caries lesions (46.9 and 56.5%, respectively). These individuals were classified as having no caries lesions when using the DMF (Table 3).

Table 3 shows that when using the DMF method, 28.1% of the individuals had at least one dentine lesion, although the severity of each lesion was not indicated. When ICDAS and CAST were used, 4.6% of the individuals showed teeth with non-cavitated dentine damage as their worst condition (these individuals are in the morbidity group).

According to the ICDAS, 23.5% of the patients had extensive or cavitated dentine lesions. CAST differentiated these lesions into two groups: the morbidity group, comprising the 18.5% of individuals who had at least one tooth with a cavitated dentine lesion and the severe morbidity group, comprising the 5% of individuals who had at least one tooth with an extensive dentine lesion with pulp involvement, which requires more complex treatment.

Comparison between methods according to the disease extent

In addition to prevalence, these methods can also reveal the extent of caries in a population. According to the results, 77.88% of the examined teeth were classified as healthy when using the DMF, 66.80% when using CAST and 59.11% when applying ICDAS (Table 4).

According to the examinations performed using ICDAS, 484 teeth (6.76%) showed the first clinical signs of caries, that is, an enamel lesion after drying the tooth; 641 (8.95%) had enamel lesions that could be observed without drying the teeth; and 190 teeth (2.65%) had cavitated enamel lesions. The last two conditions are grouped in CAST as enamel lesions, and 821 teeth were classified as having this condition (11.46%). Teeth with such lesions may be classified as being in the pre-morbidity stage.

Application of the DMF classified 136 teeth as having dentine caries lesions (1.90%), with no distinction

Table 4 Distributions of classifications of tooth conditions according to the ICDAS, CAST and DMF methods

	ICDAS N	%	CAST N	%	DMF N	%	STAGE
Healthy teeth	4235	59.11	4786	66.80	5580	77.88	Healthy
Filled teeth	1268	17.70	1205	16.82	1223	17.07	
Teeth with EL* after drying	484	6.76					Pre-morbidity
Teeth with EL without drying	641	8.95					
Teeth with cavitated EL	190	2.65					
Teeth with EL without drying + cavitated EL			821	11.46			
Teeth with non-cavitated DL**	31	0.43	35	0.49			Morbidity
Teeth with cavitated DL			74	1.03			
Teeth with cavitated DL + extensive cavitated DL	90	1.25					
Teeth with extensive DL with pulp involvement			18	0.25			Severe morbidity
Teeth with non-cavitated + cavitated DL + extensive DL with or without pulp involvement					136	1.90	
Missing teeth due to caries	226	3.15	226	3.15	226	3.15	Mortality

* *EL* Enamel lesion ** *DL* Dentine lesion

between teeth with morbidity or severe morbidity and with all being classified as decayed teeth.

According to ICDAS, 121 teeth were found to be in the morbidity stage: 31 with non-cavitated dentine lesions (0.43%) and 90 with extensive or non-cavitated dentine lesions (1.25%). When using CAST, 109 teeth were diagnosed as being in the morbidity stage; 35 teeth with non-cavitated dentine lesions (0.49%), 74 teeth with cavitated dentine lesions (1.03%) and 18 teeth (0.43%) in the severe morbidity stage with extensive dentine lesions with pulp involvement.

According to the three methods, 226 teeth extracted due to caries (3.15%) were classified as being in the mortality stage. A total of 1268 (17.70%) teeth were filled when examined by ICDAS; 1205 (16.82%) when using CAST and 1223 (17.07%) according to the DMF. The different percentages were due to differences in inter-examiner classifications.

Only 19 teeth (9 people) had sealants, justifying the decision to classify teeth in this condition as healthy. There were no teeth with abscesses or fistulae, and as such, CAST code 7 was not used.

Comparison between methods according to the mean number of decayed, missing and filled teeth

When calculating the mean DMF for the study group, a value of 6.0 was obtained, which was very similar to the mean of 5.9 calculated using the data obtained from CAST and similar to the sum of teeth classified as decayed, missing and filled according to ICDAS, which was 6.2.

Discussion

The results of this study showed that most of the individuals examined were students (70.39%) and female (74.2%).

The four examiners obtained Kendall's W values greater than 0.90. According to Silva et al. [34], a Kendall's W value equal to or greater than 0.90 indicates that the evaluators applied essentially the same standard, so the three methods presented good reproducibility. This result demonstrated that more detailed methods, including enamel lesions and various codes for dentine lesions, do not diminish reproducibility provided that a good calibration of the examiners is performed.

Regarding differences in application times of the indices, according to Cohen [32], the effect sizes show a large difference between the ICDAS and the DMF [35] and a medium difference between the CAST and the DMF; therefore, choosing the ICDAS instead of the CAST to replace the DMF will have a sizable impact on the increased time necessary to carry out the survey.

According to the literature, the DMF is simple to apply, and analysis of its results is straightforward [1, 36], as also observed in this study.

Several authors [8, 16–19] have stated that the CAST method offers a simple application and analysis. No difficulties were encountered when applying the method during calibration and clinical examinations, nor during the analysis. This method proposes 10 codes arranged in a hierarchical manner, without the need to dry the teeth, contributing to its greater ease of application. On average, it took one minute longer than the time taken to apply the DMF index.

Similar to the present work, CAST and DMF showed an equivalent time in the study by Souza et al. [8], in which an absolute and percentage difference of 1.6 and 2.5% were reported between these two methods, respectively; these are small differences despite the ability of CAST to measure lesions in enamel and distinguish the three levels of gravity of the lesions in dentin.

In a study by Braga et al. [22] using the DMF and ICDAS on the same group of 252 children, ICDAS took twice as long to use in deciduous teeth, and the data generated using this method for cavitated dentine caries lesions were comparable to those of the DMF.

According to the literature, the most complex method to use is ICDAS [18, 20, 21] because its two-digit system uses the first digit to indicate fillings and sealants and the second for the detection of caries lesions. Additionally, enamel lesions are classified according to three different levels. During the examinations, it was necessary to classify each surface in relation to these two digits and to observe each surface before and after drying the tooth, as described below. All 128 tooth surfaces of each patient were analysed without drying the surface to detect the presence of an ICDAS code 2 lesion (enamel lesion without drying). Each surface was then dried for 5 s to detect the presence of ICDAS code 1 lesions (enamel lesion after surface drying). These extra steps meant that this method took longer to apply (8.9 min), taking an average of more than 5 min longer than the DMF.

The total duration of the examinations of the 260 individuals was 4 h longer when using CAST than when using the DMF and 22 h longer when examining patients using ICDAS than when using the DMF. Assuming a hypothetical population of 2600 people, which is 10 times larger than the studied sample, application of the ICDAS would require an additional 220 h, demanding more human resources and making this diagnosis costlier and more time-consuming.

The disadvantages of ICDAS have been reported by de Amorim et al. [21] and Iranzo-Cortes et al. [4], as also verified in the present study. Use of a two-digit system and many codes made it difficult to analyse data, and the application of air to dry surfaces made the method time-consuming.

The development and use of the indicator of the most severe caries lesion per individual aimed to identify people who had enamel caries lesions and those with dentine lesions. This indicator does not include the past history of filled and extracted teeth; instead, it is reversible; that is, it can be zero if all curative and preventive needs of the studied community are met.

This indicator aims to identify the needs of each individual at the time of the examination, and if the worst condition was an enamel lesion, that individual would be identified as belonging to the group needing care for this type of lesion. If a dentine injury is present, the individual will be included in the group for which restoration should be performed. The lesion is not reversible, but the need for treatment for this lesion is reversible; therefore, after the group of individuals receive the treatment, the information related to this dental care will be provided through a more direct measure showing the changes occurring in the community after receiving dental care.

This concept of a reversible measure is employed in CAST. Upon calculating the disease prevalence, the authors [27] recommend considering filled teeth, those with sealants and those without signs of caries as healthy. Therefore, the CAST code values decrease as the population receives dental care, unlike the DMF, for which the mean value does not decrease after treatment.

CAST and ICDAS were used at the enamel level, and the DMF was used at the dentine level. Therefore, these two methods were likely to produce higher caries estimates than the DMF, not because of how they are constructed but because of the much larger number of enamel caries than dentine caries. If the DMF was used with the inclusion of enamel caries, then the difference would substantially decrease. The DMF was used in this way because caries in dentine is the diagnostic threshold commonly employed by the DMF. The different criteria used by the methods can cause variations in the prevalence. This study intends to demonstrate the consequences of the use of certain criteria in the diagnosis of caries and dental care planning.

When using the DMF, a good proportion of the individuals considered to be affected by caries was related to past history (fillings and extractions), and as these conditions were not included, it was concluded that the vast majority of individuals had no need for treatment at the time of examination. In contrast to the DMF, the use of CAST allowed the identification of individuals who had caries lesions on enamel. In addition, CAST was the only method that distinguished lesions with morbidity and severe morbidity in which caries lesions reached the tooth pulp.

The greater detailing of dentine lesions obtained when using CAST has also been described by de Souza et al. [8], who stated that a disadvantage of the DMF is its inability to distinguish between dentine lesions that can be restored and those that require more complex treatment. This limitation precludes the acquisition of an overview of the type of treatment required by a population, thus preventing proper planning with respect to the quantity of dental materials, human resources, methods and equipment required to adequately resolve the situation.

When using the tooth as the measurement unit, ICDAS and CAST showed lower percentages of healthy teeth than the DMF because these methods include enamel caries lesions among their criteria, which is why some teeth classified as healthy by the DMF would be classified as having enamel lesions by other methods.

The examined population had access to dental care at UNEB's dental service, which might explain the large percentages of teeth with fillings. In the 2010 Brazilian dental health survey, the restored component represented 43.5% of the examined teeth that were affected by caries in the adult population [36]. In the present study, the restored component, according to DMF, represented 77.6% of the teeth affected by caries, which is well above the national average. Access to dental care may also explain the small percentages of teeth with dentine caries lesions.

The ICDAS was the only one of the three methods in which caries lesions were detected in enamel after drying the teeth, which was the major difference observed between ICDAS and CAST; however, the identification of these lesions is one of the reasons for the more time-consuming and laborious nature of ICDAS. The detection of this type of lesion is questionable for use in large population groups because many of the surfaces with these lesions return to a healthy state without any type of treatment and entail a high cost due to the use of prophylaxis, good illumination and compressed air.

Comparability is an important advantage of the DMF; the DMF average can be compared with studies from the 1940s onwards and with data collected from across the world. The mean values obtained using the three methods for decayed, missing and filled teeth were very close. Therefore, to stop using CAST and ICDAS due to a lack of comparability is unreasonable, as the results obtained using these methods can be converted into the mean DMF.

Conclusions

CAST was able to classify the severity of lesions and identify preventive and curative needs without the need to dry the tooth, with a similar application time to the DMF. Therefore, CAST is suitable for use in the detection of caries in a population.

The prevalence calculated by the DMF was lower than that detected by the other methods because this index does not include enamel lesions, and DMF does not distinguish between severities of caries lesions, which is important for health planning. However, the DMF is a quick, simple and easily applied index that can be used when it is not necessary to measure enamel lesions.

Finally, the ICDAS method obtained the most detailed data regarding caries classification, but it is difficult to use in epidemiological surveys of dental caries, as it is time-consuming. Moreover, its analysis is complex because it classifies enamel lesions into three levels and uses two digits and too many codes. However, it was the only method among the three able to detect the first clinical signs of caries and can be used in conjunction with other systems to assess caries activity. Therefore, the ICDAS method is appropriate for use in clinical studies and in individual evaluations of caries lesions.

Abbreviations
CAST: Caries Assessment Spectrum and Treatment; DMF: Decayed, Missing and Filled index; ICCMS: International Caries Classification & Management System; ICDAS: International Caries Detection and Assessment System; LA: Lesion Activity; PUFA: Exposed Pulp, Ulceration, Fistula, Abscess; SMOS: Medical, Dental and Social Service; UNEB: State University of Bahia

Acknowledgements
The authors would like to thank the professors who monitored the calibration of the three methods; the examiners and note-takers who devoted themselves with such commitment and professionalism to the research; the coordinator and staff of SMOS and UNEB, who helped us during application of the methods; and the students, staff and their dependents who agreed to participate in the study.

Author's contributions
ALSC, CMCM and MIPV designed the study, ALSC organised the survey and participated as an examiner, ALSC drafted the manuscript, and ALSC and CMCM performed the statistical analyses. All authors reviewed the original draft and read and approved the final manuscript.

Competing interests
The authors declare that they have no competing interests.

Author details
[1]Department of Health, State University of Feira de Santana, Transnordestina, s/n, Novo Horizonte, Feira de Santana, Bahia CEP 44036-900, Brazil.
[2]Department of Public Oral Health, School of Dentistry, Federal University of Bahia, Araújo Pinho, 62, Canela, Salvador, Bahia CEP 40110040, Brazil.
[3]Postgraduate Studies in Interactive Processes of Organs and Systems, Health Science Institute, Federal University of Bahia, Avenida Reitor Miguel Calmon, 1272, Salvador, Bahia CEP 40231300, Brazil.

References
1. Fejerskov O, Kidd E. Dental caries: the disease and its clinical management. Hoboken, NJ: John Wiley & Sons; 2009.
2. Petersen PE, Bourgeois D, Ogawa H, Estupinan-Day S, Ndiaye C. The global burden of oral diseases and risks to oral health. Bull World Health Organ. 2005;83:661–9.
3. Baelum V, Ole F. How big is the problem? Epidemiological features of dental caries. In: Fejerskov O, Nyvad B, Kidd E, editors. Dental caries: the disease and its clinical management. Oxford, UK: Wiley; 2015. p. 21–41.
4. Iranzo-Cortés JE, Montiel-company JM, Almerich-Silla JM. Caries diagnosis: agreement between WHO and ICDAS II criteria in epidemiological surveys. Community Dent Health. 2013;30:108–11.
5. Melgar RA, Pereira JT, Luz PB, Hugo FN, Araujo FB. Differential impacts of caries classification in children and adults: a comparison of ICDAS and DMF-T. Braz Dent J. 2016;27:761–6.
6. Mount GJ, Hume WR. A revised classification of carious lesions by site and size. Quintessence Int. 1997;28:301–3.
7. Fisher J, Glick M. FDI world dental federation science committee. A new model for caries classification and management: the FDI world dental federation caries matrix. J Am Dent Assoc. 2012;143:546–51.
8. de Souza AL, Leal SC, Bronkhorst EM, Frencken JE. Assessing caries status according to the CAST instrument and WHO criterion in epidemiological studies. BMC Oral Health. 2014;14:119.
9. Nyvad B. Diagnosis versus detection of caries. Caries Res. 2004;38:192–8.
10. Castro ALS, Vianna MIP, Reis SR de A. A new index for measuring dental caries: reversible dental caries index-IRCD. Rev Fac Odontol Univ Fed Bahia. 1999;19:35–40.
11. Ismail AI, Sohn W, Tellez M, Amaya A, Sen A, Hasson H, et al. The international caries detection and assessment system (ICDAS): an integrated system for measuring dental caries. Community Dent Oral Epidemiol. 2007;35:170–8.
12. Sheiham A, Maizels J, Maizels A. New composite indicators of dental health. Community Dent Health. 1987;4:407–14.
13. Monse B, Heinrich-Weltzien R, Benzian H, Holmgren C, Helderman WP. PUFA–an index of clinical consequences of untreated dental caries. Community Dent Oral Epidemiol. 2010;38:77–82.
14. Frencken JE, de Amorim RG, Faber J, Leal SC. The caries assessment Spectrum and treatment (CAST) index: rational and development. Int Dent J. 2011;61:117–23.
15. Klein H, Palmer CE, Knutson JW. Studies on dental caries: I. Dental status and dental needs of elementary school children. Public Health Rep. 1938;53: 751–65.
16. Maciel IP. Epidemiological survey of oral health in schoolchildren using the instrument CAST. 2016. http://repositorio.unb.br/bitstream/10482/21254/1/2016_IsadoraPassosMaciel.pdf. Accessed 9 Feb 2017.
17. Baginska J, Rodakowska E, Milewski R, Kierklo A. Dental caries in primary and permanent molars in 7-8-year-old schoolchildren evaluated with caries assessment Spectrum and treatment (CAST) index. BMC Oral Health. 2014;14:74.
18. Baginska J, Rodakowska E, Wilczko M, Kierklo A. Caries assessment Spectrum and treatment (CAST) index in the primary molars of 6- to 7-year-old polish children. Oral Health Prev Dent. 2016;14:85–92.
19. Anchala K, Challa R, Vadaganadham Y, Kamatham R, Deepak V, Nuvvula S. Assessment of dental caries in primary dentition employing caries assessment spectrum and treatment index. J Orofac Sci. 2016;8:115.
20. Almerich-Silla JM, Boronat-Ferrer T, Montiel-Company JM, Iranzo-Cortés JE. Caries prevalence in children from Valencia (Spain) using ICDAS II criteria, 2010. 2014. https://www.ncbi.nlm.nih.gov/pmc/articles/PMC4259373/. Accessed 14 Mar 2017.
21. de Amorim RG, Figueiredo MJ, Leal SC, Mulder J, Frencken JE. Caries experience in a child population in a deprived area of Brazil, using ICDAS II. Clin Oral Investig. 2012;16:513–20.
22. Braga MM, Oliveira LB, Bonini GA, Bonecker M, Mendes FM. Feasibility of the international caries detection and assessment system (ICDAS-II) in epidemiological surveys and comparability with standard World Health Organization criteria. Caries Res. 2009;43:245–9.
23. Ludwig DA. Use and misuse of p-values in designed and observational studies: guide for researchers and reviewers. Aviat Space Environ Med. 2005; 76:675–80.
24. Kendall MG. Rank correlation methods. 1948[cited on march 17, 2017]; Available at: https://onlinelibrary.wiley.com/doi/abs/10.1111/j.2044-8317.1956.tb00172.x
25. Topping GVA, Hally JD, Bonner BC, Pitts NB. Training for the international caries detection and assessment system (ICDAS II): CD-room and web-based educational software. London: Smile-on; 2008.
26. Port AL da F, Zaleski V Development of a digital learning object for caries lesions detection training using ICDAS [cited on March 1, 2017]; Available at: https://www.lume.ufrgs.br/bitstream/handle/10183/153016/000938457.pdf?sequence=1.
27. Leal SCFJ, de Souza AL, Bronkhorst EM. Manual CAST: caries assessment and treatment. Ipskamp Drukkers: Holanda; 2015.

28. (MS) M da S do B. Examiner's manual. Projeto SB Brasil 2010. In: MS Brasília; 2009.

29. R Core Team. R: A language and environment for statistical computing. R Foundation for Statistical Computing, Vienna; 2014. https://stat.ethz.ch/pipermail/r-help/2014-October/422975.html.

30. Leal SC, Ribeiro APD, Frencken JE. Caries assessment Spectrum and treatment (CAST): a novel epidemiological instrument. Caries Res. 2017;51:500–6.

31. Maltz M, Alves L. S. G S, Moura M. S. Epidemiology of dental caries. In: Cariology: basic concepts, diagnosis and non-restorative treatment. São Paulo: Artes Médicas; 2016. p. 51–64. (ABENO).

32. Cohen J. Statistical power analysis for the behavioral sciences. Hillsdale NJ: Erlbaum; 1988.

33. FERGUSON CJ. An effect size primer: a guide for clinicians and researchers. Prof Pathol Res Pract. 2009;40(5):532–8.

34. Silva EMM, Sena D, Gutierres JCM, JHF G. Quantitative analysis of subjectivity: an example of attribute agreement. Curitiba: RAC; 2005. p. 299–310.

35. Conboy JE. Some typical univariate measures of magnitude of effect. Psychological Analysis. 2012;21:145–58.

36. Pinto VG. Public Oral Health. 6th ed. Santos: São Paulo; 2013.

18

Dental caries experience and associated risk indicators among Palestinian pregnant women in the Jerusalem area

Elham Kateeb[1,2,3]* ⓘ and Elizabeth Momany[2]

Abstract

Background: This study described the dental caries experience of Palestinian pregnant women and examined its relationships to their oral health knowledge, beliefs, behavior, and access to dental care.

Methods: Pregnant women receiving prenatal care at the Ministry of Health (MOH) centers in the Jerusalem Governorate were invited to participate in this study. Structured interviews were conducted to assess pregnant mothers' beliefs about oral health care and their oral hygiene practices. Screening for mothers' dental caries experience was carried out using the Decayed, Missing and Filled Teeth/Surfaces (DMFT/S) index. Univariate, bi-variate and multi-variable analysis were conducted to explain the high level of disease in this population.

Results: A total of 152 pregnant women participated in this study. Mean DMFT in this sample was 15.5 ± 4.5 and an average DMFS of 31.8 ± 21. According the World Health Organization (WHO) criteria, 89% of our sample were categorized in the "Extremely High" dental caries experience. Fifty-eight percent of the DMFT scores among this sample were due to untreated dental decay, while 22% of the same DMFT scores demonstrated restorative care received by this sample. Bivariate analysis showed that mothers who completed a degree after high school had lower DMFT scores than mothers who did not ($F = 4$, $n = 152$, $p = .024$). In addition, mothers who believed they could lose a tooth just because they are pregnant had higher DMFT scores ($t = -4$, $n = 152$, $p = .037$). The final model found that age, level of education, providers' advice on utilizing dental care during pregnancy, and the belief that a woman can lose a tooth just because she is pregnant explained 22% of the variation in DMFT scores.

Conclusions: Women in this study had a high prevalence of dental diseases and knew little about dental care during pregnancy. Faulty beliefs about dental care during pregnancy among women and health care providers were major factors in the high levels of disease.

Keywords: Access to care, Pregnant, Dental caries, Beliefs, Attitude, Knowledge

Background

The literature has demonstrated that women are more susceptible to dental caries during pregnancy. This finding could be due to the special conditions pregnant mothers suffer, such as increased acidity in the oral cavity, sugary dietary cravings, inadequate attention to oral health (OH) and delayed treatment [1]. In the literature, it is recorded that women who gave birth to more children show a higher percentage of 'decays' compared to women with only one child [2].

While pregnancy made mothers more vulnerable to OH changes, many factors independent of pregnancy may also play important roles. Three important domains presented in some conceptual models of health [3–5] include personal characteristics (e.g., demographics, socio-economic status [6]), health behaviors (e.g., health practices [7], healthcare utilization [8]), and the broader

---

* Correspondence: ekateeb@staff.alquds.edu; elhame20@gmail.com
[1]Department of Periodontology and Preventive Dentistry, Al-Quds University, Jerusalem, State of Palestine
[2]Public Policy Center, the University of Iowa, Iowa City, IA, USA
Full list of author information is available at the end of the article

social context and environment (e.g., health care system [8]). These models suggested that dental care utilization can be a mediating factor; other factors, including demographic and personal characteristics, may influence access to care, and positive health outcomes can be impacted by easier access to professional dental care [4, 5].

In other models, some psychosocial factors were suggested, such as mothers' stress levels (MSL) and social support (the support the mothers usually get from their families and friends) [9–11]. In one study [11], social support and MSL were both identified to be associated with OH status and OH behavior, and they were likely to influence both the decision-making process of when to seek dental care and the type of treatment to opt for. In another study [9], both social networks and MSL were identified as barriers to utilizing dental services.

Although there are many studies discussed factors related to OH of pregnant women, the complex and dynamic interactions among these factors and their influences on OH status for pregnant women are not yet fully understood. In addition, most of the previous literature did not relate those factors to pregnant women's clinically assessed OH [12].

The importance of this study stems from the fact that there are scarce data attempted to describe the OH status, behaviors, beliefs and attitudes of pregnant women in the Levant area in general and in Palestine in particular. Hence, the present study assessed OH status among pregnant mothers attending maternal and child health care (MCHC) programs at the Ministry of Health (MOH) and examined its relationships to mothers' OH knowledge, beliefs, behaviors, and access to dental care. These data will be helpful in planning OH prevention and intervention programs for this study population.

The current study's specific objectives were to describe the dental caries experience among a sample of low-income pregnant women and their knowledge, beliefs and attitudes towards oral health and dental care during pregnancy. In addition, guided by our conceptual model, this study examined associations between different distal (sociodemographic and psychosocial) and proximal (oral hygiene practices and beliefs, attitudes and access to dental care) factors on the mothers' dental caries experience.

Methods

This study was a cross-sectional investigation employed individual in-depth interviews using a structured questionnaire among pregnant women in their 2nd and 3rd trimesters. The study was carried out by a dental public health professional team in the Jerusalem Governorate of the State of Palestine in the period from March 2015 to December 2015.

All MCHC centers at the MOH's public clinics in the Jerusalem Governorate ($N = 15$) were included in this study. Pregnant women who attended their scheduled Obstetrician/Gynecologist (OB-GYN) appointments at the 15 clinics were invited to participate in the study. All pregnant women who were enrolled in the MCHC program in those centers were initially recruited through clinics' listings to schedule their monthly OB-GYN appointment. Mothers who showed up on the scheduled day were asked to participate in this study. Non-responses were minimal because there was a long queue to see the OB-GYN and because mothers thought that answering some questions would help them pass the time. However, if respondents chose not to answer any of the questions, that question was excluded from the analysis.

The minimal non-response bias combined with the recruiting strategy used in this study made our final sample representative of all mothers use MCHC programs in Jerusalem governorate.

Inclusion criteria for participation included healthy women who were pregnant, in their second or third trimesters, resided in the Jerusalem Governorate and used one of the 15 MCHC centers at the MOH's public clinics.

The study team consisted of a dental public health specialist, E.K., who conducted all the interviews in this study, and well-trained senior dental students at Al-Quds University Faculty of Dental Medicine, who conducted the clinical screening. A structured questionnaire was developed based on previous studies [13, 14] and checked for its cultural sensitivity in a sample of 13 pregnant women.

The final version of the questionnaire included questions about pregnant women's socio-demographic data ("Age," "Household Income," "Level of Education," "Employment Status," "Insurance Coverage," and "Number of Previous Pregnancies"), their access to dental care, their oral hygiene habits and their perception of their own OH status.

The questionnaire also included questions that assessed mothers' beliefs about the importance of dental care during pregnancy and the influence of their OH on their own general health and on their birth outcomes. Beliefs that promoted positive OH behaviors were measured using a five-point scale ("Strongly Agree," "Agree," "Neither Agree nor Disagree" "Disagree," or "Strongly Disagree").

The questionnaire also assessed some psychosocial constructs that were measured by validated scales, such as instrumental social support and MSL [13, 14]. The MSL instrument included six items scored on a Likert scale from 1 ("Never") to 5 ("Almost Always"). Scale's final score of each respondent was the mean score of the ratings of the six items; thus, higher scores indicate higher levels of stress. The social support instrument comprised four items scored "Yes" or "No." The social support instrument was calculated as a sum of the answers; each "Yes" received a "1", and each "No" received a "0". The higher the final result was, the more social support the mother received.

Mothers' dental caries experience and plaque accumulation were screened using the World Health Organization (WHO) oral health survey's community-based indices [15]. Pregnant mothers' dental caries prevalence was assessed by the DMFT index and their dental caries experience severity by the DMFS index [15]. In addition, Russell Plaque index (PI) was used to assess oral hygiene and plaque accumulation [15]. Senior dental students who attended two calibration sessions and one hands-on training session on real patients did the OH screening for all participants. The supervisor (E.K) double checked the final recording of the OH exams.

Mothers were invited to the maternal exam room at the public clinics and were seated on a patient chair. Clinical screening followed the methods specified in the WHO pathfinder survey guidelines [15]. However, tongue depressors were used instead of periodontal probes, to exclude the need for sterilization on-site. The use of tongue depressors in field screening was validated in a previous study [16]. Plaque accumulation using PI was first evaluated, and then mothers were asked to brush their teeth; dental caries indices were examined afterward. Clinical exam data were recorded in special forms and collected with the questionnaire data at the end of each session.

Participation was voluntary, and signed paper consent forms were collected from mothers who agreed to participate in this study. Consents for participants under the age of 18 were signed by their parents/guardians. All aspects of this study, including the consent forms, were approved by the Scientific Research Ethics Committee of Al-Quds University. This study has been conducted in full accordance with the World Medical Association Declaration of Helsinki.

The analysis used in this study was guided by the conceptual model shown in Fig. 1. This conceptual model was based on previous models used in the dental literature [17, 18] to explain access to dental care and OH conditions among different populations.

Independent variables included the following: social variables, demographic variables, a social support scale, employment status ("Student," "Housewife," "Part-time Job", "Full-time Job"); dental insurance ("Private," "Public," "None"); and education ("Less than High School," "High School," "Two Year College," "Four-Year College or More"). Household monthly income (less than $399, $400–$799, $800–$1199, $1200–$1599, more than

$1600) was used according to the Palestinian Central Bureau of Statistics [19].

Variables describing access to dental care were as follows: 1) last dental visit within the past "6 Months," "12 Months," "3 Years," "5 Years," "Never Been to a Dentist Office," and 2) if the mother had a dental home (a particular dentist she usually visits). Variables describing oral hygiene practices such as brushing ("Never," "Sometimes," "Once a Day or More") and flossing ("Never," "Sometimes," "Daily") were also used to describe oral hygiene habits (self-reported). In addition, we asked mothers to demonstrate the way they usually brush and floss their teeth to assess if they perform this task correctly or not (oral hygiene habits noted). Plaque accumulation measured by PI was treated as continuous variable; however, this variable was categorized according to WHO Oral Health Survey [15] criteria to describe mothers' oral hygiene.

MSL and statements that described mothers' beliefs about 1) dental care during pregnancy, 2) relationship between their oral and general health, and 3) relationship between their OH and birth outcomes were used as mediating variables, as illustrated in the conceptual model.

Dental caries experience was the dependent variable in this study, summarized by the DMFT index. DMFT index was treated as continuous data; however, for descriptive purposes, DMFT index was categorized into 4 categories according to cut points assigned by the WHO Oral Health Survey [15].

Results

One hundred fifty-two pregnant mothers completed our in-person structured questionnaire, and 151 of these mothers did the OH clinical screening. Mothers' ages ranged from 17 to 42 years old, with an average of 26 years (SD = 5.4). Table 1 presents socio-demographic characteristics and barriers to accessing dental care in our sample.

The mean score of the MSL scale in this sample was 3.4 out of 5 (SD = 0.8, range = 1.2–5.00), and the mean score of the Social Support scale was 2.6 out of 4 (SD = 1.1, range = 0–4).

Oral hygiene practices and oral hygiene scores are shown in Table 2. A total of 100% of our sample had experienced dental decay. On average, participants had a DMFT score of 15.5 (SD = 5.5, range = 1–26) and a DMFS score of 31.8 (SD = 21.8, range = 1–127), with untreated decay DT of 7.9 (SD = 4.7, range = 0–20) and DS of 12.7 (SD = 10.5, range = 0–58). The FT component, which reflects the dental treatments the mother received, was 3.0 on average (SD = 3.2, range = 0–15). Dental caries experience severities, according to the

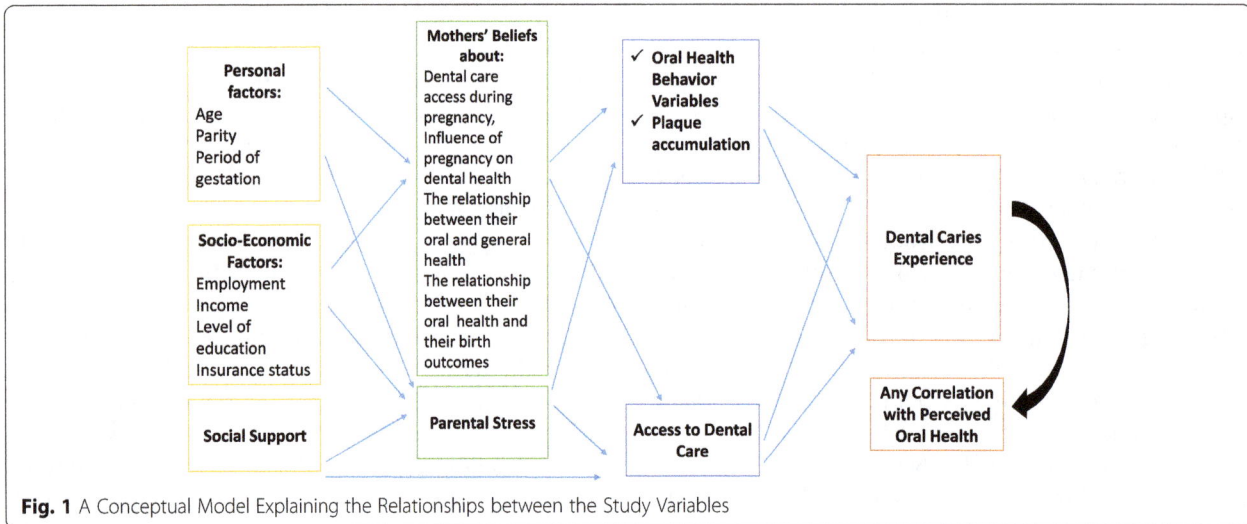

Fig. 1 A Conceptual Model Explaining the Relationships between the Study Variables

WHO Oral Health Survey [15] and mothers' perception of their own OH, are shown in Table 2.

When mothers' perceived OH was compared to clinical measures, significant correlations were found with mothers' dental caries experience (DMFT) (Spearman's Rank p = 0.305, $p < 0.000$).

A total of 51.8% of our sample believed that their dental problems might affect their general health. However, 75% of the same sample were not sure if a mother's poor OH may contribute to a low-birth-weight baby or other negative birth outcomes.

In addition, although 86.8% of the mothers "Agreed "or "Strongly Agreed" that it is important for adults to go to the dentist, even when they do not have problems with their teeth, 38% of our sample still thought it was unsafe for pregnant women to get routine dental care, such as checkups and cleanings. Moreover, 57% "Agreed "or "Strongly Agreed" that a woman can lose a tooth just because she is pregnant.

After stratifying by socio-demographic and behavioral characteristics, disparities were found in the dental caries experience in our sample. Education was a significant factor in dental caries experience; there was a statistically significant difference between groups, as determined by one-way ANOVA (F = 4.00, $p = 0.02$). A Tukey post hoc test revealed that mothers who had a post-high school diploma had lower DMFT scores than mothers who only finished their high school diploma ($p = 0.015$). In addition, mothers' level of education was a statistically significant factor in mothers demonstrating the correct way of brushing ($\Sigma^2 = 15.6$, $p = 0.048$). In turn, mothers who failed to demonstrate the correct way of brushing ($t = 2.06$, $p = 0.041$) and had more plaque accumulation ($r = .31$, $p < .0001$), scored higher on the DMFT index.

As expected, older mothers and mothers who had more than one baby had higher scores on the DMFT ($r = 0.292$, $p < 0.0001$) and ($t = 2.6$, $p = 0.01$) respectively.

Mothers who had a dental home had lower DMFT than did mothers without a dental home ($t = 2.09$, $p = 0.038$). A surprising result, although it was of borderline statistical significance, was that mothers who had never been to a dentist had lower DMFT scores compared to mothers who visited a dentist in the past 6 months, based on findings from a one-way ANOVA (F = 2.4. $p = 0.053$; Tukey post hoc test $p = 0.058$).

When we assessed barriers to utilizing dental care during pregnancy, we found that mothers who perceived dental costs and time restrictions as important challenges had higher DMFT scores ($t = 2.09$, $p = 0.038$ and $t = 2.11$, $p = 0.036$, respectively). Mothers also reported that their general health providers' advice about the lack of safety of visiting dentists while pregnant was another barrier to accessing dental care ($t = 2.09$, p = 0.038).

Mothers' beliefs about OH during pregnancy were the most important factors in their high caries experience. Pregnant mothers who thought that they could lose a tooth just because they were pregnant or that it was unsafe to visit a dentist while pregnant scored higher on the DMFT index ($t = 3.99$, $p < 0.0001$). This widespread incorrect belief was also associated with more plaque accumulation ($t = 2.372$, $p = 0.019$).

Regarding psychological factors, MSL was a significant factor in increasing DMFT scores ($r = 0.20$, $p = 0.014$). Although social support and household monthly income were not directly associated with DMFT scores, they were instrumental in increasing MSL ($r = -2.37$, $p = 0.003$ and $r = 0.232$, $p = 0.006$), respectively.

Dental caries experience and associated risk indicators among Palestinian pregnant women...

159

Table 1 Demographic and access to care characteristics of the study sample

Demographic characteristics	Percentages
Mother's employment	
Working	6.6
Stay at home	86.8
Students	6.6
Mother's education level	
Less than high school	41.1
High school diploma	25.8
Post-high school education	33.1
Monthly household income	
Less than $400	24
$400–$799	46.7
$800–$1200	19.3
More than $1200	10
Access to dental care	
Dental Insurance	
Public	4.6
Private	24.8
No insurance	70.6
Dental home	
Yes	35
No	65
Last visit to the dentist	
6 months	32.2
12 months	34.2
3 years	15.4
5 years	10.1
Never been to a dentist	8.1
Barriers to dental care (Self-reported)	
Safety concerns by family and friends	47.3
Dental costs	26.2
Time constraints	20.8
Advice by care providers not to seek treatment	32.9
Oral health is not a priority during pregnancy	25.5

Table 2 Oral hygiene practices, perceived oral health and oral health indices of the study sample

Oral hygiene practices (self-reported)	Percentages
Brushing	
At least twice a day	30
Once a day	34.6
Sometimes, irregular	32.7
Never	2.7
Flossing	
Daily	1.3
Sometimes	12
Never	86.7
Correct brushing (noted)	
Yes	73.6
No	25.7
Perceived oral health	
Poor or Fair	45.1
Average	29.1
Good or Excellent	25.8
Dental caries experience (DMFT Index)	
Very low	0.7
Low	2.0
Moderate	2.0
High	6.0
Extremely high	89.3
Oral hygiene (Plaque index)	
Good	14.6
Fair	70.1
Poor	15.3

brushing and believed that they could lose a tooth only because they were pregnant scored higher on the DMFT index ($\beta = 0.16$, $p = 0.039$; $\beta = 0.26$, $p = 0.001$ respectively). Mothers who didn't seek dental care during pregnancy because of their health care providers' advice had higher DMFT scores ($\beta = 0.16$, $p = 0.036$).

Discussion

There is enough evidence-based literature to suggest that good OH during pregnancy not only improves the quality of life of the pregnant mother but also potentially reduces complications during pregnancy and the risk of her child developing Early Childhood Caries (ECC) in the future. However, pregnant women often have misconceptions about OH during pregnancy, which prevents them from taking care of their OH or seeking professional care.

This study investigated pregnant women's OH beliefs and behaviors and assessed their dental caries experience.

All variables that were found significant in the bivariate analysis were included in the linear regression model. Stepwise linear regression was carried out, and results were then confirmed by forward and backward regression.

After controlling all other variables, five variables explained 22% of the variation in the DMFT scores in this sample. Older mothers ($\beta = 0.23$, $p = 0.004$) who did not have a degree past their high school diploma ($\beta = 0.17$, $p = 0.04$) scored higher on DMFT index. In addition, mothers who failed to demonstrate the correct way of

The sample in this study represented mothers who used MCHC programs at the Palestinian MOH public clinics. The sample was randomly selected from the 15 centers, and mothers shared many demographic characteristics. Our results showed that most of the mothers had low levels of education, low monthly household incomes, and irregular access to dental care. As a consequence, all mothers in this sample suffered from dental caries and bad oral hygiene. Although the intensity of these oral conditions varied, the numbers demonstrated a high burden of disease.

According to the classification of the WHO Oral Health Survey Basic Methods [15], 89% of our sample were categorized in the "Extremely High" dental caries experience. Moreover, 58% of the DMFT scores among this sample were due to untreated dental decay, while 22% of the same DMFT scores demonstrated restorative care received by this sample. This finding reflects the high treatment needs in this sample; however, restorative care alone will not solve the problem. The high plaque accumulation in this sample, combined with the fact that almost 85% of the sample perceived their OH as "Poor" or "Fair", suggests that oral hygiene education, motivation and raising awareness among pregnant women are necessary here.

Data from published literature showed significant differences in the caries experience among pregnant women in different areas of the world. The DMFT scores of pregnant mothers in some disadvantaged groups in Finland (DMFT = 18), Brazil (DMFT = 14) and Hungary (DMFT = 12.57) were very close to the DMFT scores in the current study [20–22]. In contrast, data from more representative samples of the general population in Iran (5.4) and India (3.6 and 4.8) indicated a lower burden of disease [23–25]. These vast differences in the caries experience between different areas in the world can be explained by the uniqueness of the socioeconomic and cultural structures of the samples in each study.

In Palestine, there is no data about dental caries experience among adults, except one study [26] that was conducted on a convenience sample of men and women in the commercial capital of the West Bank area in Palestine, Ramallah. Data from the previous study demonstrated lower DMFT scores in general for the same age group, 18–45 years old, with a DMFT mean of 9.03 ± 6.07. However, when subgroup analysis was carried out, women in this age group scored a DMFT mean of 8.5 ± 6.22, which is much lower than the numbers in the current study. This finding can be explained by the fact that the Ramallah study was conducted in a sample that had higher education attainment and lived in a wealthier part of the West Bank.

The high DMFT values found in this study were related to many factors in the current analysis. As documented in other literature, mothers' level of education was detrimental to their dental caries experience; not only did mothers with post-high school education score lower on the DMFT index, but they were also able to demonstrate the correct way of brushing and had less plaque accumulation on their teeth.

The literature shows that dental care access and utilization are influenced by factors at the personal, provider, community, and organizational levels [27]. Factors such as cost and insurance status, knowledge and beliefs, perceptions of the importance of OH, and providers' advice about dental care during pregnancy were found to be important in pregnant mothers' access to dental care [28, 29]. Interestingly, in the current study, having a dental home was a better indicator of dental care utilization than having a recent visit in the past year. Mothers who answered "yes" to having a private dentist scored lower on the DMFT, while mothers who had a recent visit during the last 6 months or one year scored higher. This finding can be explained simply by the reason for the recent visit, being mainly due to pain, which suggests that visits to dental offices were irregular and mainly to relieve pain among mothers in this sample.

Mothers' belief that OH is unrelated to general health or that it has no influence on their unborn children's general health made seeking dental care not a priority in this sample, as our results demonstrate. Cost and time were the main barriers, which is expected in a sample that showed large numbers of children per family and low monthly household incomes. However, health care providers' advice not to visit a dentist while pregnant is an unacceptable practice in light of the current understanding of the relationship between OH and general health. This finding implies that awareness needs to be extended not only to mothers but to different health care providers about the importance of OH and dental care during pregnancy.

Consistent with previous literature [30], older and multiparous mothers scored higher on the DMFT. Having more than one baby increased MSL in our sample and influenced DMFT scores directly and indirectly. In contrast, high scores on social support scale were associated with low MSL and indirectly affected DMFT in a positive way.

Mothers' beliefs about OH during pregnancy played an important role in mothers' OH status, especially dental caries experience. In line with previous literature [31], these beliefs were the strongest predictors of high levels of disease. The belief that pregnant women can lose a tooth just because they are pregnant was surprisingly embraced by many mothers and was one of the most solid beliefs they had about OH during pregnancy. Paradoxically, mothers also believed that visiting dentists during pregnancy for routine care is unsafe. These two beliefs and the failure to demonstrate the correct way of brushing were very detrimental factors in high disease levels.

The findings of this study demonstrated that pregnant women from disadvantaged backgrounds had the greatest burden of poor oral hygiene and dental caries experience, which is consistent with the findings in the current literature on OH status disparities in general [8, 32] and in pregnancy in particular [33].

This finding suggests that the current situation should be addressed at different levels. Educational campaigns targeting pregnant women and health care providers should be designed and incorporated in pre- and postnatal programs to promote the importance and safety of dental care during pregnancy. These interventions are necessary but insufficient; multilevel national programs that address the social, economic and organizational factors that influence OH status provide other important venues to alleviate this problem from its root factors.

The strengths of this study were random sampling and combining clinical screening with self-reports to assess OH status. Although we are confident of the generalizability of our results to the population of pregnant women in the Jerusalem Governorate, we cannot extrapolate beyond this geographical area. Additionally, the small sample size may underestimate the influence of some significant variables in the final analysis.

Another limitation was that oral hygiene practices were self-reported, which made them susceptible to social desirability. Moreover, methods used in this study had some limitations; periodontal conditions were only assessed by the GI index, which measures gingivitis but not periodontitis. In addition, tongue depressors were used to assess dental caries among pregnant women instead of periodontal probes. This method has high specificity but low sensitivity [16].

Conclusions

The results from this study provide evidence that emphasizes the importance of OH promotion and disease prevention programs during pregnancy. High levels of dental caries experience and poor oral hygiene practices in this sample justify the need to incorporate OH education and motivation interventions in the pre- and postnatal care programs administered by the MOH in public clinics. Findings regarding the factors that explain the high burden of disease, such as faulty beliefs, incorrect practices, access to dental care and other health care providers' perspectives on dental care during pregnancy, can be used to tailor OH programs that benefit pregnant mothers the most.

Abbreviations
DMFS: Decayed, Missing, and Filled Surfaces; DMFT: Decayed, Missing and Filled Teeth; ECC: Early Childhood Caries; MCHC: Maternal and Child Health Care; MOH: Ministry of Health (MOH); MSL: Mothers' Stress Levels; OH: Oral Health; PI: Russell's Plaque index; WHO: World Health Organization

Acknowledgements
Authors thank Mrs. Raghda Belebesi, the head of the nursing department in the Jerusalem Governorate, and all nurses working in maternal and child health care centers at the Ministry of Health public clinics for their great help and support during this study.

Funding
Data collection was funded by the 2016 FDI SMILE Award, the Zamalah University Fellowship Program and the L'Oréal-UNESCO "For Women in Science" Fellowship.

Authors' contributions
EK developed the concept and the design for this project. She collected, analyzed and interpreted the data for this publication. EK also drafted the manuscript for publication. EM helped in study design and data interpretation. Both authors read and approved the final manuscript.

Authors' information
EK, BDS, MPH, PhD is an assistant professor of Dental Public Health at Al-Quds University and the Dean of Scientific Research there. EM, PhD is a research scientist at the Public Policy Center, the University of Iowa.

Competing interests
The authors declare that they have no competing interests.

Author details
[1]Department of Periodontology and Preventive Dentistry, Al-Quds University, Jerusalem, State of Palestine. [2]Public Policy Center, the University of Iowa, Iowa City, IA, USA. [3]Department of Periodontology and Preventive Dentistry, Al-Quds University, College of Dentistry, University Main St., P.O Box 89, Jerusalem, State of Palestine.

References
1. Tadakamadla SK, Agarwal P, Jain P, Balasubramanyam G, Duraiswamy P, Kulkarni S. Dental status and its socio-demographic influences among pregnant women attending a maternity hospital in India. Rev Clín Pesq Odontol. 2007;3:183–92.
2. Molnar-Varlam C, Molnar-Varlam C, Gabriela B, Tohati A. Risk assessment of caries in pregnancy. Acta Medica Marisiensis. 2011;57(6):685–9.
3. Canada Department of National Health and Welfare, Lalonde M. A new perspective on the health of Canadians: a working document. Ottawa: ON: Ministry of Supply and Services; 1974.
4. Andersen RM. Revisiting the behavioral model and access to medical care: does it matter? J Health Soc Behav. 1995;36:1–10.
5. U.S. Department of Health and Human Services. Oral health in America: a report of the Surgeon General [Internet]. Rockville, MD: U.S. Department of Health and Human Services, National Institute of Dental and Craniofacial Research, National Institutes of Health; 2000. Available at:.

6.   Abidin R. Parenting stress index (PSI): professional manual. 3rd ed. Psychological Assessment Resources: Florida; 1995.

7.   McGrath C, Bedi R. Influences of social support on the oral health of older people in Britain. J Oral Rehabil. 2002;29(10):918–22.

8.   Grembowski D, Spiekerman C, Milgrom P. Social gradients in dental health among low-income mothers and their young children. J Health Care Poor Underserved. 2012;23:570–88.

9.   Dye BA, Tan S, Smith V, Lewis BG, Barker LK, Thornton-Evans G, et al. Trends in oral health status: United States, 1988–1994 and 1999–2004. National Center for Health Statistics. Vital Health Stat. 2007;11:1–92.

10. Christensen LB, Jeppe-Jensen D, Petersen PE. Self-reported gingival conditions and self-care in the oral health of Danish women during pregnancy. J Clin Periodontol. 2003;30:949–53.

11. Offenbacher S, Lin D, Strauss R, McKaig R, Irving J, Barros SP, et al. Effects of periodontal therapy during pregnancy on periodontal status, biologic parameters, and pregnancy outcomes: a pilot study. J Periodontol. 2006;77:2011–24.

12. McLoyd V, Jayaratne T, Ceballo R, Borquez J. Unemployment and work interruption among African American single mothers: effects on parenting and adolescent socioemotional functioning. Child Dev. 1994;65:562–89.

13. KA B, Urlaub DM, Moos MK, Polinkovsky M, El-Khorazaty J, Lorenz C. Knowledge and beliefs regarding oral health among pregnant women. J Am Dent Assoc. 2011;142(11):1275–82.

14. Finlayson TL, Siefert K, Ismail AI, Delva J, Sohn W. Reliability and validity of brief measures of oral health-related knowledge, fatalism, and self-efficacy in mothers of African American children. Pediatr Dent. 2005;27(5):422–8.

15. Petersen, Paul Erik, Baez Ramon J. Oral health surveys: basic methods – 5th ed. World Health Organization I. ISBN 978 92 4 154864 9 (NLM classification: WU 30) © World Health Organization 2013.

16. Thompson NJ, Boyer EM. Validity of oral health screening in field conditions: pilot study. J Dent Hyg. 2006 80(2):9. Epub 2006 Apr 1.

17. Jamieson LM, Parker EJ, Roberts-Thomson KF, Lawrence HP, Broughton J. Self-efficacy and self-rated oral health among pregnant aboriginal Australian women. BMC Oral Health. 2014;14:29.

18. ADLER NE, OSTROVE JM. Socioeconomic status and health: what we know and what we don't. Ann N Y Acad Sci. 1999;896:3–15.

19. Palestinian Central Bureau of Statistics. State of Palestine. Accessed at http://www.pcbs.gov.ps/site/lang__en/1008/default.aspx?lang=en on September 18th 2017.

20. Soderling E, Isokangas P, Pienihäkkinen K, Tenovuo J. Influence of maternal xylitol consumption on acquisition of Mutans streptococci by infants. J Dent Res. 2000;79:882–7.

21. Zanata RL, Navarro MF, Pereira JC, Franco EB, Lauris JR, Barbosa SH. Effect of caries preventive measures directed to expectant mothers on caries experience in their children. Braz Dent J. 2003;14:75–81.

22. Radnai M, Gorzo I, Nagy E, Urban E, Eller J, Novak T. The oral health status of postpartum mothers in south-East Hungary. Community Dent Health. 2007;24:111–6.

23. Shamsi M, Hidarnia A, Niknami S, Khorsandi M. The status of dental caries and some acting factors in a sample of Iranian women with pregnancy. World J Med Sci. 2013;9(4):190–7.

24. Acharya S, Bhat PV. Oral-health-related quality of life during pregnancy. J Public Health Dent. 2009;69:74–7.

25. Santhosh Kumar S, Tadakamadla J, Tibdewal H, Duraiswamy P, Kulkarni S. Factors influencing caries status and treatment needs among pregnant women attending a maternity hospital in Udaipur city. India J Clin Exp Dent. 2013;5(2):e72–6.

26. Kateeb E, Sarhan M, Gannam I. Oral health status among convenience sample of Palestinian adults. Int Dent J. 2015;65(Suppl. 2):55–107.

27. Kateeb ET, McKernan SC, Gaeth GJ, Kuthy RA, Adrianse NB, Damiano PC. Predicting dentists' decisions: a choice-based conjoint analysis of Medicaid participation. J Public Health Dent. 2016;76(3):171–8.

28. Kloetzel MK, Huebner CE, Milgrom P, Littell CT, Eggertsson H. Oral health in pregnancy: educational needs of dental professionals and office staff. J Public Health Dent. 2012;72:279–86.

29. Le M, Riedy C, Weinstein P, Milgrom P. Barriers to utilization of dental services during pregnancy: a qualitative analysis. J Dent Child (Chic). 2009;76:46–52.

30. Chung LH, Gregorich SE, Armitage GC, Gonzalez-Vargas J, Adams SH. Sociodemographic disparities and behavioral factors in clinical oral health status during pregnancy. Community Dent Oral Epidemiol. 2014;42:151–9.

31. Habashneh R, Guthmiller JM, Levy S, Johnson GK, Squier C, Dawson DV, Fang Q. Factors related to utilization of dental services during pregnancy. J Clin Periodontol. 2005;32:815–21.

32. Eke PI, Dye BA, Wei L, Thornton-Evans GO, Genco RJ. Prevalence of periodontitis in adults in the United States: 2009 and 2010. J Dent Res. 2012;91:914–20.

33. Lieff S, Boggess KA, Murtha AP, Jared H, Madianos PN, Moss K, et al. The oral conditions and pregnancy study: periodontal status of a cohort of pregnant women. J Periodontol. 2004. 75:116–26.

19

Somatosensory profiles of patients with chronic myogenic temporomandibular disorders in relation to their painDETECT score

C. Welte-Jzyk[1*] (iD), D. B. Pfau[2,3], A. Hartmann[4] and M. Daubländer[1]

Abstract

Background: The purpose of this study was to characterize patients with chronic temporomandibular disorders (TMD) in terms of existing hyperalgesia against cold, heat and pressure.

Methods: The extent of hyperalgesia for pressure and thermal sensation in TMD patients was determined by the use of the painDETECT questionnaire ("Is cold or heat in this area occasionally painful?" "Does slight pressure in this area, e.g., with a finger, trigger pain?") and experimental somatosensory testing against thermal and pressure stimuli (Quantitative Sensory Testing; QST). In addition, we explored psychological comorbidity among the chronic TMD patients (hospital anxiety and depression scale, HADS-D and coping strategies questionnaire, CSQ).

Results: Nineteen patients with chronic TMD and 38 healthy subjects participated in the study. $N = 12$ patients had a painDETECT score ≤ 12, $n = 3$ patients had a painDETECT score of 13–18 and $n = 4$ patients had a painDETECT score ≥ 19. TMD patients with painDETECT scores ≥ 19 had moderately, strong or very strong enhancement of thermal and pressure pain perception, whereas patients with painDETECT scores 13–18 and ≤ 12 responded these questions with "never", "hardly noticed" or "slightly painful" ($p < 0.05$–0.01). With increasing painDETECT scores we found increased hyperalgesia for pressure ($p < 0.01$) and thermal stimuli ($p < 0.05$) in QST. The patients with a painDETECT score ≥ 19 showed increased signs of anxiety ($p < 0.05$), depression ($p < 0.01$), praying and hoping ($p < 0.05$).

Conclusion: The present study has shown that the PainDETECT questionnaire can be a helpful additional diagnostic tool. Together with QST, the PainDETECT questionnaire detected hyperalgesia for pressure and thermal sensation. Therefore the PainDETECT questionnaire is helpful to decide which TMD patients should undergo QST.

Keywords: Temporomandibular disorder (TMD), Quantitative sensory testing (QST), PainDETECT questionnaire, Stress-induced hyperalgesia

Background

Temporomandibular disorder (TMD) is an umbrella term for various pathological conditions characterized by pain and/or dysfunction of the masticatory muscles and/or the temporomandibular joint [1–4]. TMD is the major cause of non-dental chronic facial pain [1, 2, 5] with an estimated prevalence of 3 to 5% in the general population [5].

Since the aetiology of TMD is multidimensional, including physiological, structural, postural, psychological and genetic factors [4, 6–8], a complex diagnostic approach for TMD is required in clinical diagnostics, treatment and research [9, 10]. Notably, the population with chronic myogenic TMD is very heterogeneous [11, 12]. Apart from "sensitive" and "insensitive" myogenic TMD pain patients, as found in a previous study [11], there were also TMD patients who respond or not to standard conservative therapy alone or in combination with cognitive behavioral therapy [12]. The characteristics of "non-responding" patients did not differ on demographics or temporomandibular joint pathology, but showed higher psychological

---
* Correspondence: claudia.welte-jzyk@unimedizin-mainz.de
[1]Department of Oral and Maxillofacial Surgery, University Medical Centre of the Johannes Gutenberg University of Mainz, Mainz, Germany
Full list of author information is available at the end of the article

comorbidity such as poorer coping strategies and higher levels of catastrophizing [12]. At the same time, psychological distress such as depression, anxiety, and somatization contribute to the progression of TMD [8, 13–15], whereby effective pain management is complicated due to the interaction of all these factors [16, 17]. Repeated episodes of pain and continuous nociceptive input may shift the balance of central modulation, contributing to sustained chronic pain [18]. For these patients, spontaneous pain most often is not only present in the area of the trigeminal nerve, but throughout the whole body. This condition is called hyperalgesia and can be interpreted as central sensitization with insufficient endogenous descending inhibition [11, 18] and is induced by persistent psychosocial stress and increased mental vulnerability [19, 20]. Stress and anxiety exert modulatory influences on pain depending on the nature, duration and intensity of the stressor and developmental influences on the maturation of the stress and pain system [21]. In this context there is a bidirectional relationship between psychological comorbidity and spontaneous myogenic pain. To reveal such stress-induced hyperalgesia, a comprehensive analysis of the medical history and a careful clinical examination is required in the diagnostic process of chronic TMD patients.

The purpose of this study was to characterize patients with chronic myogenic TMD in terms of existing hyperalgesia for pressure and thermal sensation.

With the painDETECT questionnaire it is possible to ask for the subjective rating of the patient of the extent of hyperalgesia to cold or heat and pressure. Those modalities can also be experimentally assessed with the Quantitative Sensory Testing (QST) protocol.

Furthermore, we looked for psychological comorbidity among the TMD patients as trigger factors of hyperalgesia.

Methods

The study followed the 1964 Declaration of Helsinki on medical protocol and ethics. Ethical approval was obtained from the local ethical committee (ethics committee of Rhineland-Palatinate, no.837.067.09 (6572)). The study was designed as a prospective clinical monocenter study at the Department of Oral and Maxillofacial Surgery, University Medical Centre of the Johannes Gutenberg University of Mainz, Germany. Written consent was obtained from all patients and volunteers prior to the study.

Patients

Nineteen patients with myogenic temporomandibular disorders (TMD) were selected from the pain outpatient clinic of the Department of Oral and Maxillofacial Surgery, University Medical Centre of the Johannes Gutenberg University of Mainz, Germany as diagnosed by one investigator (MD) using the Research Diagnostic

Criteria for TMD [22]. Inclusion criteria were chronic uni- or bilateral myogenic pain (duration ≥6 months). Only patients with bilateral intact or prosthetically supported occlusion were included. Diseases that interfere with pain perception or cause pain in other body regions were an exclusion criterion. Also excluded were patients consuming antidepressant or anticonvulsive drugs, as well as those having taken drugs influencing pain perception (analgesics) within the last 24 h.

TMD patients underwent careful clinical examination as stated below to reveal abnormalities in facial sensibility, muscle and temporomandibular joint sensitivity to palpation, mandibular movement and auscultation of the joint. Additionally, comprehensive medical history as well as pain history was documented on paper-based charts. QST was performed and the psychological comorbidity determined.

We first analysed the patients as a collective group (TMD all) and then divided them into 3 groups depending on the patient's painDETECT score (≤ 12, $n = 12$; 13–18, $n = 3$; ≥ 19, $n = 4$).

Control group (healthy subjects)

Patients were compared to healthy subjects who had had no temporomandibular disorder complaints during the last 6 months. Healthy subjects were recruited by an announcement in the department of Oral and Maxillofacial Surgery, University Medical Centre of the Johannes Gutenberg University of Mainz, Germany. Patients were compared related to clinical investigation, QST values and psychological comorbidity. Included were healthy subjects not having taken drugs influencing pain perception (analgesics) within the last 24 h.

Clinical investigation

Patients and healthy subjects were examined by one investigator (MD) according to dental and clinical factors to reveal abnormalities in countenance, mandibular movement, auscultation of the jaw, tension of the facial muscles, and facial sensitivity. Examination was carried out as described in Pfau et al. 2009 [11].

For intraoral dental examination, the dentition and static contacts were noted as well as signs of oral habits. We determined the total number of missing teeth, the number of missing teeth having been replaced by removable dentures or bridges, and the numbers of crowned or filled teeth. Distances of overbite, overjet and interocclusal distances were measured. For extraoral examination, we tested the functions of muscles, nerves and the movements of the temporomandibular joint. We investigated the function of the facial nerve and the sensitivity to pressure over trigeminal foramina. Signs of underlying myogenic orofacial hyperactivity were documented after checking the mimic muscles, masticatory and neck muscles. Temporalis, masseter muscle, sternocleidomas-toid muscle, muscles of the cervical spine, trapezius muscle and suprahyoidal muscles were palpated with the fingertips of the index and the third finger, using the non-dominant hand of the investigator to fix the head e.g. the mandible. For palpation of the extra oral muscles we used an approximate pressure of ~ 10 N, for intraoral muscle and joint palpation an approximate pressure of ~ 5 N. We checked if a single active mandibular move-ment (forward movements, laterotrusion and mouth opening) or an assisted backward movement was painful. The diagnostic findings (unpleasant, painful, trigger point) during palpation of temporalis, medial and lateral pterygoid and masseter muscle were also documented.

Pain history and current pain

The medical records and pain history of the patients were taken in a written form and completed verbally. Pa-tients were asked to answer different questionnaires on pain, including questions on pain intensity, pain dur-ation, and pain localisation. We used the Berne pain questionnaire (BPQ, paper-based chart) consisting of 20 groups of sensory, affective, and evaluative items to de-scribe the quality and intensity of the pain [23] and the painDETECT paper-based form [24]. The painDETECT questionnaire was developed and validated for patients with neuropathic pain and is increasingly applied to pa-tients with back pain [25, 26]. It consists of questions concerning estimation of pain intensity, pain duration, pain patterns (persistent pain and or pain attacks) and pain quality (burning, tingling or prickling sensation, numbness, and temperature and pressure hyperalgesia). We used the painDETECT questionnaire as it contains questions concerning hyperalgesia against cold or heat and pressure ("Is cold or heat in this area occasionally painful?" "Does slight pressure in this area, e.g., with a finger, trigger pain?") Patients were divided into 3 groups according to their PainDETECT score. In the group "≤ 12" a neuropathic component is unlikely, in the group "≥ 19" a neuropathic component is likely, and in the group "13–18", it is uncertain whether a neuropathic component exists. The painDETECT questionnaire demonstrated satisfactory reliability [27], showing accurate test-retest stability as a prerequisite for use in repeated measure-ments [25].

Psychological testing

In order to assess psychological comorbidity, patients and healthy subjects were asked questions relating to coping strategies (CSQ, full paper-based version), and questions on anxiety and depression disorders (HADS-D; hospital anxiety and depression scale, German version, full paper-based charts).

Quantitative sensory testing (QST)

Changes of thermal and mechanical detection and pain thresholds were examined using the Quantitative Sensory Testing protocol according to the DFNS (Deutscher Forschungsverbund Neuropathischer Schmerz), described in detail by Rolke et al. [28, 29] and Hartmann et al. [30].

The QST protocol consists of the following parameters: CDT (cold detection threshold); WDT (warm detection threshold); TSL (thermal sensory limen); PHS (paradoxical heat sensation); CPT (cold pain threshold); HPT (heat pain threshold); MDT (mechanical detection threshold); MPT (mechanical pain threshold); MPS (mechanical pain sensitivity); DMA (dynamic mechanical allodynia); WUR (wind up ratio); VDT (vibration detection threshold) and PPT (pressure pain threshold).

All patients and healthy subjects underwent the same QST protocol. They were tested on the left and on the right masseter muscles by one trained examiner within one experimental session, which took roughly 60 min.

In a first step, the patients were examined as a whole group and then divided into 3 groups according to their painDETECT score (≤ 12; 13–18; ≥ 19).

Z-transformation of QST data

To compare patients' QST data profiles with the age and gender-matched healthy subjects, reference data of healthy subjects were used to normalize test results of patients by calculating the z-transform: Z = (value (patient) − mean (healthy subjects))/ standard deviation (healthy subjects). This procedure results in a QST pro-file where all parameters are presented as standard nor-mal distributions (zero mean, unit variance). Z-values above "0" indicate a gain of function when the single pa-tient is more sensitive to the tested stimuli compared with controls (hyperalgesia, allodynia, hyperpathia), while Z-scores below "0" indicate a loss of function re-ferring to a lower sensitivity of the patient (small and large fibre functions). A Z-score of zero represents a value corresponding to the group mean of the healthy control subjects.

Statistical analysis
QST data analysis

Data evaluation was performed according to the stan-dardized protocol of the German Research Network on Neuropathic Pain [28, 29]. All data were normally dis-tributed in log-space and were transformed logarithmic-ally before statistical analysis, with the exception of the CPT, HPT and VDT number, which were normally dis-tributed as raw data. All statistical calculations were per-formed using SPSS software (IBM SPSS Statistics 23) or Excel for Windows (Microsoft Excel 2010). All data are presented as mean ± standard error of the mean (SEM). Differences of QST data between patient groups and control group (healthy subjects) were determined using an unpaired t-test, considering the Levene's test for equality of variances for comparison of TMD all with healthy subjects or analysis of variance (ANOVA) with LSD post hoc corrections of multiple comparisons for comparison of the different painDETECT subgroups with healthy subjects. The significance level was set at $p < 0.05$.

Data of clinical examination and questionnaires

All statistical calculations were performed using SPSS software (IBM SPSS Statistics 23) or Excel for Windows (Microsoft Excel 2010). All data are presented as mean ± standard deviation (SD). Differences between patient groups and control group (healthy subjects) were determined using an unpaired t-test, considering the Levene's test for equality of variances for comparison of TMD all with healthy subjects or analysis of variance (ANOVA) with LSD post hoc corrections of multiple comparisons for comparison of the different painDETECT subgroups with healthy subjects. The level of significance was set at $p < 0.05$.

Results

Patients

Nineteen patients with myogenic temporomandibular disorders (TMD) were included as diagnosed by one investigator (MD) using the Research Diagnostic Criteria for TMD [22]. The patients (13 women, 6 men) had a mean age of 52.2 ± 14.9 years. Fifteen patients had unilateral symptoms of temporomandibular disorder, 7 patients on the left side, 8 patients on the right side and 4 patients had bilateral findings.

Control group (healthy subjects)

Thirty-eight healthy subjects (33 women, 5 men) with a mean age of 46.7 ± 13.3 years were included.

Clinical findings

TMD patients (TMD all)

Regarding the patients with chronic TMD in its entirety (TMD all) we found no changes in the function of mimic muscle. TMD patients (TMD all) showed increased sensitivity towards palpation of the trigeminal foramina, but only palpation of the left infraorbital foramen was significantly more painful ($p < 0.05$). TMD patients (TMD all) showed increased sensitivity towards palpation of the masticatory muscles. In particular, the pain values for the temporalis (left $p < 0.05$; right $p < 0.001$), the masseter (left $p < 0.05$; right $p < 001$, masseter left + right $p < 0.01$, Fig. 1a) and the sternocleidomastoid muscle (left $p < 0.05$; right $p < 0.01$) were increased. It should be noted that, with regards to the palpation of the masticatory muscles, particularly the masseter, that also the healthy subjects ($n = 12$, 31%) showed pain upon palpation. TMD patients (TMD all)

showed increased sensitivity to palpation of the temporomandibular joint ($p < 0.01$), particularly during dorsal palpation. Furthermore, TMD patients (TMD all) showed pain when opening the mouth ($p < 0.01$) and during laterotrusion ($p < 0.01$).

TMD subgroups as a function of painDETECT scores

Examining the patients with chronic TMD according to their painDETECT scores, we found patients within the "painDETECT ≥ 19" subgroup showing notably increased sensitivity towards palpation of the temporalis (left $p < 0.001$; right $p < 0.001$), the sternocleidomastoid muscle (left $p < 0.05$; right $p < 0.01$) and the masseter muscle (left $p < 0.01$; right $p < 0.001$; masseter left + right $p < 0.001$, Fig. 1a). Furthermore, sensitivity towards palpation of the temporomandibular joint was enhanced in the "painDETECT ≥ 19" subgroup (lateral $p < 0.05$ and dorsal $p < 0.01$). In addition, opening the mouth was painful ($p < 0.05$) and forward movements (protrusion; $p < 0.001$) in the TMD subgroup with painDETECT scores ≥ 19.

QST findings

TMD patients (TMD all)

The significant differences in masseter pressure pain sensitivity found in clinical examination for the TMD patients in its entirety (TMD all), compared to the healthy subjects (Fig. 1a), $p < 0.01$), could not be confirmed in QST pressure pain thresholds (PPT) (Fig. 1b, Table 1). Furthermore, there were no differences for all other QST parameter, except for VDT, whereby the TMD patients showed a higher sensitivity than the healthy subjects (Table 1, $p < 0.05$).

TMD subgroups as a function of painDETECT scores

When analysing the results of patients with chronic TMD according to their painDETECT scores, we found similar results for palpation of the masseter muscle (Fig. 1a), whereas totally different results emerged for the QST PPT values. In QST we found the TMD patients with a painDETECT score ≥ 19 showing significant higher sensitivity to pressure (PPT) compared to healthy subjects (Fig. 1b, Table 1, $p < 0.01$). Patients with a painDETECT score ≥ 19 were also significantly more sensitive to painful cold (CPT) and painful heat (HPT) compared to healthy subjects (Fig. 2, Table 1, $p < 0.05$; $p < 0.05$), whereas patients showing painDETECT scores ≤ 12 were less sensitive to cold (CPT) than healthy subjects (Fig. 2, Table 1, $p < 0.05$). The results underline the finding that TMD pain patients appear to be a heterogeneous group.

Findings of the painDETECT questionnaire

An analysis of the individual answers from the painDETECT questionnaire revealed similar variation in

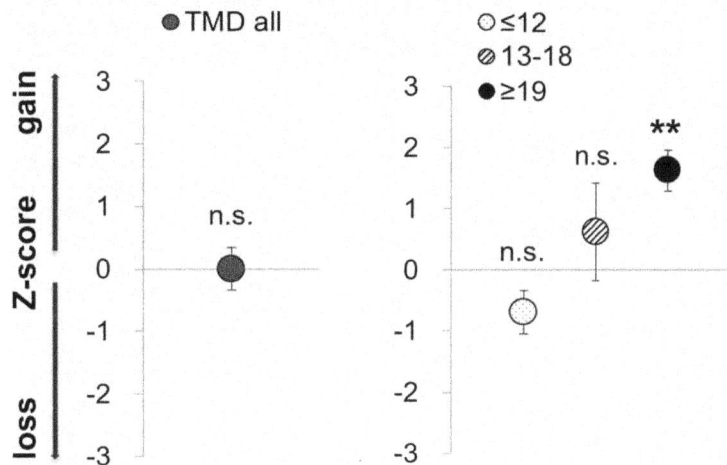

Fig. 1 a Increase of pressure pain from unpleasant over painful to trigger point on masseter muscle palpation in patients with TMD (TMD all, $n = 19$; TMD subgroups concerning their painDETECT score (≤ 12, $n = 12$; 13–18, $n = 3$; ≥ 19, $n = 4$); mean $\pm$ SD (masseter left $+$ right); **b** QST-pressure pain threshold (PPT) presented as z-score values (mean value of patients (masseter left $+$ right) - mean controls (masseter left $+$ right)/SD controls). A z-score of 0 means the score is the same as for the mean of healthy subjects. It can also be negative or positive indicating a loss or gain of function; p-value for TMD all as results of unpaired t-test as related to healthy subjects considering the Levene's test for equality of variances; p-value according to the painDETECT scores as results of analysis of variance (ANOVA) with LSD post hoc correction of multiple comparison; (n.s. = not significant, $* = p < 0.05$, $** = p < 0.01$, $*** = p < 0.001$)

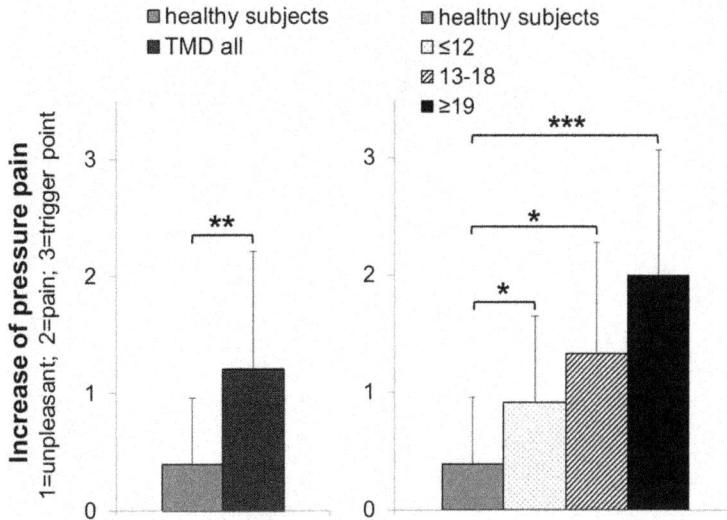

severity of pain perceptions for the distinct TMD groups (painDETECT ≤ 12; 13–18; ≥ 19). Particularly answers to questions concerning hyperalgesia, such as, "Is cold or heat in this area occasionally painful?", "Does slight pressure in this area, e.g., with a finger, trigger pain?" [24] revealed that TMD patients with painDETECT scores ≥ 19 had moderately, strong or very strong enhancement of pain perception, whereas patients with painDETECT scores 13–18 and ≤ 12 answered these questions with "never", "hardly noticed" or "slightly painful" ($p < 0.05$–0.01, Fig. 3).

Pain history and current pain

All TMD patients with painDETECT scores ≥ 19 reported additional pain in other body regions already lasting for years (Table 2). On a numeric rating scale (NRS 0–10), the group with painDETECT scores ≥ 19 quoted the lowest present pain (1.8 ± 0.9) and the lowest pain maximum during the last week (1.8 ± 0.7) among all TMD groups. In contrast, the painDETECT 13–18 group with pain lasting for only 6–12 months showed the highest pain estimation for present pain (3.7 ± 1.2)

Table 1 QST data of the masseter of patients with TMD (TMD all and according to their painDETECT scores ($\leq$ 12., n = 12; 13-18, n = 3; $\geq$ 19, n = 4)); CPT, HPT, VDT (Data in original unit as mean ± SEM); CDT, WDT, TSL, MDT, MPT, MPS, WUR, PPT (retransformed log data (mean log ± SEM))

masseter	Healthy subjects (n = 38)	TMD all (n = 19)		TMD - painDETECT ≤ 12 (n = 12)		13-18 (n = 3)		≥ 19 (n = 4)	
	QST data raw mean ± SEM or log retransformed (mean$_{log}$ ± SEM)	QST data raw mean ± SEM or log retransformed (mean$_{log}$ ± SEM)	p-value	QST data raw mean ± SEM or log retransformed (mean$_{log}$ ± SEM)	p-value	QST data raw mean ± SEM or log retransformed (mean$_{log}$ ± SEM)	p-value	QST data raw mean ± SEM or log retransformed (mean$_{log}$ ± SEM)	p-value
CDT (Δ°C)	1.2 (0.078 ± 0.024)	1.39 (0.142 ± 0.0579)	0.327	1.62 (0.209 ± 0.082)	0.041*	1.08 (0.033 ± 0.058)	0.691	1.05 (0.022 ± 0.031)	0.565
WDT (Δ°C)	1.84 (0.265 ± 0.029)	2.23 (0.348 ± 0.056)	0.164	2.63 (0.420 ± 0.079)	0.027*	1.82 (0.259 ± 0.041)	0.959	1.58 (0.199 ± 0.067)	0.541
TSL (°C)	2.78 (0.443 ± 0.031)	3.42 (0.534 ± 0.069)	0.181	4.22 (0.625 ± 0.093)	0.02*	3.07 (0.487 ± 0.059)	0.752	1.97 (0.294 ± 0.067)	0.218
CPT(°C)	16.54 ± 1.35	14.59 ± 2.44	0.500	10.53 ± 2.63	0.043*	15.23 ± 6.1	0.804	26.3 ± 2.15	0.038*
HPT (°C)	42.99 ± 0.74	43.62 ± 1.26	0.655	45.92 ± 1.38	0.062	43.09 ± 2.68	0.972	37.14 ± 0.56	0.02*
MDT (mN)	0.42 (−0.375 ± 0.053)	0.34 (−0.469 ± 0.058)	0.290	0.31 (−0.507 ± 0.065)	0.209	0.56 (−0.253 ± 0.189)	0.509	0.3 (−0.518 ± 0.079)	0.388
MPT (mN)	41.44 (1.617 ± 0.067)	51.33 (1.710 ± 0.108)	0.458	39.94 (1.601 ± 0.122)	0.909	204.46 (2.311 ± 0.130)	0.009**	38.67 (1.587 ± 0.20)	0.893
MPS (0–100)	0.34 (−0.471 ± 0.099)	0.36 (−0.447 ± 0.136)	0.883	0.36 (−0.440 ± 0.114)	0.851	0.08 (−1.119 ± 0.114)	0.073	1.08 (0.034 ± 0.387)	0.116
WUR (0–100)	3.96 (0.598 ± 0.061)	3.35 (0.526 ± 0.063)	0.565	3.25 (0.512 ± 0.080)	0.539	not evaluable		3.73 (0.572 ± 0.133)	0.911
VDT (x/8)	6.02 ± 0.11	6.56 ± 0.2	0.014*	6.86 ± 0.25	0.001**	5.83 ± 0.21	0.684	6.21 ± 0.36	0.622
PPT (kPa)	191 (2.281 ± 0.025)	191 (2.281 ± 0.052)	0.920	244 (2.387 ± 0.054)	0.066	154 (2.186 ± 0.120)	0.305	108 (2.034 ± 0.051)	0.004**

CDT Cold detection treshold, *WDT* Warm detection threshold, *TSL* Thermal sensory lumen, *CPT* Cold pain threshold, *HPT* Heat pain threshold, *MDT* Mechanical detection threshold, *MPT* Mechanical pain threshold, *MPS* Mechanical pain sensitivity, *WUR* Wind up ratio, *VDT* Vibration detection threshold, *PPT* Pressure pain threshold, *p*-value for TMD all as results of unpaired t-test as related to healthy subjects considering the Levene's test for equality of variances; *p*-value according to the painDETECT scores as results of analysis of variance (ANOVA) with LSD post hoc correction of multiple comparison; (*$p < 0.05$; **$p < 0.01$; ***$p < 0.001$)

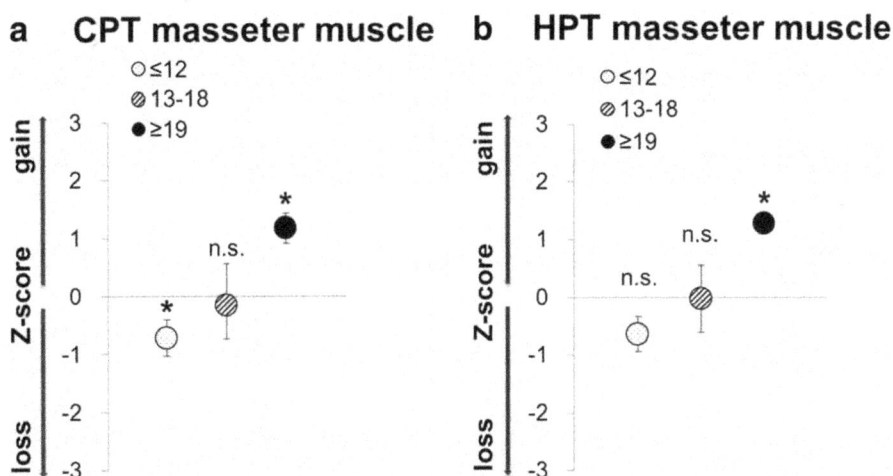

Fig. 2 Thermal hyperalgesia in patients with myogenic TMD concerning their painDETECT score (≤ 12, n = 12; 13–18, n = 3; ≥ 19, n = 4) **a** QST-Cold pain threshold (CPT) and **b** QST-Heat pain threshold (HPT) presented as z-score values (mean value of patients-mean controls/SD controls). A z-score of 0 means the score is the same as for the mean of healthy subjects. It can also be negative or positive indicating loss or gain of function; Significance as results of analysis of variance (ANOVA) with LSD post hoc correction of multiple comparison; (n.s. = not significant, * = $p < 0.05$, ** = $p < 0.01$, *** = $p < 0.001$)

and maximal pain of the last week (6.7 ± 1.1). In addition, this group showed the highest score for days per year when they were unable to work (> 50) (Table 2).

Psychological comorbidity

The patients with a painDETECT score ≥ 19 showed the highest values for anxiety (mean 9.3 ± 7.0, $p > 0.05$, 50% > 10) and depression (mean 7.0 ± 3.2, $p < 0.01$) in the HADS-D among the TMD painDETECT groups (≤ 12, 13–18, ≥ 19) compared to healthy subjects (Table 3). Significant differences were found for the painDETECT ≥ 19 group for praying and hoping (CSQ5) (mean 4.1 ± 0.9, $p < 0.05$). The painDETECT group ≤ 12 showed significant values for catastrophizing (CSQ6) (mean 3.6 ± 2.1, $p < 0.05$) and the painDETECT group 13–18 showed significant values for increased behaviour activities (CSQ7) (5.4 ± 0.8, $p < 0.05$) (Table 3).

Discussion

The present study disclosed pronounced somatosensory changes in a subgroup of TMD patients identified by their scores in the painDETECT questionnaire.

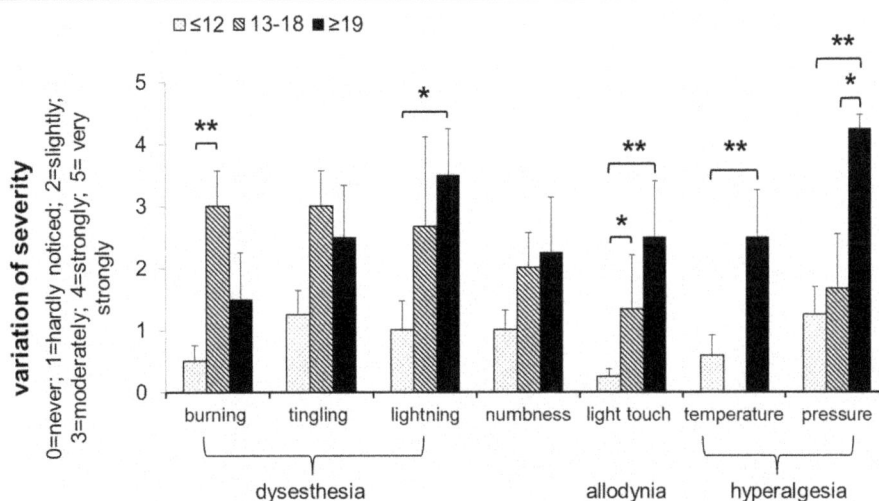

Fig. 3 Variation of sensorial and pain perception in patients with myogenic TMD concerning their painDETECT score (≤ 12, n = 12; 13–18, n = 3; ≥ 19, n = 4); Variation of severity of sensational (dysaesthesia, numbness) and pain perception (allodynia, hyperalgesia) as revealed by the painDETECT questionnaire (1 = never, 2 = hardly noticed, 3 = slightly, 4 = moderately, 5 = strongly, 6 = very strongly); mean ± SD; Significance as results of analysis of variance (ANOVA) with LSD post hoc correction of multiple comparison (*$p < 0.05$; **$p < 0.01$; ***$p < 0.001$)

Table 2 Pain estimation of TMD patients (TMD all and according to their painDETECT scores (≤ 12, $n = 12$; 13–18, $n = 3$; ≥ 19, $n = 4$)); pain estimation in mean value ± SD or in mean % of 100%

Pain estimation (mean ± SD)	TMD	TMD - painDETECT		
	all ($n = 19$)	≤ 12 ($n = 12$)	13–18 ($n = 3$)	≥ 19 ($n = 4$)
present pain (NRS)	2.9 ± 0.5	3.2 ± 0.7	3.7 ± 1.2	1.8 ± 0.9
maximal pain - last week (NRS)	4.3 ± 0.6	4.6 ± 0.7	6.7 ± 1.1	1.8 ± 0.7
minimal pain - last week (NRS)	2.4 ± 0.4	2.7 ± 0.6	2.3 ± 0.7	1.5 ± 0.8
pain estimation BPQ 25 (1–13)/ sensory	8.1 ± 1.6	4.8 ± 1.1	18.3 ± 3.1	9.3 ± 2.9
pain estimation BPQ 25 (14–17)/ affective	3.5 ± 0.7	3.5 ± 1.0	3.7 ± 1.4	3.5 ± 1.3
pain estimation BPQ 25 (18–19)/ evaluative	2.7 ± 0.5	2.3 ± 0.6	4.3 ± 0.7	2.8 ± 1.2
pain estimation BPQ 25 (18 + 19 + 20/2)/ affective-evaluative	1.6 ± 0.3	1.4 ± 0.4	2.3 ± 0.3	1.5 ± 0.7
pain since	1–2 y	1–2 y	6–12 m	2–5 y
inability to work due to pain	12% (1–2 d)	45% (1d)	67% (> 50 d)	25% (1–5 d)
reduction of activity due to pain (work)	39%	36%	43%	48%
reduction of activity due to pain (leisure)	44%	46%	43%	40%
additonal pain in other body regions	67%	55%	67%	100%
pain-free time	min-h	min	h	d

NRS Numeric rating scale, *BPQ* Berne pain questionnaire (number 1–13 comprising sensory adjectives, maximum value 50; 14–17 comprising affective adjectives, maximum value 17; 18–19 comprising evaluative adjectives, maximum value 7; 20 comprising affective-evaluative adjectives, maximum value 5.5)

Somatosensory changes in this subgroup with painDE-TECT scores ≥ 19 consisted of lowered thresholds for pressure pain as well as for cold and heat stimuli in the Quantitative Sensory Testing (QST). Additionally, in the painDETECT questionnaire, the questions concerning sensory gain (hyperalgesia) in particular were answered with high values. Similarly, Herpich et al. found that patients with more severe signs and symptoms of TMD had a lower pressure pain threshold [31]. Such somatosensory changes result in amplification of nociception, which promotes and sustains chronic pain states [18]. As we believe stress-induced sensitisation to be one

Table 3 Psychological Comorbidity of TMD patients (TMD all and according to their painDETECT scores (≤ 12, $n = 12$; 13–18, $n = 3$; ≥ 19, $n = 4$))

Psychological comorbidity		Healthy subjects ($n = 38$)	TMD all ($n = 19$)	p-value	≤ 12 ($n = 12$)	p-value	13–18 ($n = 3$)	p-value	≥ 19 ($n = 4$)	p-value
anxiety (HADS-D)	mean ± SD	5.0 ± 3	7.3 ± 5	0.082	7.1 ± 4.5	0.102	5.3 ± 3.1	0.865	9.3 ± 7.0	0.034*
	< 8	$n = 32$	$n = 12$		$n = 8$		$n = 2$		$n = 2$	
	8–10	$n = 4$	$n = 0$		$n = 0$		$n = 0$		$n = 0$	
	> 10	$n = 2$	$n = 6$		$n = 3$		$n = 1$		$n = 2$	
depression (HADS-D)	mean ± SD	2.2 ± 2.5	6.4 ± 4.3	0.001**	6.6 ± 5.1	0.000***	5.3 ± 3.1	0.105	7.0 ± 3.2	0.006**
	< 8	$n = 37$	$n = 10$		$n = 6$		$n = 2$		$n = 2$	
	8–10	$n = 1$	$n = 5$		$n = 2$		$n = 1$		$n = 2$	
	> 10	$n = 0$	$n = 3$		$n = 3$		$n = 0$		$n = 0$	
diverting attention (CSQ1)	mean ± SD	2.9 ± 1.1	3.3 ± 0.3	0.335	3.3 ± 1.4	0.423	3.4 ± 2	0.592	3.3 ± 1.6	0.634
reinterpreting pain sensation (CSQ2)	mean ± SD	2.2 ± 1	2.0 ± 0.2	0.584	2.2 ± 1.1	0.983	1.7 ± 1.1	0.499	1.7 ± 0.5	0.434
coping self-statement (CSQ3)	mean ± SD	3.7 ± 1.1	4.3 ± 0.4	0.157	4.2 ± 2	0.306	3.8 ± 0.5	0.932	4.9 ± 0.8	0.108
ignoring sensation (CSQ4)	mean ± SD	3.3 ± 1.2	3.3 ± 0.3	0.960	3.5 ± 1.8	0.783	2.3 ± 1.2	0.229	3.8 ± 1	0.497
praying and hoping (CSQ5)	mean ± SD	2.6 ± 1.3	3.0 ± 0.3	0.314	2.5 ± 1.4	0.872	3.1 ± 0.8	0.481	4.1 ± 0.9	0.030*
catastrophizing (CSQ6)	mean ± SD	2.0 ± 1.1	3.3 ± 0.4	0.022*	3.6 ± 2.1	0.006**	3.2 ± 2.1	0.193	2.6 ± 1.8	0.503
increased behaviour activities (CSQ7)	mean ± SD	3.5 ± 1.5	4.3 ± 0.3	0.080	4.1 ± 1.5	0.328	5.4 ± 0.8	0.044*	4.3 ± 1.6	0.320
pain behaviour (CSQ8)	mean ± SD	4.0 ± 1	3.7 ± 0.3	0.473	3.2 ± 1.2	0.055	5.1 ± 1.5	0.089	4.0 ± 0.6	0.967

HADS-D Hospital anxiety and depression scale, anxiety in mean value ± SD or divided in subgroups concerning their severity (< 8, 8–10, > 10), depression in mean value ± SD CSQ = Coping strategies in mean value ± SD; p-value for TMD all as results of unpaired t-test as related to healthy subjects considering the Levene's test for equality of variances; p-value according to the painDETECT scores as results of analysis of variance (ANOVA) with LSD post hoc correction of multiple comparison (*$p < 0.05$; **$p < 0.01$; ***$p < 0.001$)

reason for chronification of TMD [18, 32], we focused our attention not only on the signs of sensory gain (pressure, cold and heat hyperalgesia), but on psychological comorbidity of the TMD patients. We found that the patients with painDETECT scores ≥ 19 also showed the highest values for anxiety, depression, praying and hoping among all TMD patients.

In clinical examination we revealed no abnormalities in facial mimic expression for all TMD patients, but found pain sensitivity for mandibular movement and upon palpation of different muscles, the temporomandibular joint and the trigeminal foramina. Relating to clinical examination, we found a positive relationship between the increased sensitivity during masseter palpation and higher painDETECT scores. In the "painDETECT ≥ 19" group, the higher pain upon masseter palpation could be confirmed by measurement of pressure pain thresholds (PPT) in the Quantitative Sensory Testing (QST).

Our findings are supported by other studies in which several patients with chronic temporomandibular disorder were found to be more sensitive to painful stimuli than other patients or healthy subjects. Pfau et al., for example, distinguished a "sensitive" and an "insensitive" TMD subgroup with regard to their tenderness on palpation of orofacial muscles and trigeminal foramina and could confirm this hyperalgesia using QST [11]. Likewise, de Sequeira et al. assessed sensory characteristics of patients with chronic pain involving a combination of thermal, mechanical pain stimuli and found the majority of patients (73.3%) with pain upon craniofacial muscle palpation [33]. Several other research groups perceived the diagnostic value of pressure pain threshold analysis for TMD as well [14, 34–36]. QST is a method to investigate pressure pain thresholds and, therefore, is a useful component in mechanism-based classification of TMD. It is frequently mentioned for pain assessment and diagnosis in the orofacial region [36–40].

The fact that only the "painDETECT ≥ 19" group showed significantly decreased QST pressure pain thresholds (PPT), underlines the effective use of the painDETECT questionnaire in the differentiated analysis of TMD subgroups.

Until now the painDETECT questionnaire has not been validated for the trigeminal region. In accordance with our study, the painDETECT questionnaire was assessed for detecting neuropathic pain in patients with post-traumatic inferior alveolar nerve injury (IANI) and lingual nerve injury (LNI) [41]. The authors concluded the painDETECT questionnaire not to be suitable for screening IANI or LNI. Heo et al. 2015 found the painDETECT questionnaire, although not being an ideal principal screening tool for burning mouth syndrome (BMS), could still be useful to identify a substantial proportion of neuropathic symptoms in primary BMS patients [42].

In addition to the significantly increased PPT, a significant hyperalgesia against cold and heat painful stimuli could be revealed for patients with chronic TMD and painDETECT scores ≥ 19. Such an increased sensitivity against cold and heat pain, in addition to pressure hyperalgesia, was also found for the "sensitive" TMD pain group as distinguished by Pfau et al. 2009 [11], showing more than 11/18 tender points according to the former diagnostic criteria for FMS. As results from both the "sensitive" and the "painDETECT ≥ 19" TMD subgroup show that the pain is not only present in the area of the trigeminal nerve, but throughout the whole body, changes involving the central nervous system should be considered [43]. Central sensitisation might arise as a result of insufficient endogenous descending inhibition [18–20]. Persistent psychosocial stress and increased mental vulnerability, as found within the patients with painDETECT scores ≥ 19, may, therefore, be the cause [21, 32, 44]. This can explain the spreading of pain throughout the body and the increase during examination. The low subjective pain rating of these patients can be interpreted as adaption to the chronic pain state, although habituation to pain is not known. In addition, the "sensitive" and "painDETECT ≥ 19" group both show high levels of anxiety and depression, further evidence for central sensitisation. Therefore, we assume psychosocial factors to be one reason for chronification in both groups.

In our study, the painDETECT questionnaire enables the identification of subgroups of patients with chronic TMD showing different severity in induced pressure, cold and heat pain. Nevertheless, the neurobiological basis for this is not fully elucidated, but as we found psychological comorbidity for the patients, we assume stress-induced hyperalgesia to be the reason [45, 46]. Thermal hyperalgesia may be triggered by a stimulation of the dorsomedial hypothalamic nucleus, whereby the rostral ventromedial medulla plays an important role by activating so-called "ON-cells" that amplify the nociceptive input. This part of the brain is also responsible for allodynia and hyperalgesia in neuropathic pain [19]. Moreover, a number of other long-lasting changes in the neural system are probably involved in brain activity. The dysfunction of the hypothalamic-pituitary-adrenal axis (HPA axis) and various neurotransmitter systems in the brain, including the endogenous opioid system and the serotonergic and noradrenergic systems, have been demonstrated in animal experiments to be relevant factors [20]. Chronic TMD might be caused by hypersensitivity of the nervous system and central sensitization [47].

In our study we found all TMD patients showing signs of depression and anxiety. The scores were higher in TMD patients with increased painDETECT scores (≥ 19). In contrast to our findings, Reiter et al. analysed a less significant role of anxiety in patients with chronic

TMD compared to depression and somatization [48]. Yu et al. 2015, however, detected high anxiety (OR 2.48; 95% CI 1.25–4.90) as the most significant factor associated with TMD. Among other publications indicating psychological stress to be significantly associated with TMD [49], Ismail et al. 2015 found clinical symptoms of depression in 16% of the TMD patients. They recommend the use of screening tools for psychological disorders on a regularly basis when evaluating TMD patients. Psychological stress is a risk factor for the development of a painful TMD [50]. The effects of stress on pain vary according to duration of exposure, mental and biological vulnerability of the individual and age at exposition. Effects are most pronounced in individuals whose genetic susceptibility increases responsiveness to catecholamine neurotransmitters [50]. Furthermore the large prospective OPPERA (Orofacial Pain: Prospective Evaluation and Risk Assessment) study found psychological variables to predict first onset of TMD [51]. Therefore, informing and educating patients about pain perception and functional jaw opening becomes essential in order to decrease fear and depression concerning TMD and to improve jaw function and quality of life [52].

Conclusion

In our study we were able to prove the painDETECT questionnaire to be helpful as an additional diagnostic tool, which, together with QST, can reveal hyperalgesia for pressure (PPT) and thermal sensation (CPT, HPT) in chronic TMD patients. High painDETECT scores (≥ 19) correlate with decreased pain levels for pressure and thermal sensation in QST. As TMD patients of the painDETECT group ≥ 19 have additional pain in other parts of the body, suggesting central sensitization [53], we would recommend testing also an extra oral site when performing QST in these patients, for example the dorsum of the hand. An obvious limitation in the present study was the small number of patients, especially in the painDETECT 13–18 ($n = 3$) and ≥ 19 ($n = 4$) group.

Abbreviations

ANOVA: Analysis of variance; BMS: Burning mouth syndrome; BPQ: Berne pain questionnaire; CDT: Cold detection threshold; CPT: Cold pain threshold; CSQ: Coping strategies questionnaire; DFNS: German Research Network on Neuropathic Pain; DMA: Dynamic mechanical allodynia; HADS-D: Hospital anxiety and depression scale; HPT: Heat pain threshold; IANI: Inferior alveolar nerve damage; LNI: Lingual nerve impairment; MDT: Mechanical detection threshold; MPS: Mechanical pain sensitivity; MPT: Mechanical pain threshold; PHS: Paradoxical heat sensation; PPT: Pressure pain threshold; QST: Quantitative Sensory Testing; SD: Standard deviation; SEM: Standard error of the mean; TMD: Temporomandibular disorders; TSL: Thermal sensory limen; VDT: Vibration detection threshold; WDT: Warm detection threshold

Acknowledgements

The authors thank all patients, nurses and physicians involved for their support. We especially thank Carolin Holländer for QST measurements. The authors report no conflict of interest.

Authors' contributions

Conception and design: MD, DBP, AH. Development of methodology: MD, DBP, AH. Analysis and interpretation of data (statistical analysis, biostatistics): CW-J. Writing, review, and/or revision of the manuscript: CW-J, AH. Administrative, technical, or material support: MD. Study supervision: MD, DBP. All authors read and approved the final manuscript.

Competing interests

The authors declare that they have no competing interests.

Author details

[1]Department of Oral and Maxillofacial Surgery, University Medical Centre of the Johannes Gutenberg University of Mainz, Mainz, Germany. [2]Mannheim Institute of Public Health (MIPH), Social and Preventive Medicine, University of Heidelberg, Heidelberg, Germany. [3]Department of Neurophysiology, Centre of Biomedicine and Medical Technology Mannheim (CBTM), University of Heidelberg, Heidelberg, Germany. [4]Private Practice Dr. Seiler and colleagues, Filderstadt, Germany.

References

1. Kothari SF, Baad-Hansen L, Oono Y, Svensson P. Somatosensory assessment and conditioned pain modulation in temporomandibular disorders pain patients. Pain. 2015;156(12):2545–55.
2. Ettlin D, Gaul C. Myoarthopathie des Kausystems (Craniomandibuläre Dysfunktion). In: Brandt T, Diener HC, Gerloff C, editors. Therapie und Verlauf neurologischer Erkrankungen. Kohlhammer (Stuttgart, Germany). 2012.
3. List T, Jensen RH. Temporomandibular disorders: old ideas and new concepts. Cephalalgia. 2017; https://doi.org/10.1177/0333102416686302.
4. Slade GD, Ohrbach R, Greenspan JD, Fillingim RB, Bair E, Sanders AE, Dubner R, Diatchenko L, Meloto CB, Smith S, et al. Painful temporomandibular disorder: decade of discovery from OPPERA studies. J Dent Res. 2016;95(10): 1084–92.
5. Zakrzewska JM. Temporomandibular disorders, headaches and chronic pain. J Pain Palliat Care Pharmacoter. 2015;29(1):61–3. discussion 63
6. Chisnoiu AM, Picos AM, Popa S, Chisnoiu PD, Lascu L, Picos A, Chisnoiu R. Factors involved in the etiology of temporomandibular disorders - a literature review. Clujul Med (1957). 2015;88(4):473–8.
7. Melis M, Di Giosia M. The role of genetic factors in the etiology of temporomandibular disorders: a review. Cranio. 2016;34(1):43–51.
8. Alrashdan MS, Alkhader M. Psychological factors in oral mucosal and orofacial pain conditions. Eur J Dent. 2017;11(4):548–52.
9. Schiffman E, Ohrbach R, Truelove E, Look J, Anderson G, Goulet JP, List T, Svensson P, Gonzalez Y, Lobbezoo F, et al. Diagnostic criteria for temporomandibular disorders (DC/TMD) for clinical and research applications: recommendations of the international RDC/TMD consortium network* and orofacial pain special interest Groupdagger. J Oral Facial Pain Headache. 2014;28(1):6–27.
10. Ohrbach R, Dworkin SF. The evolution of TMD diagnosis: past, present, future. J Dent Res. 2016;95(10):1093–101.
11. Pfau DB, Rolke R, Nickel R, Treede RD, Daublaender M. Somatosensory profiles in subgroups of patients with myogenic temporomandibular disorders and fibromyalgia syndrome. Pain. 2009;147(1–3):72–83.
12. Litt MD, Porto FB. Determinants of pain treatment response and nonresponse: identification of TMD patient subgroups. J Pain. 2013;14(11):1502–13.

13. Maixner W, Diatchenko L, Dubner R, Fillingim RB, Greenspan JD, Knott C, Ohrbach R, Weir B, Slade GD. Orofacial pain prospective evaluation and risk assessment study--the OPPERA study. J Pain. 2011;12(11 Suppl):T4–11.e11–12.

14. Greenspan JD, Slade GD, Bair E, Dubner R, Fillingim RB, Ohrbach R, Knott C, Diatchenko L, Liu Q, Maixner W. Pain sensitivity and autonomic factors associated with development of TMD: the OPPERA prospective cohort study. J Pain. 2013;14(12 Suppl):T63–74.e61–66.

15. Muzalev K, Visscher CM, Koutris M, Lobbezoo F. Long-term variability of sleep bruxism and psychological stress in patients with jaw-muscle pain: report of two longitudinal clinical cases. J Oral Rehabil. 2018;45(2):104–9.

16. Galli U, Ettlin DA, Palla S, Ehlert U, Gaab J. Do illness perceptions predict pain-related disability and mood in chronic orofacial pain patients? A 6-month follow-up study. Eur J Pain (London, England). 2010;14(5):550–8.

17. Maisa Soares G, Rizzatti-Barbosa CM. Chronicity factors of temporomandibular disorders: a critical review of the literature. Braz Oral Res. 2015;29(1):1–6.

18. Chichorro JG, Porreca F, Sessle B. Mechanisms of craniofacial pain. Cephalalgia. 2017;37(7):613–26.

19. Martenson ME, Cetas JS, Heinricher MM. A possible neural basis for stress-induced hyperalgesia. Pain. 2009;142(3):236–44.

20. Jennings EM, Okine BN, Roche M, Finn DP. Stress-induced hyperalgesia. Prog Neurobiol. 2014;121:1–18.

21. Egle UT, Egloff N, von Kanel R. Stress-induced hyperalgesia (SIH) as a consequence of emotional deprivation and psychosocial traumatization in childhood: implications for the treatment of chronic pain. Schmerz (Berlin, Germany). 2016;30(6):526-36.

22. Dworkin SF, LeResche L. Research diagnostic criteria for temporomandibular disorders: review, criteria, examinations and specifications, critique. J Craniomandib Disord. 1992;6(4):301–55.

23. Radvila A, Adler RH, Galeazzi RL, Vorkauf H. The development of a German language (Berne) pain questionnaire and its application in a situation causing acute pain. Pain. 1987;28(2):185–95.

24. Freynhagen R, Baron R, Gockel U, Tolle TR. painDETECT: a new screening questionnaire to identify neuropathic components in patients with back pain. Curr Med Res Opin. 2006;22(10):1911–20.

25. Keller T, Freynhagen R, Tolle TR, Liwowsky I, Moller P, Hullemann P, Gockel U, Stemmler E, Baron R. A retrospective analysis of the long-term test-retest stability of pain descriptors of the painDETECT questionnaire. Curr Med Res Opin. 2016;32(2):343–9.

26. Mathieson S, Lin C. painDETECT questionnaire. J Phys. 2013;59(3):211.

27. Mathieson S, Maher CG, Terwee CB, Folly de Campos T, Lin CW. Neuropathic pain screening questionnaires have limited measurement properties. A systematic review. J Clin Epidemiol. 2015;68(8):957–66.

28. Rolke R, Baron R, Maier C, Tolle TR, Treede RD, Beyer A, Binder A, Birbaumer N, Birklein F, Botefur IC, et al. Quantitative sensory testing in the German research network on neuropathic pain (DFNS): standardized protocol and reference values. Pain. 2006;123(3):231–43.

29. Rolke R, Magerl W, Campbell KA, Schalber C, Caspari S, Birklein F, Treede RD. Quantitative sensory testing: a comprehensive protocol for clinical trials. Eur J Pain (London, England). 2006;10(1):77–88.

30. Hartmann A, Seeberger R, Bittner M, Rolke R, Welte-Jzyk C, Daublander M. Profiling intraoral neuropathic disturbances following lingual nerve injury and in burning mouth syndrome. BMC Oral Health. 2017;17(1):68.

31. Herpich CM, Gomes C, Dibai-Filho AV, Politti F, Souza CDS, Biasotto-Gonzalez DA. Correlation between severity of temporomandibular disorder, pain intensity, and pressure pain threshold. J Manip Physiol Ther. 2018;41(1):47–51.

32. Daubländer M, Welte-Jzyk C. Craniomandibuläre Dysfunktion und stressinduzierte Hyperalgesie. Ärtzliche Psychotherapie. 2016;3:150–4.

33. de Siqueira SR, Teixeira MJ, de Siqueira JT. Orofacial pain and sensory characteristics of chronic patients compared with controls. Oral Surg Oral Med Oral Pathol Oral Radiol. 2013;115(6):e37–45.

34. Wieckiewicz W, Wozniak K, Piatkowska D, Szyszka-Sommerfeld L, Lipski M. The diagnostic value of pressure algometry for temporomandibular disorders. Biomed Res Int. 2015;2015:575038.

35. Sanches ML, Juliano Y, Novo NF, Guimaraes AS, Rodrigues Conti PC, Alonso LG. Correlation between pressure pain threshold and pain intensity in patients with temporomandibular disorders who are compliant or non-compliant with conservative treatment. Oral Surg Oral Med Oral Pathol Oral Radiol. 2015;120(4):459–68.

36. Ramalho D, Macedo L, Goffredo Filho G, Goes C, Tesch R. Correlation between the levels of non-specific physical symptoms and pressure pain

37. thresholds measured by algometry in patients with temporomandibular disorders. J Oral Rehabil. 2015;42(2):120–6.

37. Svensson P, Baad-Hansen L, Pigg M, List T, Eliav E, Ettlin D, Michelotti A, Tsukiyama Y, Matsuka Y, Jaaskelainen SK, et al. Guidelines and recommendations for assessment of somatosensory function in oro-facial pain conditions--a taskforce report. J Oral Rehabil. 2011;38(5):366–94.

38. Baad-Hansen L, Pigg M, Yang G, List T, Svensson P, Drangsholt M. Reliability of intra-oral quantitative sensory testing (QST) in patients with atypical odontalgia and healthy controls - a multicentre study. J Oral Rehabil. 2015;42(2):127–35.

39. Juhl GI, Jensen TS, Norholt SE, Svensson P. Central sensitization phenomena after third molar surgery: a quantitative sensory testing study. Eur J Pain (London, England). 2008;12(1):116–27.

40. Eberhard L. Quantitative sensory testing in the facial area: a review. Z Evid Fortbild Qual Gesundhwes. 2013;107(4–5):291–6.

41. Elias LA, Yilmaz Z, Smith JG, Bouchiba M, van der Valk RA, Page L, Barker S, Renton T. PainDETECT: a suitable screening tool for neuropathic pain in patients with painful post-traumatic trigeminal nerve injuries? Int J Oral Maxillofac Surg. 2014;43(1):120–6.

42. Heo JY, Ok SM, Ahn YW, Ko MY, Jeong SH. The application of neuropathic pain questionnaires in burning mouth syndrome patients. J Oral Facial Pain Headache. 2015;29(2):177–82.

43. Campi LB, Jordani PC, Tenan HL, Camparis CM, Goncalves DA. Painful temporomandibular disorders and central sensitization: implications for management-a pilot study. Int J Oral Maxillofac Surg. 2017;46(1):104–10.

44. Maisa Soares G, Rizzatti-Barbosa CM. Chronicity factors of temporomandibular disorders: a critical review of the literature. Braz Oral Res. 2015;29(1):1-6.

45. Zhao YJ, Liu Y, Li Q, Zhao YH, Wang J, Zhang M, Chen YJ. Involvement of trigeminal astrocyte activation in masseter hyperalgesia under stress. Physiol Behav. 2015;142:57–65.

46. Lorduy KM, Liegey-Dougall A, Haggard R, Sanders CN, Gatchel RJ. The prevalence of comorbid symptoms of central sensitization syndrome among three different groups of temporomandibular disorder patients. Pain Pract. 2013;13(8):604–13.

47. Robinson LJ, Durham J, Newton JL. A systematic review of the comorbidity between temporomandibular disorders and chronic fatigue syndrome. J Oral Rehabil. 2015;43(4):306-16.

48. Reiter S, Emodi-Perlman A, Goldsmith C, Friedman-Rubin P, Winocur E. Comorbidity between depression and anxiety in patients with temporomandibular disorders according to the research diagnostic criteria for temporomandibular disorders. J Oral Facial Pain Headache. 2015;29(2):135–43.

49. Yu Q, Liu Y, Chen X, Chen D, Xie L, Hong X, Wang X, Huang H, Yu H. Prevalence and associated factors for temporomandibular disorders in Chinese civilian pilots. Int Arch Occup Environ Health. 2015;88(7):905–11.

50. Slade GD, Sanders AE, Ohrbach R, Bair E, Maixner W, Greenspan JD, Fillingim RB, Smith S, Diatchenko L. COMT Diplotype amplifies effect of stress on risk of temporomandibular pain. J Dent Res. 2015;94(9):1187–95.

51. Fillingim RB, Ohrbach R, Greenspan JD, Knott C, Diatchenko L, Dubner R, Bair E, Baraian C, Mack N, Slade GD, et al. Psychological factors associated with development of TMD: the OPPERA prospective cohort study. J Pain. 2013;14(12 Suppl):T75–90.

52. Jochum H, Baumgartner-Gruber A, Brand S, Zeilhofer HF, Keel P, Leiggener CS. Chronic myofacial pain. Reduced pain through psychoeducation and physiotherapy. Schmerz (Berlin, Germany). 2015;29(3):285–92.

53. Blumenstiel K, Gerhardt A, Rolke R, Bieber C, Tesarz J, Friederich HC, Eich W, Treede RD. Quantitative sensory testing profiles in chronic back pain are distinct from those in fibromyalgia. Clin J Pain. 2011;27(8):682–90.

20

Polymer-based dental filling materials placed during pregnancy and risk to the foetus

Trine Lise Lundekvam Berge[1,2]* (iD), Gunvor Bentung Lygre[1], Stein Atle Lie[3] and Lars Björkman[1,3]

Abstract

Background: Tooth-coloured polymer-based dental filling materials are currently the first choice for dental restorative treatment in many countries. However, there are some concerns about their safety. It has been shown that substances known as endocrine disrupters, which might pass through the placental barrier, are released from these materials within the first hours after curing. Thus, the placement of polymer-based dental fillings in pregnant women may put the vulnerable foetus at risk. Large epidemiological studies exploring the risk of having polymer-based dental materials placed during pregnancy are lacking. The aim of this study was to investigate the association between the placement of polymer-based dental fillings during pregnancy and adverse birth outcomes.

Methods: This study is based on data from the large Norwegian Mother and Child Cohort Study (MoBa). The information about dental treatment during pregnancy was obtained from questionnaires sent to the participating women during weeks 17 and 30 of pregnancy. Reported placement of "white fillings" was used as exposure marker for having received polymer-based dental filling materials. Only singleton births were included in the present study. Data were linked to the Medical Birth Registry of Norway. Logistic regression models that included the mother's age, level of education, body mass index, parity, and smoking and alcohol consumption during pregnancy were used to estimate the odds ratio (OR) and 95% confidence interval (CI). Different adverse birth outcomes were of interest in the present study.

Results: Valid data were available from 90,886 pregnancies. Dentist consultation during pregnancy was reported by 33,727 women, 10,972 of whom had white fillings placed. The adjusted logistic regression models showed no statistically significant association between having white dental fillings placed during pregnancy and stillbirth, malformations, preterm births, and low or high birth weight.

Conclusions: In this study, women who reported white fillings placed during pregnancy had no increased risk for adverse birth outcomes compared with women who did not consult a dentist during pregnancy. Thus, our findings do not support the hypothesis of an association between placement of polymer-based fillings during pregnancy and adverse birth outcomes.

Keywords: Polymer-based dental filling materials, Pregnancy, Adverse birth outcomes, Congenital malformation, Birth weight, Stillbirth, Premature birth, Bisphenol A, BPA, The Norwegian mother and child cohort study

* Correspondence: trbe@norceresearch.no
[1]Dental Biomaterials Adverse Reaction Unit, Uni Research Health, Bergen, Norway
[2]Oral Health Centre of Expertise in Western Norway, Bergen, Hordaland, Norway
Full list of author information is available at the end of the article

Background

Tooth-coloured polymer-based materials are the first choice for dental restorative treatment in many countries [1, 2]. However, there are concerns about the safety of these materials [3]. Results of in vitro and in vivo studies have shown that substances that potentially could lead to adverse effects in the patient are released from these materials within 24 h after curing [4–8]. Elution may initially be due to incomplete polymerization [9, 10] and contaminants [11, 12]. The local adverse effects [13] caused by the leachable components are rare [14]. However, the possibility of systemic adverse effects could not be ruled out [15].

The elution of bisphenol A (BPA) has been of particular concern [16]. BPA is a chemical known to be an endocrine disruptor, mimicking oestrogen [17, 18]. Polymer-based dental filling materials may contain BPA as an impurity from the production process of bisphenol-A glycidyl dimethacrylate (Bis-GMA) [8, 11, 19, 20] or, less probable, a degradation product of monomers [12, 21, 22]. Results from animal studies have indicated that BPA has reproductive, developmental and systemic toxic effects [23, 24]. It has been shown that newly placed composite restorations in humans may be associated with short-term elevated BPA levels in both saliva and urine [4, 7].

The impact of exposure to BPA on human health remains uncertain. However, data from the literature indicate that exposure to BPA, even at relatively low doses, could potentially result in adverse health effects [15]. Moreover, studies suggest that BPA might pass through the placental barrier [25], and thus, maternal exposure to BPA may offer a potential risk to the vulnerable foetus.

Even though substances with potential toxicity are released from dental polymer-based materials [4, 5], studies exploring the risk of having these materials placed during pregnancy are lacking.

The aim of the present study was to investigate whether the placement of polymer-based dental fillings during pregnancy is associated with adverse birth outcomes including stillbirth, preterm birth, malformations and low or high birth weight.

Methods

Data from the ongoing Norwegian Mother and Child Cohort Study (MoBa), a prospective population-based cohort study conducted by the Norwegian Institute of Public Health, were used. From 1999 to the end of 2008, pregnant women in Norway were invited to MoBa through a postal invitation in connection with their first routine ultrasound examination. The participation rate was approximately 41%, and the cohort currently comprises more than 108,000 pregnancies, 114,000 children, 95,000 mothers and 75,000 fathers. Written informed consent was obtained from each participant upon recruitment [26, 27].

In the present study, data were gathered from two questionnaires that were sent to the participating women in weeks 17 and 30 of pregnancy [28]. Each woman could participate with multiple pregnancies. Only singleton births were included in the present study.

Information about white fillings placed during pregnancy was obtained from the questionnaires sent to the participants in week 30. Reported placement of white fillings was used as exposure marker. The participants reported if they had consulted a dentist during pregnancy ("Have you been to the dentist during this pregnancy? Yes/No") and if so, whether they had received white fillings ("If, yes, did the dentist put in new white fillings? Yes/No").

Women without valid information about dental treatment during pregnancy and those with missing data on birth outcomes were excluded, leaving a study population that included 90,886 pregnancies (Fig. 1).

Information about gender, preterm delivery, stillbirth, malformations, birth weight and mother's age at delivery was obtained from the Medical Birth Registry of Norway (MBRN) [29]. The mother's 11-digit unique personal identification number assigned to every citizen in Norway was used to link data sources. Gestational age was based on ultrasound examination in the 17th week of pregnancy.

Infants were classified as late preterm if they were born between gestational week 33 and 37, and very preterm if they were born before or during the 32nd gestational week [30, 31]. Infants with a birth weight less than 2500 g at birth were classified as low-birth weight infants, and infants with a birth weight more than 4000 g were classified as high-birth weight infants [32].

Maternal body mass index (BMI; kg/m^2) was calculated from self-reported pre-pregnancy height and weight. The BMI was categorized according to the WHO classification [33].

Information about parity, defined as the number of former births with a gestational age of 12 weeks or more, was based on data reported by the mothers in the MoBa study and from the MBRN.

Information about education, smoking habits and alcohol consumption during pregnancy was obtained from the first questionnaire completed at approximately the 17th week.

The present study is based on version 8 of the quality-assured MoBa data files. We defined dental treatment during pregnancy as follows: participants who did not consult a dentist during pregnancy (reference category); participants who consulted a dentist but had no white fillings placed; and participants who consulted a dentist and had white fillings placed (Fig. 1).

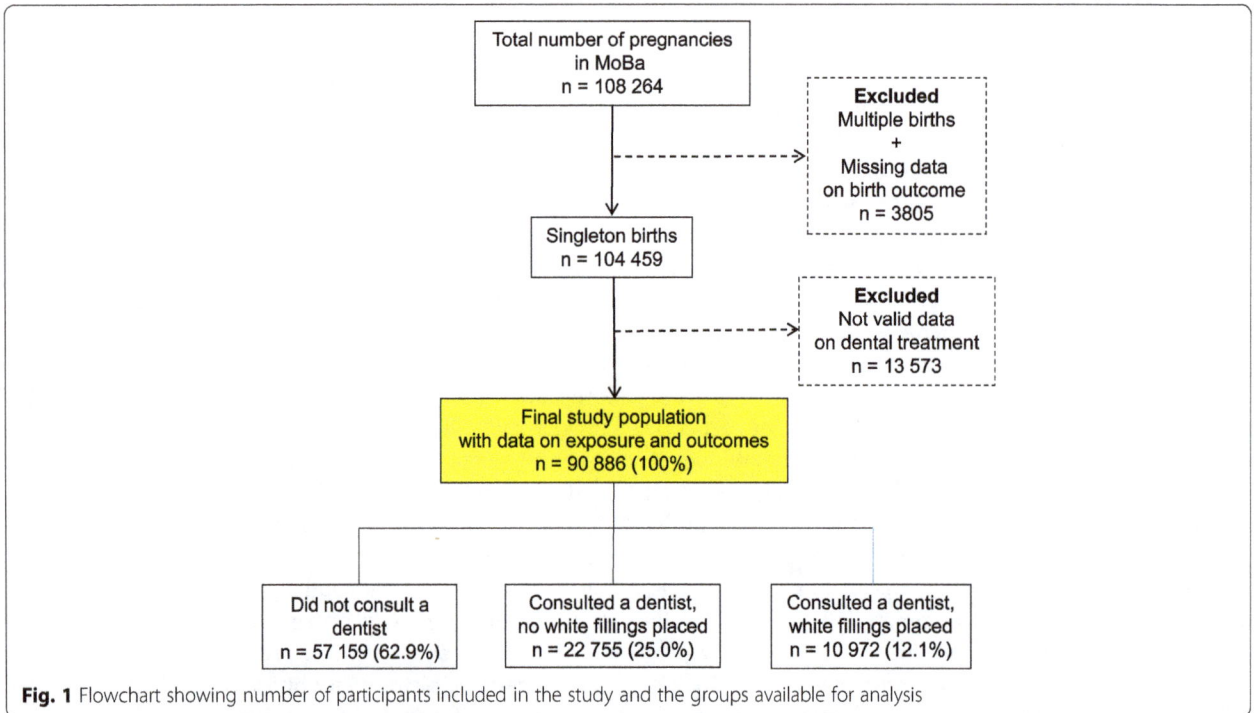

Fig. 1 Flowchart showing number of participants included in the study and the groups available for analysis

Infants were defined as small for gestational age (SGA) if the weight at birth was less than the 10th percentile for gestational age and large for gestational age (LGA) if they were larger than the 90th percentile. Very small for gestational age was defined as weight below the 2.5th percentile [34].

The odds ratio (OR) with a 95% confidence interval was calculated using logistic regression. The OR was adjusted for maternal age (≤19, 20–24, 25–29, 30–34, 35–39, 40+ years), length of education (≤12, 13–16, ≥17 years), pre-pregnancy BMI (< 18.5, 18.5–24.9, 25.0–29.9, 30.0–34.9, 35.0–39.9, ≥ 40 kg/m^2), parity (first, second and more), smoking during pregnancy (never, occasionally, daily) and alcohol consumption during pregnancy (never, less than once a week, once a week, more than once a week).

Analyses were performed using IBM-SPSS (IBM Corp. Released 2016. IBM SPSS Statistics for Windows, Version 24.0, Armonk, NY, USA: IBM Corp.). *p*-values less than 0.05 were considered statistically significant.

The MoBa cohort study obtained a license from the Norwegian Data Inspectorate, and this research project was approved by the Regional Ethics Committee for Medical Research (REC South-East D, 2011/727).

Results

Dentist consultation during pregnancy was reported by 33,727 women, and of these, 10,972 had white fillings placed (Fig. 1). Detailed descriptive information regarding the characteristics of the participants is included in

Table 1. Of the included pregnancies, 204 (0.2%) resulted in a stillbirth. The overall proportion of malformation was 4.8%, and the proportion of very preterm births and late preterm births was 0.6 and 3.8%, respectively (Table 2).

Compared to the reference group, there was no statistically significant increased risk for any adverse birth outcomes for participants who had consulted a dentist during pregnancy without having white fillings placed or for those who had white fillings placed (Table 3).

Separate analyses by gender showed that girls born to mothers who had white fillings placed during pregnancy had an increased risk of being small for gestational age (below the 10th percentile) compared to the reference group. The unadjusted OR was 1.14 (95% CI 1.01–1.28; *p* = 0.029) while after adjustment for potential confounders, the OR was reduced and not statistically significant (OR = 1.10, 95% CI 0.97–1.24; Table 3).

Boys born to mothers who received white fillings during pregnancy had a slightly increased risk of being born late preterm compared to the boys born in the reference group. The unadjusted OR was 1.16 (95% CI 1.01–1.34; *p* = 0.041), and the adjusted OR was 1.13 (95% CI 0.98–1.31; *p* = 0.082; Table 3).

Discussion

The aim of the present study was to investigate whether the placement of polymer-based dental fillings during pregnancy was associated with outcomes including stillbirth, preterm delivery, malformations, and low or high

Table 1 Characteristics of the participants related to dental treatment during pregnancy ($n = 90{,}886$)

	Did not consult a dentist	Consulted a dentist, no white fillings placed	Consulted a dentist, white filling placed	Total
Number of participating pregnancies, n (%)	57,159 (62.9)	22,755 (25.0)	10,972 (12.1)	90,886 (100)
Maternal age (years), n (%)				
≤ 19	525 (0.9)	207 (0.9)	127 (1.2)	859 (0.9)
20–24	6056 (10.6)	1767 (7.8)	1195 (10.9)	9018 (9.9)
25–29	19,288 (33.7)	7159 (31.5)	3686 (33.6)	30,133 (33.2)
30–34	21,928 (38.4)	9273 (40.8)	3990 (36.4)	35,191 (38.7)
35–39	8315 (14.5)	3856 (16.9)	1711 (15.6)	13,882 (15.3)
≥ 40	1047 (1.8)	493 (2.2)	263 (2.4)	1803 (2.0)
Maternal pre-pregnant Body Mass Index, n (%)				
< 18.5	1663 (2.9)	660 (2.9)	319 (2.9)	2642 (2.9)
18.5–24.9	36,021 (63.0)	14,956 (65.7)	6655 (60.7)	57,632 (63.4)
25.0–29.9	12,003 (21.0)	4542 (20.0)	2443 (22.3)	18,988 (20.9)
30.0–34.9	3837 (6.7)	1402 (6.2)	842 (7.7)	6081 (6.7)
35.0–39.9	1091 (1.9)	354 (1.6)	232 (2.1)	1677 (1.8)
≥ 40	341 (0.6)	124 (0.5)	68 (0.6)	533 (0.6)
Missing	2203 (3.9)	717 (3.2)	413 (3.8)	3333 (3.7)
Parity, n (%)				
Para 0 (first pregnancy)	25,428 (44.5)	10,897 (47.9)	4836 (44.1)	41,161 (45.3)
Para 1+ (second pregnancy or more)	31,731 (55.5)	11,858 (52.1)	6136 (55.9)	49,725 (54.7)
Maternal education, n (%)				
≤ 12 years	18,849 (33.0)	6831 (30.0)	4177 (38.1)	29,857 (32.9)
13–16 years	22,042 (38.6)	9226 (40.5)	4018 (36.6)	35,286 (38.8)
≥17 years	12,725 (22.3)	5366 (23.6)	2097 (19.1)	20,188 (22.2)
Missing	3543 (6.2)	1332 (5.9)	680 (6.2)	5555 (6.1)
Smoking during pregnancy, n (%)				
Never	45,831 (80.2)	18,208 (80.0)	8420 (76.7)	72,459 (79.7)
Occasionally	1421 (2.5)	567 (2.5)	374 (3.4)	2362 (2.6)
Daily	2848 (5.0)	968 (4.3)	821 (7.5)	4637 (5.1)
Missing	7059 (12.3)	3012 (13.2)	1357 (12.4)	11,428 (12.6)
Alcohol during pregnancy, n (%)				
Never	42,203 (73.8)	16,731 (73.5)	7834 (71.4)	66,768 (73.5)
Less than once a week	5709 (10.0)	2512 (11.0)	1251 (11.4)	9472 (10.4)
Once a week	233 (0.4)	100 (0.4)	46 (0.4)	379 (0.4)
More than once a week	39 (0.1)	25 (0.1)	6 (0.1)	70 (0.1)
Missing	8975 (15.7)	3387 (14.9)	1835 (16.7)	14,197 (15.6)

Body Mass Index = weight (kg)/height^2 (m)^2

birth weight. No evidence of an increased risk of adverse birth outcomes after placement of white fillings during pregnancy was found. Gender-specific analyses showed generally similar results for girls and boys analysed together.

The main strengths of the present study are the overall large sample size and the large number of participants who had white fillings placed. These large numbers enabled us to study even rare birth outcomes. Furthermore, the prospective design of the study reduced the risk for recall bias. Additionally, the information on health-related and lifestyle data that was derived from both the MBRN and the MoBa questionnaires enabled us to control for some potential confounding factors.

To the best of our knowledge, the present study is the first to investigate potential associations between

Table 2 Birth outcomes by dental treatment during pregnancy (n = 90,886)

	Did not consult a dentist	Consulted a dentist, no white fillings placed	Consulted a dentist, white filling placed	Total
Number of boys, n (%)	29,387 (51.4)	11,607 (51.0)	5582 (50.9)	46,576 (51.2)
Number of preterm births, n (%)				
Very preterm births (≤ 32 weeks)	337 (0.6)	124 (0.5)	65 (0.6)	526 (0.6)
Late preterm births (33–36 weeks)	2150 (3.8)	884 (3.9)	454 (4.1)	3488 (3.8)
Mean birth weight (g)				
Mean birth weight (SD)	3611 (546)	3603 (538)	3607 (549)	3608 (544)
Number of children with low birth weight, n (%)				
Low birth weight (< 2500 g)	1465 (2.6)	576 (2.5)	290 (2.6)	2331 (2.6)
Small for gestational age (SGA) 10 percentile	3660 (6.4)	1475 (6.5)	726 (6.6)	5861 (6.5)
Small for gestational age (SGA) 2.5 percentile	793 (1.4)	293 (1.3)	145 (1,3)	1231 (1.4)
Number of children with high birth weight, n (%)				
High birth weight children (> 4000 g)	12,515 (21.9)	4905 (21.6)	2390 (21.8)	19,810 (21.8)
Large for gestational age (LGA) 10 percentile	6633 (11.7)	2557 (11.3)	1285 (11.8)	10,475 (11.6)
Large for gestational age (LGA) 2.5 percentile	2110 (3.7)	809 (3.6)	418 (3.8)	3337 (3.7)
Number of children with malformation, n (%)	2697(4.7)	1108 (4.9)	519 (4.7)	4324 (4.8)
Number of stillbirths, n (%)	125 (0.2)	49 (0.2)	30 (0.3)	204 (0.2)

polymer-based fillings placed during pregnancy and birth outcomes. Michalowicz et al. found no significant associations between adverse pregnancy outcomes and periodontal treatment, the use of anaesthetic during nonsurgical periodontal treatment, treatment including temporary and permanent restorations, endodontic therapy, and extractions [35]. These results are in agreement with our findings. However, in the study of Michalowicz et al., the type of restorative material was not specified. Thus, the results are not directly comparable.

A limitation of the MoBa study is the low response rate, with a possible self-selection of the healthiest women. The MoBa has an underrepresentation of young mothers (< 25 years). The participants have a higher level of education and are more likely to be non-smokers than the general population of pregnant women in Norway [36].

However, self-selection to the cohort is not a validity problem in studies of associations between exposure and outcomes [36].

The MoBa study is based on questionnaires filled in by the participating women. To achieve reliable answers from all participants in this large cohort, an effort was made to make the questions as easy and achievable as possible. Thus, information about dental treatment is sparse. Detailed information about the type and manufacturer of the polymer-based filling material and size and number of fillings placed, would be of interest. However, to obtain accurate information about this, access to dental records would be needed. In large epidemiological studies, like the MoBa study, access to updated dental records would be unfeasible. Accordingly, reliable knowledge about the number and size of possible pre-existing composite restorations is lacking. Since leakage of BPA from existing polymer-based restorative materials is very low compared with other sources [37], this information would most likely be of minor importance.

The participants were asked if they had received "white fillings" during pregnancy. In Norway, white fillings would practically be the same as polymer-based restorative fillings or so called polymer-based or resin-based composites. However, the term "white fillings" may include materials like resin-modified cements, compomers and water-based glass ionomer cements (GIC). In the period of this study, the vast majority of Norwegian dentists used polymer-based filling materials when restoring cavities in adults. Kopperud et al. described management of occlusal caries in adults by Norwegian dentists in 2009 and stated that polymer-based composite was the preferred restorative material (91.9%) [38]. In the same study the use of other filling materials was reported to be less than 4%. This is in accordance with another study examining treatment concept for approximal caries in Norway [39]. In 2009 polymer-based filling material was preferred by 94.9% of the responding dentists. Preference for other filling materials was: 1.1% compomer, 1.1% GIC, 0.5% resin-modified GIC and 1.8% a combination of resin composite and GIC [39]. In 1997, 2 years before recruitment started in MoBa, Norwegian data showed that approximately 70% of the tooth-coloured fillings placed in adults were polymer-based [40].

Table 3 Crude and adjusted odds ratio (OR) and confidence interval (CI) for adverse birth outcomes related to dental treatment during pregnancy. (Reference category: Women who did not consult a dentist, OR = 1)

		Consulted a dentist, no white fillings placed OR (95% CI)	Consulted a dentist, white filling placed OR (95% CI)
Very preterm birth (≤ 32 weeks)			
Girls	Crude	0.96 (0.71–1.30)	0.91 (0.60–1.37)
	Adjusted	0.94 (0.69–1.27)	0.88 (0.58–1.33)
Boys	Crude	0.91 (0.69–1.21)	1.08 (0.76–1.53)
	Adjusted	0.88 (0.67–1.17)	1.02 (0.72–1.45)
All	Crude	0.92 (0.75–1.14)	1.01 (0.77–1.31)
	Adjusted	0.90 (0.73–1.11)	0.97 (0.74–1.26)
Late preterm birth (33–36 weeks)			
Girls	Crude	1.00 (0.89–1.13)	1.05 (0.90–1.22)
	Adjusted	1.00 (0.89–1.12)	1.03 (0.88–1.19)
Boys	Crude	1.06 (0.95–1.18)	1.16*(1.01–1.34)
	Adjusted	1.05 (0.94–1.18)	1.14 (0.99–1.31)
All	Crude	1.03 (0.96–1.12)	1.10 (1.00–1.23)
	Adjusted	1.03 (0.95–1.11)	1.08 (0.97–1.20)
Low birth weight (< 2500 g)			
Girls	Crude	1.01 (0.88–1.51)	1.03 (0.86–1.23)
	Adjusted	0.98 (0.86–1.12)	0.99 (0.83–1.18)
Boys	Crude	0.96 (0.84–1.11)	1.03 (0.86–1.24)
	Adjusted	0.94 (0.82–1.09)	0.99 (0.83–1.19)
All	Crude	0.99 (0.90–1.09)	1.03 (0.91–1.17)
	Adjusted	0.96 (0.87–1.06)	0.99 (0.87–1.13)
Small for gestational age (SGA) 10 percentile			
Girls	Crude	1.07 (0.97–1.17)	1.14*(1.01–1.28)
	Adjusted	1.03 (0.94–1.13)	1.10 (0.97–1.24)
Boys	Crude	0.97 (0.89–1.05)	0.95 (0.85–1.07)
	Adjusted	0.92 (0.84–1.00)	0.93 (0.83–1.04)
All	Crude	1.01 (0.95–1.08)	1.04 (0.95–1.13)
	Adjusted	0.97 (0.91–1.03)	1.00 (0.92–1.09)
Very small for gestational age (SGA) 2.5 percentile			
Girls	Crude	0.86 (0.71–1.06)	1.04 (0.81–1.34)
	Adjusted	0.84 (0.68–1.03)	0.97 (0.75–1.25)
Boys	Crude	0.98 (0.82–1.17)	0.88 (0.68–1.13)
	Adjusted	0.93 (0.77–1.11)	0.84 (0.65–1.08)
All	Crude	0.93 (0.81–1.06)	0.95 (0.80–1.14)
	Adjusted	0.89 (0.77–1.02)	0.90 (0.75–1.08)
High birth weight (> 4000 g)			
Girls	Crude	0.99 (0.94–1.05)	0.98 (0.91–1.06)
	Adjusted	1.03 (0.97–1.09)	0.98 (0.91–1.06)
Boys	Crude	0.98 (0.93–1.03)	1.01 (0.94–1.07)
	Adjusted	1.01 (0.96–1.06)	1.00 (0.93–1.07)
All	Crude	0.98 (0.94–1.02)	0.99 (0.95–1.04)
	Adjusted	1.01 (0.98–1.05)	0.99 (0.94–1.04)

Table 3 Crude and adjusted odds ratio (OR) and confidence interval (CI) for adverse birth outcomes related to dental treatment during pregnancy. (Reference category: Women who did not consult a dentist, OR = 1) *(Continued)*

		Consulted a dentist, no white fillings placed OR (95% CI)	Consulted a dentist, white filling placed OR (95% CI)
Large for gestational age (LGA) 10 percentile			
Girls	Crude	0.96 (0.90–1.02)	0.99 (0.91–1.08)
	Adjusted	1.00 (0.93–1.07)	0.98 (0.90–1.08)
Boys	Crude	0.97 (0.90–1.04)	1.03 (0.94–1.13)
	Adjusted	1.01 (0.94–1.08)	1.01 (0.93–1.11)
All	Crude	0.96 (0.92–1.01)	1.01 (0.95–1.08)
	Adjusted	1.01 (0.96–1.06)	1.00 (0.94–1.06)
Large for gestational age (LGA) 2.5 percentile			
Girls	Crude	0.97 (0.87–1.09)	1.01 (0.87–1.17)
	Adjusted	1.02 (0.91–1.15)	0.99 (0.86–1.15)
Boys	Crude	0.95 (0.84–1.07)	1.06 (0.90–1.24)
	Adjusted	0.98 (0.87–1.11)	1.03 (0.88–1.20)
All	Crude	0.96 (0.88–1.04)	1.03 (0.93–1.15)
	Adjusted	1.00 (0.92–1.09)	1.01 (0.91–1.12)
Malformation			
Girls	Crude	1.02 (0.92–1.14)	0.99 (0.86–1.15)
	Adjusted	1.00 (0.90–1.12)	1.00 (0.86–1.15)
Boys	Crude	1.05 (0.95–1.15)	1.01 (0.89–1.15)
	Adjusted	1.03 (0.94–1.14)	1.00 (0.88–1.14)
All	Crude	1.03 (0.96–1.11)	1.00 (0.91–1.10)
	Adjusted	1.02 (0.95–1.09)	1.00 (0.91–1.10)
Stillbirth			
Girls	Crude	0.96 (0.59–1.55)	1.20 (0.67–2.15)
	Adjusted	0.92 (0.57–1.50)	1.16 (0.64-2.07)
Boys	Crude	0.97 (0.61–1.54)	1.30 (0.75–2.24)
	Adjusted	0.95 (0.60–1.51)	1.22 (0.70–2.11)
All	Crude	0.98 (0.71–1.37)	1.25 (0.84–1.86)
	Adjusted	0.96 (0.69–1.33)	1.18 (0.79–1.76)

The OR was adjusted for mothers age (≤19, 20–24, 25–29, 30–34, 35–39, 40+), parity (0, 1 or more previous viable pregnancies), education (≤ 12 years, 13–16 years, ≥ 17 years), pre-pregnancy body mass index (< 18.5, 18.5–24.9, 25.0–29.9, 30.0–34.9, 35.0–39.9, ≥ 40), smoking (never, occasionally, daily) and alcohol consumption during pregnancy (never, less than once a week, once a week, more than once a week). *$p < 0.05$

The participants answered questions regarding dental treatment during the first 30 weeks of pregnancy but were not asked to specify in which week of pregnancy they visited the dentist. Hence, a limitation is that we could not study if treatment with polymer-based filling materials could be a factor of importance at specific time windows during pregnancy. The severity of the effects of prenatal exposure to toxic agents appears to be influenced by the degree and timing of the exposure during gestation [41]. Some teratogens cause damage only during specific days or weeks early in pregnancy, when a particular part of the body is formed [41]. A well-known example is the thalidomide-tragedy in the late 1950s

and the early 1960s, where the medication taken during days 20–36 after fertilization resulted in serious malformations of the foetus [42, 43].

Some women with the need for dental treatment do not seek or do not receive dental care during pregnancy [44]. This may, in part, be due to their concerns about the potential risk to the foetus, as well as dentists and other health care providers' attitudes and beliefs about the safety of dental treatment during pregnancy [44].

The findings from the present study, including more than 90,000 pregnancies, are reassuring. However, taken the limitations of a prospective cohort study into account, these findings could be corroborated in case control studies. Thus, access to dental records and thereby accurate and detailed information regarding dental treatment could be possible to obtain.

Conclusion

In this study, women who had white fillings placed during pregnancy had no increased risk for adverse birth outcomes compared with women who did not consult a dentist during pregnancy. Thus, our findings do not support the hypothesis of an association between placement of polymer-based fillings during pregnancy and adverse birth outcomes.

Abbreviations

Bis-GMA: Bisphenol-A glycidyl dimethacrylate; BMI: Body mass index; BPA: Bisphenol A; LGA: Large for gestational age; MBRN: Medical Birth Registry of Norway; MoBa: the Norwegian Mother and Child Cohort Study; SGA: Small for gestational age; WHO: World Health Organization

Acknowledgements

The Norwegian Mother and Child Cohort Study is supported by the Norwegian Ministry of Health and Care Services and the Ministry of Education and Research, NIH/NINDS (grant no.1 UO1 NS 047537-01 and grant no.2 UO1 NS 047537-06A1). We are grateful to all the participating families in Norway who take part in this on-going cohort study.

Funding

The Norwegian Dental Biomaterials Adverse Reaction Unit and the Oral Health Centre of Expertise in Western Norway are funded by the Norwegian Ministry of Health and Care Services.

Authors' contributions

GBL and LB conceptualized the study, critically reviewed the results of the analyses, reviewed and revised the manuscript. TLLB carried out the analyses, drafted the initial manuscript and coordinated the editing. SAL critically reviewed the results of analyses, reviewed and revised the manuscript. All authors approved the final manuscript as submitted.

Competing interests

The authors declare that they have no competing interests.

Author details

[1]Dental Biomaterials Adverse Reaction Unit, Uni Research Health, Bergen, Norway. [2]Oral Health Centre of Expertise in Western Norway, Bergen, Hordaland, Norway. [3]Department of Clinical Dentistry, University of Bergen, Bergen, Norway.

References

1. Alexander G, Hopcraft MS, Tyas MJ, Wong RH. Dentists' restorative decision-making and implications for an 'amalgamless' profession. Part 1: a review. Aust Dent J. 2014;59:408–19. https://doi.org/10.1111/adj.12209.

2. Eklund SA. Trends in dental treatment, 1992 to 2007. J Am Dent Assoc. 2010;141:391–9. https://www.ncbi.nlm.nih.gov/pubmed/20354088

3. SCENIHR (Scientific Committee on Emerging and Newly-Identified Health Risks). Opinion on the safety of dental amalgam and alternative dental restoration materials for patients and users (update), 29 April. European commission. DG Health and Food Safety. 2015:2015. http://ec.europa.eu/health/sites/health/files/scientific_committees/emerging/docs/scenihr_o_046.pdf. Accessed 14 Dec 2017

4. Kingman A, Hyman J, Masten SA, Jayaram B, Smith C, Eichmiller F, et al. Bisphenol A and other compounds in human saliva and urine associated with the placement of composite restorations. J Am Dent Assoc. 2012;143:1292–302. http://www.ncbi.nlm.nih.gov/pubmed/23204083

5. Michelsen VB, Kopperud HB, Lygre GB, Bjorkman L, Jensen E, Kleven IS, et al. Detection and quantification of monomers in unstimulated whole saliva after treatment with resin-based composite fillings in vivo. Eur J Oral Sci. 2012;120:89–95. https://doi.org/10.1111/j.1600-0722.2011.00897.x.

6. Sevkusic M, Schuster L, Rothmund L, Dettinger K, Maier M, Hickel R, et al. The elution and breakdown behavior of constituents from various light-cured composites. Dent Mater. 2014;30:619–31. https://doi.org/10.1016/j.dental.2014.02.022.

7. Maserejian NN, Trachtenberg FL, Wheaton OB, Calafat AM, Ranganathan G, Kim HY, et al. Changes in urinary bisphenol a concentrations associated with placement of dental composite restorations in children and adolescents. J Am Dent Assoc. 2016; https://doi.org/10.1016/j.adaj.2016.02.020.

8. Van Landuyt KL, Nawrot T, Geebelen B, De Munck J, Snauwaert J, Yoshihara K, et al. How much do resin-based dental materials release? A meta-analytical approach. Dent Mater. 2011;27:723–47. https://doi.org/10.1016/j.dental.2011.05.001.

9. Durner J, Obermaier J, Draenert M, Ilie N. Correlation of the degree of conversion with the amount of elutable substances in nano-hybrid dental composites. Dent Mater. 2012;28:1146–53. https://doi.org/10.1016/j.dental.2012.08.006.

10. Ferracane JL. Elution of leachable components from composites. J Oral Rehabil. 1994;21:441–52. https://www.ncbi.nlm.nih.gov/pubmed/7965355

11. American Dental Association Council on Scientific Affairs. Determination of bisphenol a released from resin-based composite dental restoratives. American Dental Association Professional Product Review. 2014;9(3). http://www.ada.org/en/publications/ada-professional-product-review-ppr. Accessed 5 Sept 2014.

12. Schmalz G, Preiss A, Arenholt-Bindslev D. Bisphenol-A content of resin monomers and related degradation products. Clin Oral Investig. 1999;3:114–9. https://www.ncbi.nlm.nih.gov/pubmed/10803121

13. Schedle A, Ortengren U, Eidler N, Gabauer M, Hensten A. Do adverse effects of dental materials exist? What are the consequences, and how can they be diagnosed and treated? Clin Oral Implants Res. 2007;18(Suppl 3):232–56. https://doi.org/10.1111/j.1600-0501.2007.01481.x.

14. Bakopoulou A, Papadopoulos T, Garefis P. Molecular toxicology of substances released from resin-based dental restorative materials. Int J Mol Sci. 2009;10:3861–99. https://doi.org/10.3390/ijms10093861.

15. Rochester JR. Bisphenol a and human health: a review of the literature. Reprod Toxicol. 2013;42:132–55. https://doi.org/10.1016/j.reprotox.2013.08.008.

16. Fleisch AF, Sheffield PE, Chinn C, Edelstein BL, Landrigan PJ. Bisphenol a and related compounds in dental materials. Pediatrics. 2010;126:760–8. https://doi.org/10.1542/peds.2009-2693.

17. Schug TT, Janesick A, Blumberg B, Heindel JJ. Endocrine disrupting chemicals and disease susceptibility. J Steroid Biochem Mol Biol. 2011;127:204–15. https://doi.org/10.1016/j.jsbmb.2011.08.007.

18. Crain DA, Eriksen M, Iguchi T, Jobling S, Laufer H, LeBlanc GA, et al. An ecological assessment of bisphenol-a: evidence from comparative biology. Reprod Toxicol. 2007;24:225–39. https://doi.org/10.1016/j.reprotox.2007.05.008.

19. Soderholm KJ, Mariotti A. BIS-GMA--based resins in dentistry: are they safe? J Am Dent Assoc. 1999;130:201–9. https://www.ncbi.nlm.nih.gov/pubmed/10036843

20. Olea N, Pulgar R, Perez P, Olea-Serrano F, Rivas A, Novillo-Fertrell A, et al. Estrogenicity of resin-based composites and sealants used in dentistry. Environ Health Perspect. 1996;104:298–305. http://www.ncbi.nlm.nih.gov/pubmed/8919768

21. Imai Y, Watanabe M, Ohsaki A. Analysis of major components and bisphenol a in commercial Bis-GMA and Bis-GMA-based resins using high performance liquid chromatography. Dent Mater J. 2000;19:263–9. https://www.ncbi.nlm.nih.gov/pubmed/11218846

22. Atkinson JC, Diamond F, Eichmiller F, Selwitz R, Jones G. Stability of bisphenol a, triethylene-glycol dimethacrylate, and bisphenol a dimethacrylate in whole saliva. Dent Mater. 2002;18:128–35. http://www.ncbi.nlm.nih.gov/pubmed/11755591

23. Vandenberg LN, Colborn T, Hayes TB, Heindel JJ, Jacobs DR Jr, Lee DH, et al. Hormones and endocrine-disrupting chemicals: low-dose effects and nonmonotonic dose responses. Endocr Rev. 2012;33:378–455. https://doi.org/10.1210/er.2011-1050.

24. Richter CA, Birnbaum LS, Farabollini F, Newbold RR, Rubin BS, Talsness CE, et al. In vivo effects of bisphenol a in laboratory rodent studies. Reprod Toxicol. 2007;24:199–224. https://doi.org/10.1016/j.reprotox.2007.06.004.

25. Miyakoda HT, Masako T, Onodera SO, Takeda K. Passage of bisphenol a into the fetus of pregnant rat. J Health Sci. 1999;45:318–23.

26. Magnus P, Irgens LM, Haug K, Nystad W, Skjaerven R, Stoltenberg C, et al. Cohort profile: the Norwegian mother and child cohort study (MoBa). Int J Epidemiol. 2006;35:1146–50. https://doi.org/10.1093/ije/dyl170.

27. Magnus P, Birke C, Vejrup K, Haugan A, Alsaker E, Daltveit AK, et al. Cohort profile update: the Norwegian mother and child cohort study (MoBa). Int J Epidemiol. 2016; https://doi.org/10.1093/ije/dyw029.

28. Norwegian Institute of Public Health. Questionnaires from MoBa. 2005 [updated 15 September 2016]. https://www.fhi.no/en/studies/moba/for-forskere-artikler/questionnaires-from-moba/. Accessed 15 Dec 2017.

29. Irgens LM. The medical birth registry of Norway. Epidemiological research and surveillance throughout 30 years. Acta Obstet Gynecol Scand. 2000;79:435–9. https://www.ncbi.nlm.nih.gov/pubmed/10857866

30. Fleischman AR, Oinuma M, Clark SL. Rethinking the definition of "term pregnancy". Obstet Gynecol. 2010;116:136–9. https://doi.org/10.1097/AOG.0b013e3181e24f28.

31. Blencowe H, Cousens S, Oestergaard MZ, Chou D, Moller AB, Narwal R, et al. National, regional, and worldwide estimates of preterm birth rates in the year 2010 with time trends since 1990 for selected countries: a systematic analysis and implications. Lancet. 2012;379:2162–72. https://doi.org/10.1016/S0140-6736(12)60820-4.

32. World Health Organization. WHO: recommended definitions, terminology and format for statistical tables related to the perinatal period and use of a new certificate for cause of perinatal deaths. Modifications recommended by FIGO as amended October 14, 1976. Acta Obstet Gynecol Scand. 1977; 56:247–53. https://www.ncbi.nlm.nih.gov/pubmed/560099

33. World Health Organization. Global Database on Body Mass Index. BMI classification 2007. 2007. http://www.who.int/. Accessed 22.11.2017.

34. Skjaerven R, Gjessing HK, Bakketeig LS. Birthweight by gestational age in Norway. Acta Obstet Gynecol Scand. 2000;79:440–9. https://www.ncbi.nlm.nih.gov/pubmed/10857867

35. Michalowicz BS, DiAngelis AJ, Novak MJ, Buchanan W, Papapanou PN, Mitchell DA, et al. Examining the safety of dental treatment in pregnant women. J Am Dent Assoc. 2008;139:685–95. https://www.ncbi.nlm.nih.gov/pubmed/18519992

36. Nilsen RM, Vollset SE, Gjessing HK, Skjaerven R, Melve KK, Schreuder P, et al. Self-selection and bias in a large prospective pregnancy cohort in Norway. Paediatr Perinat Epidemiol. 2009;23:597–608. https://doi.org/10.1111/j.1365-3016.2009.01062.x.

37. Berge TL, Lygre GB, Jonsson BA, Lindh CH, Bjorkman L. Bisphenol a concentration in human saliva related to dental polymer-based fillings. Clin Oral Investig. 2017; https://doi.org/10.1007/s00784-017-2055-9.

38. Kopperud SE, Tveit AB, Opdam NJ, Espelid I. Occlusal caries management: preferences among dentists in Norway. Caries Res. 2016;50:40–7. https://doi.org/10.1159/000442796.

39. Vidnes-Kopperud S, Tveit AB, Espelid I. Changes in the treatment concept for approximal caries from 1983 to 2009 in Norway. Caries Res. 2011;45:113–20. https://doi.org/10.1159/000324810.

40. Wang NJ. Tannhelseutvikling og bruk av tannrestaureringsmaterialer. In: Bruk av tannrestaureringsmaterialer i Norge IK-2652. 98–8. Oslo: Statens helsetilsyn; 1998. p. 69–74.

41. Selevan SG, Kimmel CA, Mendola P. Identifying critical windows of exposure for children's health. Environ Health Perspect. 2000;108(Suppl 3):451–5. https://www.ncbi.nlm.nih.gov/pubmed/10852844

42. Miller MT, Ventura L, Stromland K. Thalidomide and misoprostol: ophthalmologic manifestations and associations both expected and unexpected. Birth Defects Res A Clin Mol Teratol. 2009;85:667–76. https://doi.org/10.1002/bdra.20609.

43. Rogers JM, Kavlok RJ. Developmental toxicology. In: Klaassen CD, editor. Casarett and Doull's toxicology: the basic science of poisons. 7th ed. New York: McGraw-Hill; 2008. p. 417–8.

44. Gaffield ML, Gilbert BJ, Malvitz DM, Romaguera R. Oral health during pregnancy: An analysis of information collected by the pregnancy risk assessment monitoring system. J Am Dent Assoc. 2001;132:1009–16. https://www.ncbi.nlm.nih.gov/pubmed/11480627

45. Norwegian Institute of Public Health. Research and data access from the Norwegian Mother and Child Cohort Study. 2010 [updated 11 January 2018]. https://www.fhi.no/div/datatilgang/. Accessed 19 Jan 2018.

46. Norwegian Institute of Public Health. MoBa study protocol. 2010 [updated October 2012]. https://www.fhi.no/globalassets/dokumenterfiler/moba/dokumenter/moba-protokoll-norsk-versjon-oktober-2012-pdf.pdf. Accessed 19 Jan 2018.

21

The knowledge and use of population-based methods for caries detection

Ana Luiza Sarno Castro[1]*, Maria Isabel Pereira Vianna[2] and Carlos Maurício Cardeal Mendes[3]

Abstract

Background: Since the 1980s, a wide variety of methods have been proposed to measure dental caries in the population, demonstrating a lack of consensus regarding the procedure that should be used for this purpose. The current study investigated the methods that are known and used by public oral health researchers and professors as well as the reasons that lead to the choice of a particular method.

Method: In the context of an interview, a questionnaire was administered to public oral health researchers and professors who used caries indices and worked in Salvador and Feira de Santana, Bahia, Brazil from 2005 to 2015. A quantitative and descriptive approach was applied that adopted the multiple correspondence analysis (MCA) technique to assess the associations among responses.

Results: The decayed, missing, and filled index (DMF) was the only measurement known by all respondents, and although 45 of the 47 professors/researchers were dissatisfied with this index, only six had used other methods. This index was chosen because of its comparability and ease of application. The MCA revealed response associations among older, male participants who graduated from the Federal University of Bahia (UFBA) and who continued to use this index because of its comparability and because it is the index recommended by the World Health Organization (WHO) and the Brazilian Ministry of Health (MS). Another group was also observed that consisted of younger females who graduated from the State University of Feira de Santana (UEFS) or another university and who used the DMF because it is well-known, simple, and easy to apply.

Conclusions: The DMF index was the most known and used method. Many respondents demonstrated a desire for change and were critical of the DMF; however, they did not know of and had not used newer methods for measuring dental caries. Greater importance should be placed on the problem of dental caries assessment in the population.

Keywords: Epidemiology, DMF, New indexes, Use, Knowledge, Surveys, Oral health

Background

The use of effective methods to assess caries in a population determines the quality of information obtained from epidemiological surveys, which in turn affects the diagnostic accuracy of this condition and is the basis for the planning, monitoring, and assessment of oral health prevention and disease control actions [1].

Several methods are used to measure dental caries in the population. The most widely used index is the decayed, missing, and filled (DMF) assessment described by Klein and Palmer in 1937 [2]. However, this index was created before the decrease in the incidence of caries and the advances in cariology that have occurred over the past decades that emphasises the importance of early diagnosis and early treatment for initial caries lesions. For these reasons, the DMF does not include non-cavitated enamel caries lesions among its components [3].

The use of the DMF has been questioned because of its limitations [3]. Since the 1980s, several authors have proposed different methods to assess caries lesions, such as the NYVAD System [4], the Significant Caries Index (SIC) [5], the Sound-Equivalent Teeth (T-Health) [6], the Filled and Sound Teeth (FS-T) [6], the Reversible Dental Caries Index (IRCD; *Índice Reversível de Cárie Dental*), the Caries Activity Index (IAC; *Índice de Atividade de Cárie*) [7], and many others [8–10]. Among the new methods used to assess caries in a population is the International Caries

---

* Correspondence: alscastro@yahoo.com.br
[1]Department of Health, State University of Feira de Santana, Transnordestina, s/n, Novo Horizonte, Feira de Santana, Bahia CEP 44036-900, Brazil
Full list of author information is available at the end of the article

Detection and Assessment System (ICDAS) [11] and the Caries Assessment Spectrum and Treatment (CAST) [12], which have both been internationally validated by several studies [13–15].

The number of methods proposed in recent decades demonstrates that the diagnosis of caries in a population is an important topic and that no consensus exists among researchers with regard to the most appropriate method for making a diagnosis [3]. As such, the current study aimed to identify the caries assessment systems that are known among public oral health researchers and professors, what methods they currently use, and the reasons behind their method of choice.

Methods

The present study employed an exploratory cross-sectional opinion poll with convenience sampling (Additional file 1). Through an interview, a semi-structured questionnaire was developed by the authors and administered to public oral health researchers and professors who used caries indices in Salvador and Feira de Santana, Bahia, Brazil, from 2005 to 2015.

The regions of Feira de Santana and Salvador were chosen for this study because they contain 43.8% of the dental schools in Bahia (14 of the 32 dental schools that existed in Bahia at the time of the interview) [16], and Salvador is among the 10 cities in Brazil with the most specialists registered in the Federal Council of Dentistry of Brazil [17].

Two search procedures were conducted to identify the study population: First, professors who teach public oral health at dental institutions in Salvador and Feira de Santana were identified; second, a search was performed using the PubMed, Lilacs, SciELO, and Google Scholar databases for researchers who had published articles describing their use of caries assessment methods during the stated period. Ultimately, 50 individuals met the study's eligibility criteria.

The respondents formalised their acceptance by signing informed consent documents. This study was approved by the Research Ethics Committee of the Sciences Institute of the Federal University of Bahia, under CAAE number 48500115.2.0000.5662.

Instrument pre-testing was conducted with six dental professors who were subsequently excluded from the sample. This pre-test was performed from October 10 to 15, 2015, and the interviews were conducted from October 16, 2015 to March 8, 2016. The principal researcher conducted face-to-face interviews at the universities, offices, or houses of the interviewees based on their preference. The interviews lasted an average of 20 min and were recorded and then transcribed. The data were entered into the EPIDATA program and analysed using R statistical software [18].

A quantitative and descriptive analysis was conducted. The multivariate analysis technique known as a multiple correspondence analysis (MCA) was used. This tool allows for a set of categorical variables to be assessed based on both their intensity and degree of association [19].

Results

Of the 50 individuals who were identified based on the search procedures, 47 agreed to participate. Their mean age was 46 years, with a standard deviation of 8 years. The mean time since graduation was 22 years, with a standard deviation of 8 years. Most participants were female (70.2%). Moreover, 28 individuals had graduated from UFBA (59.6%), 13 from UEFS (27.7%), and six (12.7%) from other universities (see Table 1).

Of the interviewees, 39 (83%) were public oral health professors, and 27 (57.4%) reported having performed research using caries assessment methods between 2005 and 2015. Of the individuals who were not university professors, five (10.6%) worked in the private sector (in offices), and three (6.4%) worked in the public sector (i.e., state organisations).

With regard to the specialties of the interviewees, 23 (48.9%) had postgraduate degrees in public health, three in health management (6.4%), and six (12.8%) in teaching methodology. The remaining 15 (32%) had specialties in other areas.

Table 1 The distribution of professors and researchers by their personal characteristics, academic training, and place of work

VARIABLES	Number	Percent
SEX		
Female	13	70.2
Male	14	29.8
AGE		
Between 30 and 50 years	35	75.4
Between 51 and 70 years	12	24.6
TIME SINCE GRADUATION		
Between 8 and 17 years	12	24.6
Between 18 and 47 years	35	75.4
PLACE OF GRADUATION		
UFBA	28	59.6
UEFS	13	27.7
Other universities	6	12.7
PLACE OF WORK [a]		
UEFS	19	40.4
UFBA	18	38.3
Other universities	10	21.3
Municipal or state health agency	8	17.0
Private practice	5	10.6

[a]The total number of responses is greater than the number of respondents because some respondents worked at more than one institution

Table 1 shows that most professors worked at UEFS (40.4%) or UFBA (38.3%); the other 10 respondents (21.3%) worked at six different private universities or at the State University of Bahia (UNEB).

In response to the question about the indices that they knew, all respondents reported that they knew of the DMF and DMF with other indices, whereas 25 individuals (53.19%) knew of only the DMF. In addition, 22 respondents mentioned other indices (46.81%); of these participants, 16 (34%) knew of the ICDAS, five (10.6%) recalled the T-Health and FS-T, four (8.5%) mentioned the NYVAD, three (6.4%) recalled the SIC, IRCD, and IAC, and two (4.3%) knew the CAST (see Fig. 1 and Table 2).

All of the professors taught the DMF index in their theory- (lectures) and practice-based classes. In addition to the DMF, three lectured on the ICDAS, and two addressed prevalence and incidence density measures. In practical classes, only one professor used the ICDAS, and one applied the prevalence coefficient (see Table 2).

According to Table 2, all respondents reported having had lectures and practical classes on the DMF during their degree programme. Only one respondent claimed to have learned about a different index during their programme. Most taught only the DMF in lectures (87.2%) and practical classes (94.9%).

All respondents said they had used the DMF index; of this group, 41 participants (87.2%) used only the DMF, and six used other indices (12.7%). Only the ICDAS, NYVAD, SIC, and incidence density measurements were used in practice at any time by the professionals (see Fig. 2 and Table 2).

The main reason given by respondents regarding their index of choice was the possibility of later data comparisons (66.0%), followed by the WHO and Brazilian Ministry of Health (MS) recommendations (55.3%), and

Table 2 The distribution of professors and researchers by knowledge and use of indices

VARIABLES	Number	Percent
KNOWN INDICES		
DMF and DMF with other indices	47	100.0
Only DMF	25	53.2
DMF index and other indices	22	46.8
USED INDICES		
DMF and DMF with other indices	47	100.0
Only DMF	41	87.2
DMF index and other indices	06	12.8
INDICES LEARNED IN THE DEGREE PROGRAMME		
DMF and DMF with other indices	47	100.0
Only DMF	46	97.9
DMF index and other indices	01	2.1
INDICES TAUGHT IN LECTURES		
DMF and DMF with other indices	39[a]	100.0
Only DMF	34	87.2
DMF index and other indices	05	2.8
INDICES TAUGHT IN PRACTICAL CLASSES		
DMF and DMF with other indices	39[a]	100.0
Only DMF	37	94.9
DMF index and other indices	02	5.1

[a] The total number of public oral health professors was 39 individuals

because it is the most widely known index (29.8%). Ten respondents (21.3%) cited its ease of application (see Table 3).

According to Table 3, all participants said they had used the DMF index. The most cited advantages of this index were its ease of application (40.4%), comparability

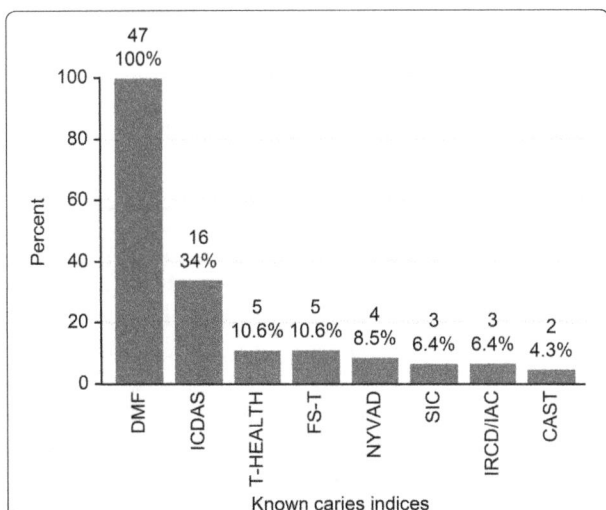

Fig. 1 Knowledge of caries detection methods among public oral health professors and researchers

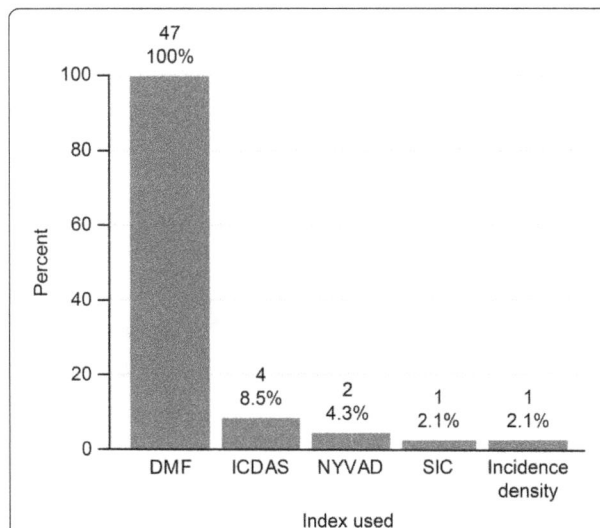

Fig. 2 Use of caries detection methods among public oral health professors and researchers

(38.3%), and the fact that it is widely known (19.1%). The most cited disadvantage of this index was that it does not allow for the detection of enamel lesions (40.4%). The second most cited disavantage was that it underestimates the prevalence of caries (19.1%), and the fact that the mean DMF value does not discriminate among decayed, missing, and filled teeth (14.9%).

As Table 3 shows, being difficult to apply (31.9%) and complex (27.7%) were the most frequently reported reasons for not using an index. Comparability (21.3%) was the second most mentioned reason to prefer an index, which was also described as the main reason for choosing one (66.0%).

Table 3 The distribution of professors and researchers by their reason for choosing an index

VARIABLES	Number	Percent
REASON FOR CHOOSING AN INDEX [a]		
Comparability	31	66.0
WHO or MS recommended	26	55.3
Very well known	14	29.8
Easy to apply	10	21.3
ADVANTAGES OF THE DMF		
Easy to apply	19	40.4
Comparability	18	38.3
Very well known	9	19.1
Others	1	2.2
DISADVANTAGES OF THE DMF		
Does not assess enamel lesions	19	40.4
Underestimates caries prevalence	9	19.2
Mean value does not discriminate components	7	14.9
Others	12	25.5
REASONS FOR NOT USING AN INDEX		
Difficult to apply	15	31.9
Complex	13	27.7
Difficult calibration	7	14.9
Time consuming	7	14.9
Others	5	10.6
REASONS FOR PREFERRING AN INDEX		
Ease of application	2	25.5
Comparability	10	21.3
More accurately evaluates caries	7	14.9
Speed	6	12.8
Others	12	25.5
WOULD USE AN INDEX OTHER THAN THE DMF		
Yes	42	89.4
No	5	10.6

[a] The total number of responses is greater than the number of respondents because some of the respondents provided more than one answer

In the sample analysed, 45 of the 47 respondents claimed to be dissatisfied with the DMF index (95.7%). Nevertheless, the DMF was the most widely used index and was known by all respondents. When criticisms of the indices were surveyed, respondents said that new indices should be used (36.2%), that these indices should overcome the limitations of the DMF (21.3%), and that the latter needs be replaced with other caries assessment methods (17%; see Table 4).

Five respondents stated that they would not use new indices; these participants were over 40 years of age. Two participants said that they were satisfied with the DMF, and three stated that they did not know other methods to measure caries and therefore would not use new indices.

According to the respondents' suggestions, the methods used to assess caries must be easy to understand (36.2%) and apply (19.1%). They believe that it is necessary to overcome the accommodation of using only the DMF (14.9%) and that enamel lesions should be included (12.8%; see Table 4).

Figure 3 displays a graphical representation of the MCA on a two-dimensional plane. This method jointly assesses how the responses are presented, without dependency relationships or prior assumptions; similar responses are presented graphically on the opposite side to dissimilar ones.

By analysing the point projections on the axes, the responses are categorised into four different groups so that the variables belonging to each group are close together and therefore associated. The groups in opposite quadrants have large distances between their projections, thereby indicating great dissimilarity among these responses.

In the upper left quadrant group, the proximity of the points indicates associations among those who graduated from UFBA; they were older (45–60 years), male, knew indices other than the DMF, recognised the disadvantages of the DMF with regard to underestimating caries but continued to use the index because of its comparability and because it is the index recommended by the World Health Organisation (WHO) and the Brazilian Ministry of Health (MS), and would not accept using an index that was complex, difficult to apply, or time consuming.

In the lower right quadrant, the variables associated form a group composed of females who graduated from UEFS or another university; they were younger (20–45), did not know indices other than the DMF, thought new research should be conducted to find new indices to assess caries, and suggested that these new indices should be simple. They used the DMF because it is widely known; however, they did not mention that this index is recommended by the WHO or MS, and their main reason for preferring an index was its ease of application.

The lower left quadrant shows a group consisting of those mentioning comparability as an advantage of the DMF and who also cited comparability as a reason for

Table 4 Distribution of professors and researchers by their suggestions and most frequent index criticisms

VARIABLES	Number	Percent
SATISFIED WITH THE DMF		
Yes	2	4.3
No	45	95.7
SUGGESTIONS		
Simple and easy to understand	17	36.2
Easy to apply	9	19.1
Overcome the accommodation of using only the DMF	7	14.9
Assesses enamel lesions	6	12.8
Others	8	17.0
CRITICISMS		
New indices should be used	17	36.2
Should overcome the DMF's limitations	10	21.3
Replace the DMF with another index	8	17.0
Research how to improve indices	7	14.9
Others	5	10.6

choosing or preferring an index. In the upper right quadrant, an association was found regarding responses indicating ease of application as an advantage of the DMF, who tended not to mention comparability as a reason to choose or prefer an index, and who did not mention comparability as an advantage of the DMF.

Discussion

According to the results presented, most people interviewed were female (70.2%), these results are in line with several studies that have shown the increasing participation of women in dental schools in Brazil [20–23].

All of the participants interviewed knew of the DMF index, but only 22 knew other caries assessment methods. Interestingly most professors taught only this index, reproducing what they had learned during their own training. Consequently, new generations of professionals will likely continue to be unaware of alternative methods.

The DMF was also the index most used by respondents, even though the vast majority of individuals surveyed claimed to be dissatisfied with it (only two people reported satisfaction). The explanation for this discrepancy lies in the reasons that led the respondents to choose an index. According to the correspondence analysis, the group who was older, male, and trained at UFBA, chose the DMF because of its comparability and

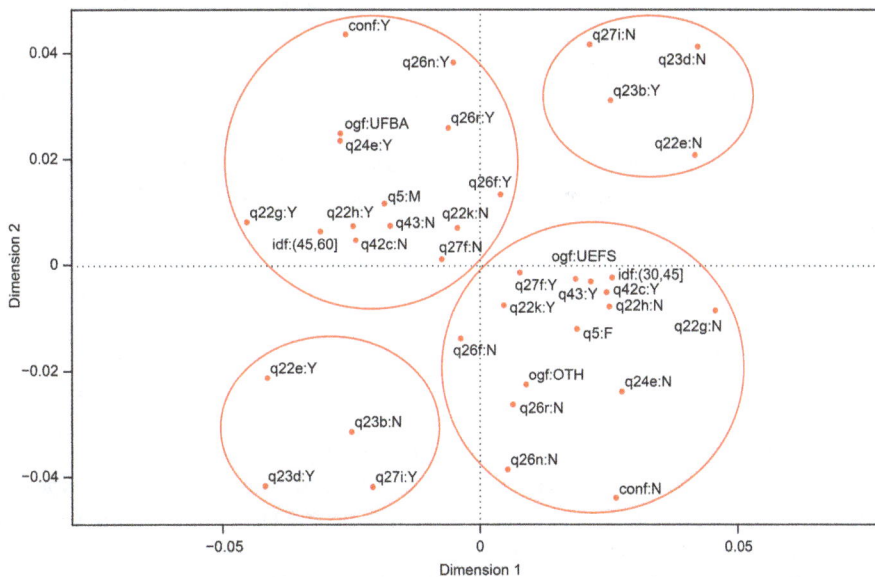

Fig. 3 The MCA of the responses of public oral health professors and researchers. legend: ogf - place of graduation, idf – age, qusof - used an index other than DMF, q5 – sex, indf - individual knows an index other than DMF, q22g - reason for choice was WHO recommendation, q22e - reason for choosing index was comparability, q22h - reason for choice was MS recommendation, q22k - reason for choosing index was it is well known, q23b - DMF's advantage is ease of application, q23d - DMF's advantage is comparability, q24a - DMF's disadvantage is not measuring enamel lesions, q24e - DMF's disadvantage is it underestimates caries, q26f - reason for not choosing index is difficult to apply, q26n - reason for not choosing index is its complexity, q26r - reason for not choosing index is it is time consuming, q27f - prefers index due to its ease of application, q27i - prefers index due to comparability, q28 - whether would use an index other than DMF, q42c - index should be simple, q43 - whether research should be conducted to find new indices, q42m - index should be easy to apply

because it was recommended by the WHO and MS. The younger female group who were trained at UEFS and other universities used the DMF because it was well known and easy to apply.

UFBA is the oldest university in the region, with a higher average age of the respondents, which may explain the greater concern to follow the norms of the WHO and MS, while the UEFS has a lower average age of those interviewed who were more concerned with the ease of application of the method.

Comparability was the most cited reason for choosing an index and the second most commonly reported advantage of the DMF. A concern with being able to later compare one's findings in an oral health survey is commendable because every well-trained researcher does so. However, this preference might be establishing a vicious cycle because only the DMF index is used. The only data available for comparison are those in this index; if other methods developed to detect caries in a population are never used, then other comparisons are not possible.

Difficulties in calibration and time consumption were the reasons mentioned not to use an index, suggesting that the use of a large-scale index depends on its simplicity. This finding is in accordance with the most frequently cited reason by the group interviewed for preferring an index (i.e., its ease of application), so the respondents are concerned about using a method that is quick and easy to apply.

Ease of application was cited as the main reason for preferring an index and the most frequently cited advantage of the DMF. However, if an index is used because it is the easiest but not because it is the best, then new methods that more accurately assessing this disease will never be developed [7]. A new method to assess caries might be more difficult to use; however, its results might be better as demonstrated by other studies [4, 24]. To assess whether a change is necessary, studies that compare indices and perform cost-benefit analyses are essential.

Most respondents would use a new method to detect dental caries. It was suggested that new indices should be simple, easy to apply, and overcome the DMF's limitations. These findings show that much of this academic community was open to accepting changes in the paradigm of how to assess caries in a population, contrary to Ismail's [3] criticism of the dental community, for being extremely conservative and slow to accept changes.

Several interviewees noted the need to use indices that assess non-cavitated enamel lesions, which is in accordance with what many authors have made this argument in the literature [3, 25]; they believe that this change is fundamental to improve the planning of health actions based on oral health surveys.

According to Pitts [26], complex and strong barriers prevent the implementation of new caries detection methods. In the present study, the potential barriers detected, in the studied group, included a lack of knowledge of new possibilities for measuring caries in a population, the prospect of being unable to compare data after using new indices, and a belief in the possibility that new indices would be more complex and difficult to apply to measure enamel lesions. It is essential to break down these barriers and use the best tools in teaching and research because it is through caries assessment methods that the presence of this disease is assessed and strategies outlined to combat it and prevent its occurrence in a population.

Using the DMF to diagnose caries lesions leads to underestimation of caries because non-cavitated enamel lesions are ignored, thereby obstructing earlier diagnoses of the disease, which might enable planning health actions more focused on dental caries prevention.

The current study revealed some of the barriers that exist regarding the implementation of new methods, indicating the necessity of a greater discussion on the subject and showing a dissatisfaction with the current methods that are often chosen for convenience because they are easy and known. Despite the local nature of this study, it can be assumed that many other regions and cities would show similar results.

Thus far, we have not found another study that has investigated the knowledge and reasons leading to the choice of caries measurement methods in the population; as such, this information is new and should stimulate reflection on this important subject. The professionals of the area should know about the advantages and disadvantages of the various methods so that they can seek better methods to measure dental caries.

According to Ismail [3], the dental community has paid little or no attention to the complex problem of caries assessment and diagnosis. However, it is necessary to change the paradigm of caries detection levels because detecting caries at an early stage, before cavitation, can have a significant effect on the population's oral health.

Conferences, panel discussions, and other activities should occur at universities and public oral health congresses to provide further discussion of the reasons for teaching and using a particular caries detection method to discuss the best way to assess caries in a population.

Study limitations

This exploratory study aimed to unveil the reasons why professionals do not use new methods to measure caries. It is a local study, and therefore, its results cannot be generalised, and inferences cannot be made because the answers might differ across other cities and countries. Studies in different places should be conducted to verify whether other reasons exist for resistance to the implementation of new indices and whether the level of knowledge of the indices differs from that found in the present study.

Conclusions

The DMF index was the best-known method and used by all respondents in teaching, research, and epidemiological caries surveys. The interviewed professionals had little knowledge of, and had seldomly used, other caries assessment methods.

Some professionals at major universities such as UFBA remain conservative because they knew of other indices but preferred to continue using the DMF because of its comparability and the fact that it is recommended by the WHO and MS. Another group composed of females who graduated from UEFS or other universities and who were younger used the DMF because it is well-known, simple, and easy to apply.

Many of the respondents demonstrated a desire for change and were critical of the DMF, although they neither knew nor used many of the current alternatives that seek to overcome the limitations of this index.

Acknowledgements
The authors thank the interviewed professors and researchers who generously donated their valuable time to be interviewed.

Authors' contributions
ALSC, CMCM, and MIPV designed the study; ALSC conducted the interviews; ALSC drafted the manuscript; and ALSC and CMCM performed the statistical analyses. All authors reviewed the original draft as well as read and approved the final manuscript.

Competing interests
The authors declare that they have no competing interests to disclose.

Author details
[1]Department of Health, State University of Feira de Santana, Transnordestina, s/n, Novo Horizonte, Feira de Santana, Bahia CEP 44036-900, Brazil.
[2]Department of Public Oral Health, School of Dentistry, Federal University of Bahia, Araújo Pinho, 62, Canela, Salvador, Bahia CEP 40110040, Brazil.
[3]Postgraduate Studies in Interactive Processes of Organs and Systems, Health Science Institute, Federal University of Bahia, Avenida Reitor Miguel Calmon, 1272, Salvador, Bahia CEP 40231300, Brazil.

References
1. Leal SC, Ribeiro APD, Frencken JE. Caries assessment Spectrum and treatment (CAST): a novel epidemiological instrument. Caries Res. 2017;51:500-6.

2. Klein H, Palmer CE, Knutson JW. Studies on dental caries: I. Dental status and dental needs of elementary school children. Public Health Rep 1896-1970. 1938:751-65.

3. Baelum F, Ole V. How big is the problem? Epidemiological features of dental caries. Dent caries dis its Clin Manegement. 3rd ed. UK: Oxfort, Wiley Blackwell; 2015. p. 21-41.

4. Nyvad B, Machiulskiene V, Baelum V. Reliability of a new caries diagnostic system differentiating between active and inactive caries lesions. Caries Res. 1999;33:252-60.

5. Bratthall D. Introducing the significant caries index together with a proposal for a new global oral health goal for 12-year-olds. Int Dent J. 2000;50:378-84.

6. Sheiham A, Maizels J, Maizels A. New composite indicators of dental health. Community Dent Health. 1987;4:407.

7. Castro ALS, Vianna MIP, de Reis SRA. A new index for measuring dental caries: a reversible index of dental caries-IRCD. Rev Fac Odontol Univ Fed Bahia. 1999;19:35-40.

8. Monse B, Heinrich-Weltzien R, Benzian H, Holmgren C, van Palenstein Helderman W. PUFA–an index of clinical consequences of untreated dental caries. Community Dent Oral Epidemiol. 2010;38:77-82.

9. Cruz RKS. Dental caries severity index: construction and validation [Internet]. Brasil; 2016 [cited 2017 Feb 9]. Available from: http://repositorio.ufrn.br:8080/jspui/bitstream/123456789/21756/1/RayanneKarinaSilvaCruz_DISSERT.pdf

10. Mount GJ, Hume WR. A revised classification of carious lesions by site and size. Quintessence Int. 1997;28:301-3.

11. Ismail AI, Sohn W, Tellez M, Amaya A, Sen A, Hasson H, et al. The international caries detection and assessment system (ICDAS): an integrated system for measuring dental caries. Community Dent Oral Epidemiol. 2007;35:170-8.

12. Frencken JE, de Amorim RG, Faber J, Leal SC. The caries assessment Spectrum and treatment (CAST) index: rational and development. Int Dent J. 2011;61:117-23.

13. Souza AL, Bronkhorst EM, Creugers NH, Leal SC, Frencken JE. The caries assessment Spectrum and treatment (CAST) instrument: its reproducibility in clinical studies. Int Dent J. 2014;64:187-94.

14. Braun A, Guiraud LMJC, Frankenberger R. Histological validation of ICDAS II and radiological assessment of occlusal carious lesions in permanent teeth. Odontology. 2017;105:46-53.

15. de Souza AL, Leal SC, Bronkhorst EM, Frencken JE. Assessing caries status according to the CAST instrument and WHO criterion in epidemiological studies. BMC Oral Health. 2014;14:119.

16. e-MEC - 2 v.3.262.0-2775 [Internet]. [cited 2017 Dec 14]. Available from: http://emec.mec.gov.br/

17. Arouca R, Pereira H, Alves L. Demographic Census of the Labor Force in Dental Specialties: Brazil, vol. 1; 2010. p. 2012.

18. R Core Team. R.: A language and environment for statistical computing. Vienna: R Foundation for Statistical Computing; 2013. URL https://www.r-project.org/

19. Hair JF, Black WC, Babin BJ, Anderson RE, Tatham RL. Multivariate data analysis (vol 6). Porto Alegre: Brazil Bookman; 2009.

20. de Melo Costa S, Prado MCM, Andrade TN, Araújo EPP, de Souza W, Junior S, et al. Profile of the professional of higher level in the teams of the family health strategy in Montes Claros, Minas Gerais, Brasil. Rev Bras Med Fam E Comunidade. 2013;8:90-6.

21. Morita MC, Haddad AE, Araújo ME. Current profile and trends of the Brazilian dental surgeon. Dental Press. 2010;

22. Baldissera R dos S, Grecca FS, dos Santos RB. The woman in dentistry: from Ohio to Rio Grande do Sul. Rev Fac Odontol Porto Alegre Porto Alegre RS; 2010. p. 27-30.

23. Vasconcellos E da CC, Brisolla SN, others. Female presence in the study and work of science at Unicamp. Cad Pagu. 2009;32:215-265.

24. Frencken JE, de Souza AL, van der Sanden WJ, Bronkhorst EM, Leal SC. The caries assessment and treatment (CAST) instrument. Community Dent Oral Epidemiol. 2013;41:e71-7.

22

The impact of anticipatory guidance on early childhood caries

Azhani Ismail[1,2], Ishak A. Razak[1,3] and Norintan Ab-Murat[1]* (ID)

Abstract

Background: This study evaluated the impact of anticipatory guidance on the caries incidence of 2–3-year-old preschool children and their 4–6-year-old siblings, as well as on their mothers' oral health literacy, as compared to the conventional Ministry of Health (MOH) programme.

Methods: This quasi-experimental study was conducted at two government dental clinics in Batu Pahat District, Malaysia. The samples comprised of 478 mother-child-sibling trios (233 families in the intervention group, and 245 families in the control group). An oral health package named the Family Dental Wellness Programme (FDWP) was designed to provide dental examinations and oral health education through anticipatory guidance technique to the intervention group at six-month intervals over 3 years. The control group received the standard MOH oral health education activities. The impact of FDWP on net caries increment, caries prevented fraction, and mother's oral health literacy was assessed after 3 years of intervention.

Results: Children and siblings in the intervention group had a significantly lower net caries increment ($0.24 \pm SD0.8$; $0.20 \pm SD0.7$) compared to the control group ($0.75 \pm SD1.2$; $0.55 \pm SD0.9$). The caries prevented fraction for FDWP was 68% for the younger siblings and 63.6% for the older children. The 2–3-year-old children in the intervention group had a significantly lower incidence of white spot lesions than their counterpart (12% vs 25%, $p < 0.05$). At three-year follow-up, there were significant increments in the oral health literacy scores of mothers in the intervention group compared to the control group.

Conclusion: The FDWP is more effective than the standard MOH programme in terms of children's and siblings' caries incidence and mother's oral health literacy.

Keywords: Anticipatory guidance, Oral health education, Early childhood caries, Oral health literacy

Background

Early Childhood Caries (ECC) is one of the most prevalent chronic childhood diseases [1, 2] and is characterized by the presence of one or more decayed (non-cavitated or cavitated), missing (because of caries), or filled tooth surfaces in any primary tooth in a child up to 6 years of age [3]. The effects of ECC extend beyond the child's individual level as their health is also influenced by family and community factors [4]. Childhood often takes place at home, and parents, being the primary role models, have a major influence on their children's oral hygiene and dietary practices. Indeed, studies have shown that oral health education (OHE) that targets parents, especially mothers, is beneficial in the prevention of ECC [5, 6]. One technique that has been suggested to increase the effectiveness of OHE is targeting the parents through anticipatory guidance. This proactive method, which is widely used in pediatric health care, is the process of providing practical, repeated rounds of developmentally appropriate health information about children to their parents, consequently maximizing parents' roles in protecting their children from oral diseases [7, 8]. It avoids the use of paternalistic approach as in the traditional OHE, but instead involves interaction with parents in developing individualized OHE strategies. The American Academy of Pediatric Dentistry (AAPD) [3] recommends that parents with young children be provided with an anticipatory

* Correspondence: norintan@um.edu.my
[1]Department of Community Oral Health and Clinical Prevention, Faculty of Dentistry, University of Malaya, 50603 Kuala Lumpur, Malaysia
Full list of author information is available at the end of the article

guidance programme that imparts information on the elimination of bottles in bed, early use of soft-bristled toothbrushes (with parental supervision), and limitation of a high-carbohydrate food intake after teeth have been brushed, with the first round scheduled within 6 months of the eruption of the first primary tooth [7, 8]. The use of this technique on first-time mothers, with information about the oral health of their infants, has been found to decrease the incidence of ECC [8].

The Ministry of Health (MOH), which is the main provider of oral health care in Malaysia, initiated the Preschool Oral Health Programme in 1984 with the aim of preventing ECC and maintaining a caries-free deciduous dentition among young children [9]. However, after more than three decades of implementing the programme, dental caries continues to be a major oral health problem among preschool children in Malaysia [10, 11]. One reason could be that the OHE given is mostly based on standard generic advice, and parental involvement is mostly ignored. This is despite the fact that interventions targeting parental empowerment towards their child's oral health have been found to be beneficial in the prevention of ECC [12]. Another possible reason is that the intervention starts very late when some of these children are already experiencing high level of caries. Children age between 1 and 3 years old is most susceptible to caries [13]; it is therefore critical that early identification of risk factors and early dental interventions are carried out to these young children to help change their trajectory of oral health [14]. A new initiative is required to achieve the MOH target of having 50% caries-free children by the year 2020 and hence the Family Dental Wellness Programme (FDWP) was initiated. This oral health package that targets both mothers and their young children, comprises of tailor-made OHE messages delivered using anticipatory guidance technique at dental clinics at six-month intervals during a three-year period. This technique which adopts a wellness and self-care concept has been reported to be effective in the developed nations, but has yet to be tested in Malaysia which has a different sociocultural setting.

The aim of this study was to evaluate the effectiveness of the FDWP in reducing the incidence of ECC in children aged 2–3 years old, and their 4–6-year-old siblings who had high risk for caries, as well as the impact to their mothers' oral health literacy. The outcome measures were net caries increment, caries prevented fraction, the incidence of white spot lesions, and mothers' oral health literacy.

Methods
Participants
The sample size of this quasi-experimental study design was estimated based on the prediction that the FDWP would be able to reduce caries prevalence in children below 6 years old by at least 27% after 3 years' implementation [15]. The only data available for caries prevalent in Batu Pahat district was on 6-year-olds children, which was 65.6% in 2012. In order to detect such a reduction at a significance level of 5% and a statistical power of 80%, and accounting for a 20% attrition rate, the minimum sample size required for the test group was 136. To overcome the cluster effect or sampling errors in selecting the control, a design effect by a factor of 1.8 was inflated to the control group. The design effect of 1.8 was assumed because of the variance in location of residences [16]. Hence, the minimum sample size required for the control group was 245.

The inclusion criteria for this study which comprised of mother-child-sibling trios were (i) children between the age of 2–3 years old, (ii) older sibling aged 4 to 6 years categorized as having high caries risk based on a Caries Risk Assessment tool adapted from the AAPD [17], and (iii) mothers who were willing to participate in the study. The older siblings were used as a proxy to depict caries trajectory of the younger children. If all risk and protective factors of caries remain the same or in other words, if no effective dental intervention was provided, the younger children will most likely develop caries experience as their older siblings when they reach preschool age. Children with medical conditions requiring special consideration as regards to their dental management and families with a high-mobility tendency were excluded from this study.

The samples for the intervention group were recruited from Batu Pahat Dental Clinic, where the FDWP was first initiated. However, the register of 2–3 year old receiving care at this clinic was very low, hence the register for preschool children (4–6 year-old) was used. A total of 1805 preschool children received dental care from this clinic. Of these, 245 children fulfilled the inclusion criteria and all were included as samples in the intervention group. The control group was recruited from preschool children under the care of a nearby dental clinic, and possible samples were matched to the 245 samples in the intervention group in terms of socio-demographic background (age, ethnicity, and family income) and other potential confounders such as family size and function. Four hundred preschool-aged children and their siblings were screened and the 245 children who fulfilled the inclusion criteria were included in the control group.

Intervention
The FDWP is an OHE package that covers the following aspects: (i) cognitive component (for example, the provision of basic oral health knowledge using an anticipatory guidance technique); (ii) psychomotor component (for example, the demonstration of basic oral health skills such as toothbrushing skills with a hands-on practical); and (iii) attitude component (activities that help to improve the children's attitude towards oral health). Children (along with their older

siblings and mothers) who participated in the FDWP were required to make six-monthly visits to the dental clinic in the three-year study period.

We created Family Dental Wellness Zones in the clinic, which consist of six different zones with different OHE activities (Table 1). This was where children and their families were given a one-hour OHE session at each visit, by either the dentists or dental therapists. At baseline, subjects and their older siblings underwent oral examination and caries risk assessment procedures, and mothers were requested to complete the oral health literacy questionnaire. They then took part in activities conducted in the Family Wellness Zones. The activities conducted at each six-monthly visit were dental examination and OHE through anticipatory guidance technique. At three-year follow-up, the final dental examination was performed again on both the children and their siblings, and the mothers completed the same questionnaire on oral health literacy again.

During the activities conducted in the aforementioned OHE zones, mothers were provided with practical, developmentally appropriate oral health information that would empower them to take the appropriate action to promote and maintain their children's oral health. The anticipatory guidance process was guided by some trigger questions and based on the answers given by the mothers, relevant advices were provided. Repeated rounds of anticipatory guidance were given at the following six-monthly visits, using different trigger questions to mothers, based on the activities that they participated in during the visits. Samples in the control group received the standard MOH programme that focuses mainly on OHE at child level.

Study instruments

At each visit, the children were examined on a dental chair using a disposable plane mouth mirror and a Community Periodontal Index probe. The oral health examination protocol followed the World Health Organization (WHO) guidelines [18]. However, some modifications were made to the WHO protocol, whereby Nyvad et al.'s

[19] caries diagnostic criteria were incorporated to assess the presence of active white spot lesions. Only the status of the deciduous teeth was recorded. The examiner (AI) and two dental therapists who were involved in clinical examinations were trained and calibrated on the dft index and white spot lesion with a gold standard, who is a dental public health specialist and a recognized benchmark examiner based at the Malaysian Ministry of Health. The overall kappa scores were 0.89, 0.85, and 0.83 respectively for the dentist and the dental therapists. During data collection, intra- and inter-examiner re-calibration was performed on 20 children aged 5 years on successive days, and the kappa score obtained was above 0.8.

Mothers' oral health literacy was assessed using the Dental Health Literacy Assessment instrument [20]. This instrument has been cross-culturally adapted for used on Malaysian population and was reported to be valid and reliable with a Cronbach alpha of 0.67 [21]. The questionnaire consists of three sections; Section 1 has 12 items that assess oral health knowledge; Section 2 consists of five questions testing mothers' ability to comprehend healthcare instructions; and Section 3 evaluates mothers' skills and motivation to care for their children's oral health (39 items). The oral health literacy scores were calculated by summing up all items in Sections 1, 2 and 3 that range from 0 to 12, 0–5, and 0–39 respectively. Thus, the total scores for oral health literacy range from 0 to 56, with the higher score indicating better oral health literacy.

Statistical analysis

Descriptive statistical analyses were performed to compare the sociodemographic characteristics of participants in both the intervention and control groups using chi square test and independent t-test, where appropriate. The mean dft, dt and ft between child and sibling group were analysed using Mann Whitney U, as the data were not normally distributed based on Kolmogorov-Smirnov test ($p < 0.05$). Comparison of net caries increment and the incidence of white spot lesion between child and sibling groups were analysed using independent-t-test. The

Table 1 Family Dental Wellness Zones and their respective oral health education activities

Zone	Activities
Zone 1	Drawing of own teeth to assess the children's knowledge of their own teeth and their associated tissues. Mothers and children were advised on the normal appearance of the child's teeth so they can identify any oral problems should they occur in the future. Mothers were also trained to diagnose white spot lesions and were advised to do home oral exams about once a month.
Zone 2	Healthy snack games to assess mothers' and children's food preferences and to advise them about the effect of sugar on oral health, the importance of reading food labels, and age-appropriate healthy meals.
Zone 3	A wide range of toothbrushes and toothpastes were displayed and children were requested to choose, and state the reasons for their choices. Mothers and children were then advised on the appropriate usage of toothbrush and toothpaste, and the benefits of fluoride
Zone 4	Mothers were asked to apply plaque-disclosing solutions to their children's teeth. A dental surgery assistant helped to explain about plaque to both mothers and children, and assisted mothers in calculating the plaque score.
Zone 5	Toothbrushing demonstrations and smiling contests amongst the samples and the younger siblings.
Zone 6	Multimedia interactive games on toothbrushing to highlight the importance of an effective brushing technique.

total mean scores for mothers' oral health literacy and the three respective domains (knowledge; comprehension; skills and motivation) were calculated based on Ludke et al.'s [20] recommendations. The mean differences of the OHL scores between groups were analysed using independent t-test as the data was normally distributed.

During dental examination, if a deciduous tooth was found to be missing at any follow-up, the score recorded during their last examination was used to denote its current status for that respective tooth. Caries prevented fraction was calculated based on the difference of the mean dft increment between the intervention and control groups over the mean increment of caries in the control groups. The mean dft increment was calculated by deducting the mean caries scores at baseline from those obtained after 3 years within the groups.

Results

A total of 233 families in the intervention group and 245 families in the control group participated in the study. The response rate was 95.1 and 100% respectively for the intervention and control group (for both children and mothers). The overall response rate was 97.6%. There were no significant differences between the intervention and control group in terms of socio-demographic variables and caries status at baseline, as the samples for both groups were matched for their individual and family profiles, as well as possible potential confounders. The proportion of boys and girls was almost equal for both children and their older siblings. The majority was of Malay ethnicity, and most of their mothers were secondary school graduates (Table 2).

The FDWP children and siblings had a significantly ($p < 0.01$) lower net caries increment (0.24, SD = 0.8; 0.20, SD = 0.7) than the control group (0.75, SD = 1.2; 0.55, SD = 0.9) at three-year follow-up (Table 3). At the end of the study period, a large proportion of the caries experience is accounted for by the filled component which is significantly higher among the 4–6 year old siblings in the FDWP group. The caries prevented fraction for FDWP was 68 and 63.6% for the younger and older siblings respectively. Children aged 2–3 years old who underwent the FDWP had

Table 2 Socio-demographic distribution at baseline for intervention and control group ($N = 478$)

Variable	Overall	Intervention	Control	p-value
	N (%)	n (%)	n (%)	
Gender of child:				
Male	215 (45.0)	103 (44.2)	112 (45.7)	0.740[a]
Female	263 (55.0)	130 (55.8)	132 (53.9)	
Age of child:				
2 years	240 (50.2)	118 (50.6)	122 (49.8)	0.853[a]
3 years	238 (49.8)	115 (49.4)	123 (50.2)	
Mean age of child*	2.5 ± 0.5	2.5 ± 0.5	2.5 ± 0.5	0.853[b]
Ethnicity of child:				
Malay	432 (90.4)	206 (88.4)	226 (92.2)	0.156[a]
Chinese	46 (9.6)	27 (10.6)	19 (7.8)	
Gender of older sibling:				
Male	237 (49.6)	111 (47.6)	126 (51.4)	0.408[a]
Female	241 (50.4)	122 (52.4)	119 (48.6)	
Age of older sibling:				
4 years	117 (24.5)	53 (22.7)	64 (26.1)	0.506[a]
5 years	155 (32.4)	81 (34.8)	74 (30.2)	
6 years	206 (43.1)	99 (42.5)	107 (43.7)	
Mean age of older sibling*	5.2 ± 0.8	5.2 ± 0.7	5.2 ± 0.8	0.765[b]
Mother's highest education:				
Never been to school	13 (2.7)	5 (2.2)	8 (3.3)	0.222[a]
Primary school	43 (9.0)	19 (8.2)	24 (9.8)	
Secondary school	295 (61.7)	138 (59.2)	157 (64.1)	
Diploma, degree and above	127 (26.6)	71 (30.5)	56 (22.8)	

[a]Chi-square test; [b]Independent t-test; significance level $p < 0.05$ *Mean and standard deviation

Table 3 Net caries increment and caries prevented fraction of 2–3-year-old children and their older siblings in control and intervention group (N = 478)

	Intervention (n = 233)			Control (n = 245)			p-value[a]	Caries prevented fraction (%)
	Baseline Mean ± SD	Follow-up	Net increment	Baseline Mean ± SD	Follow-up	Net increment		
2–3-year-old								
dft	0.94 (1.6)	1.18 (1.8)	0.24(0.8)	1.15 (1.6)	1.90 (1.9)	0.75 (1.2)	< 0.001	68.0
dt	0.76 (1.2)	0.34 (0.8)	−0.42 (0.9)	0.91 (1.4)	0.87 (1.4)	0.04 (1.2)	< 0.001	
ft	0.18 (0.6)	0.84 (1.3)	0.66 (1.1)	0.24(0.8)	1.04 (1.2)	0.79 (1.3)	0.021	
4–6-year-old								
dft	2.45 (2.1)	2.60 (3.0)	0.20 (0.7)	2.08 (2.3)	2.63 (2.4)	0.55 (0.9)	< 0.001	63.6
dt	2.07 (2.6)	0.97 (1.7)	−1.17 (1.8)	1.57 (1.8)	1.29 (1.5)	− 0.28 (1.3)	< 0.001	
ft	0.33 (0.9)	1.70 (2.0)	1.37 (1.7)	0.51 (1.1)	1.34 (1.5)	0.83 (1.2)	< 0.001	

[a]Mann-Whitney U; significance level $p < 0.05$

significantly lower incidence rates of white spot lesion (12%) than their counterpart in the control group (25%) at three-year follow-up ($p < 0.05$). However, there was not much difference in the incidence rate of white spot lesion among the older siblings in the intervention and control groups (3% versus 4%), and the result was not statistically significant (Table 4).

Table 5 shows the effect of anticipatory guidance on mothers' oral health literacy at baseline and follow-up between the two groups. There was baseline equivalence of mothers in the control and intervention group for all oral health literacy variables prior to intervention ($p > 0.001$). However, at the end of the intervention, there were significant increments of scores in the knowledge, comprehension, skills, and motivation sections, as well as the overall oral health literacy scores of mothers in the intervention group, as compared to the control group. The magnitude of change in the mean scores for the overall oral health literacy of mothers in the intervention group pre and post intervention was significantly higher (7.70 ± 0.4) than that of the control group (0.46 ± 0.5).

Discussion

This study assessed the effect of anticipatory guidance provided to mothers in the FDWP on their children's caries increment and caries prevented fraction, and their own oral health literacy. The main findings showed that

the intervention not only resulted in reduced caries increment among the younger children in the intervention group but the positive effect was also seen in the older siblings who were already diagnosed as having high caries risk. Children in the intervention group and their siblings also had a higher prevented fraction of 63.6 and 68.0% respectively than the control group at follow-up. The values of the prevented fraction in the present study are considered high compared to findings from the systematic reviews of OHE intervention aimed to reduce ECC [22], which ranged from 18 to 93%. These findings suggest that anticipatory guidance provided to mothers is beneficial in the prevention of ECC amongst their 2–3-year-old children, as well as the caries-prone older siblings in the family.

Mothers, being the primary role model in shaping children's behavior, have major influences on their children's oral habits and practices. Particularly, their education level is one of the important socioeconomic indicators that affect the incidence of ECC of their children. Highly educated mothers were reported to have higher positive attitudes and stronger intentions to control children's sugar intake, as compared to low-educated parents [23]. Hallet and Rourke [24] also proved that the prevalence and severity of ECC is linked to decreasing level of mother's education. The OHE activities provided in the Family Wellness Zones and the trigger questions and

Table 4 Incidence of white spot lesions of 2–3-year-old children and their older siblings in the control and intervention group (N = 478)

	Group	Number of new cases of white spot	Number of children at risk	Incidence of white spot lesions	Incidence rate (%)	p-value [a]
2–3 year-old children	Intervention	24	196	0.12	12	< 0.001
	Control	53	211	0.25	25	
4–6 year-old children	Intervention	5	159	0.03	3	0.621
	Control	6	166	0.04	4	

[a]Independent T-test; significance level $p < 0.05$

Table 5 Mean differences of mothers' oral health literacy scores between the intervention and control groups

Variable	Intervention Mean (SD)	Control Mean (SD)	Mean differences between group, Mean (SD)	95% CI	p-value[a]
Knowledge:					
Baseline	6.73 (1.9)	6.47 (2.1)	0.25 (0.2)	−0.11-0.62	0.167
Post-intervention	9.07 (1.6)	6.80 (2.1)	2.26 (1.7)	1.93–2.59	< 0.001
Comprehension:					
Baseline	4.27 (1.0)	4.04 (1.1)	0.23 (0.01)	0.04–0.41	0.006
Post-intervention	4.71 (0.5)	4.17 (1.0)	0.57 (0.7)	0.43–0.70	< 0.001
Skills & motivation:					
Baseline	26.13 (4.5)	26.15 (5.2)	1.94 (2.1)	−0.90- 1.86	0.968
Post-intervention	32.92 (2.5)	28.09 (4.4)	4.87 (0.3)	4.23–5.5	< 0.001
Oral health literacy:					
Baseline	37.13 (5.7)	36.67 (6.5)	0.46 (0.5)	−0.64 – 1.57	0.411
Post-intervention	46.74 (3.4)	39.05 (5.7)	7.70 (0.4)	6.85–8.55	< 0.001

[a]Independent t test; significance level $p < 0.05$

related advice given to mothers in this study have been shown to improve their knowledge, comprehension, skills, and motivation to care for their child's oral health. The knowledge and skills that they acquired may translate into their own positive oral health behaviors, which have been shown to exert a significant positive influence on children's toothbrushing habits and caries experience [25]. Although parental-related factors have been acknowledged to influence the development of ECC, studies that assessed the association of individual factors and social determinants seem to attract more attention in the ECC research areas [12]. Children's greatest social support initially comes from their family; hence it is important to empower families, especially mothers, to take control of their children's oral health.

Anticipatory guidance assists mothers or parents to anticipate any changes or potential oral health problems that may occur in relation to their children's health and oral development. The AAPD [3] advocates that anticipatory guidance be given to expectant mothers and parents of infants and young children and age-appropriate advice is provided to prevent or control oral diseases. For young children aged between 2 and 6 years old, appropriate oral health advice should include counseling sessions on oral hygiene, dietary, injury-prevention, and non-nutritive habits. In our study, we focused only on oral hygiene and dietary advice, as this information is related to caries incidence, which is our main study objective.

Recently, there have been initiatives to replicate the FDWP in other government dental clinics in Malaysia. The recently initiated FDWP can be strengthened by including anticipatory guidance initiatives that are advocated by the AAPD, as mentioned above. However, the uptake of anticipatory guidance in dental clinics globally has been lukewarm as compared to that by their medical counterparts, and the impact of this method on children's oral health has not been well studied [26]. Ramazani et al. [27] found that anticipatory guidance improved Iranian expectant mothers' knowledge about maternal, infant, and toddler's oral health. Plutzer and Spencer [8] evaluated the effect of anticipatory guidance provided to expectant mothers and found that the incidence of ECC among their children in the intervention group (1.7%) is significantly lower than in the control group (9.6%). It is not possible to compare the incidence rate of ECC among children in our study to that of the latter study, as they assessed ECC at the relatively early age of 20 months old, which could partly explain the lower incidence observed. In addition, interventions started early in that study with expectant mothers being provided with oral health information during pregnancy, which may assist them to set up proper oral health habits for their children earlier.

The strength of using anticipatory guidance is that it does away with the standard generic advice that most dentists usually offer in their clinic. Instead, this technique forces interaction between dentists and parents in obtaining the children's oral health-related development information [7], which is then used to provide oral health anticipatory advice matched to each child's characteristics. This customization of OHE has been shown to increase clients' interest and positively affect their cognitive responses to the information received [28]. Cognitive responses stimulated by tailored health messages have been shown to significantly lead to subsequent behavioral intention and actual behavior change [29]. In our intervention, the anticipatory guidance was delivered by a verbal face-to-face technique, without any printed health education take-home messages. There is some evidence that anticipatory guidance provided by a face-to-face technique has a better outcome than information given using pamphlets [27]. Most new mothers now are from the millennial generations and are users of social technology; hence, it would be interesting to assess the potential of using social media in enhancing personalized oral health communication amongst these web-savvy generations.

Although the effectiveness of the FDWP in reducing caries incidence among young children and the improvement in their mothers' oral health literacy has been proven in this study, its incorporation into the mainstream Ministry of Health programme will be strongly dependent on the political will of the Ministry. As it involved individualized strategies of intervention which is labour intensive, the cost of its application may deem to be prohibitive and may discourage its formal adoption. A possible trade off would be that this programme be restricted to high caries risk communities which would make it to be cost effective.

Several limitations restrict the interpretability of the present study. Firstly, the influence of social and mass media in the dissemination of information cannot be ignored. This may result in mothers in the control group also obtaining the oral health-related information received by mothers in the intervention group. Hence, if this influence is disregarded, the impact of the anticipatory guidance would have been more significant. Secondly, the control group was recruited from a dental clinic under the same administration of Batu Pahat Oral Health Division, which means that the clinics are in close proximity to one another. This was done to ensure that subjects in both intervention and control groups had similar socio-demographic characteristics. Hence, the occurrence of a halo effect or diffusion could exist, as mothers in the control group may have received the anticipatory guidance from mothers in the test group or they may also have visited the clinic involved in the interventions and obtained the information indirectly. Thirdly, the FDWP children and siblings had a significantly lower net caries increment than the control group at three-year follow-up with a large proportion of the caries experience being accounted for by the filled component. It cannot be discounted that both groups may be exposed to different criteria of restorative dental care. However this is unlikely as both groups come under the management of the same Senior Dental Officer in charge of the administrative district. The use of a quasi-experimental study design also limited the generalizability of the findings and reduced its internal validity. Equality of the two groups was a concern because random assignment (randomization) is absent. We tried to minimize participant differences by selecting participants as similar as possible in terms of socio-demographic and oral health status at baseline. Barring these limitations, the results of this pilot study show that anticipatory guidance provided to mothers assists in reducing the prevalence of caries of the children, and improved the mothers' oral health literacy. To ensure the FDWP remains relevant and sustainable, both dentists and dental therapists must undergo continuous training to increase and update their knowledge, to improve their oral health promotion skills, and to maintain their motivation in ensuring the success of this programme.

Conclusions

The anticipatory guidance technique used in the FDWP was effective in reducing caries incidence among young children aged six and below, and improved mothers' oral health literacy after 3 years of implementation. It is recommended that this technique is incorporated in OHE activities targeting children.

Abbreviations
AAPD: The American Academy of Pediatric Dentistry; ECC: Early childhood caries; FDWP: Family Dental Wellness Programme; MOH: Ministry of Health; OHE: Oral health education; WHO: World Health Organization

Acknowledgements
The authors would like to thank Professor Dr. Nasruddin Jaafar for his ideas and valuable input during the conception of the study.

Funding
This study obtained financial support from University of Malaya's Postgraduate by Coursework Research Fund (Vote No: NMRR-14-1680-23783). The funders had no role in the design of the study and collection, analysis, and interpretation of data and in writing the manuscript.

Authors' contributions
AI, IAR and NA made substantial contributions to the conception and design of the study. AI collected, analysed and interpreted the data and drafted the initial manuscript. IAR and NA revised the manuscript critically for important intellectual content. All authors approved the final version of the manuscript to be published.

Competing interests
The authors declare that they have no competing interests.

Author details
[1]Department of Community Oral Health and Clinical Prevention, Faculty of Dentistry, University of Malaya, 50603 Kuala Lumpur, Malaysia. [2]Klang Dental Clinic, Jalan Tengku Kelana, 41000 Klang, Selangor, Malaysia. [3]Faculty of Dentistry, MAHSA University, 42610 Bandar Saujana Putra, Selangor, Malaysia.

References

1. Colak H, Dulgergil CT, Dalli M, Mehmet MH. Early childhood caries update: a review of causes, diagnoses, and treatments. J Nat Sci Biol Med. 2013;4:29–38.
2. Isong IA, Zuckerman KE, Rao SR, Kuhlthau KA, Winickoff JP, Perrin JM. Association between parents' and children's use of oral health services. Pediatrics. 2010;125:502–8.
3. American Academy of Pediatric Dentistry. Policy on early childhood caries (ECC): classifications, consequences, and preventive strategies. Pediatr Dent. 2016;38:52–4.
4. Fisher-Owens SA, Gansky SA, Platt LJ, Weintraub JA, Soobader MJ, Bramlett DM, Newacheck PW. Influences on children's oral health: a conceptual model. Pediatrics. 2007;120:e510–20.
5. Kobayashi M, Chi D, Coldwell SE, Domoto P, Milgrom P. The effectiveness and estimated costs of the access to baby and child dentistry program in Washington state. J Am Dent Assoc. 2005;136:1257–63.
6. Medeiros PB, Otero SA, Frencken JE, Bronkhorst EM, Leal SC. Effectiveness of an oral health program for mothers and their infants. Int J Paediatr Dent. 2015;25:29–34.
7. Nowak AJ, Casamassimo PS. Using anticipatory guidance to provide early dental intervention. J Am Dent Assoc. 1995;126:1156–63.
8. Plutzer K, Spencer AJ. Efficacy of an oral health promotion intervention in the prevention of early childhood caries. Community Dent Oral Epidemiol. 2008;36:335–46.
9. Ministry of Health Malaysia. Guidelines on oral healthcare for preschool children. Oral Health Division: Ministry of Health; 2003.
10. Ministry of Health Malaysia. Dental epidemiological survey of preschool children in Malaysia. Dental Services Division: Ministry of Health; 1995.
11. Ministry of Health Malaysia. The national oral health survey of preschool children. Oral Health Division: Ministry of Health; 2005.
12. Hooley M, Skouteris H, Boganin C, Satur J, Kilpatrick N. Parental influence and the development of dental caries in children aged 0–6 years: a systematic review of the literature. J Dent. 2012;40:873–85.
13. Hiremath SS, Caries D. In: Hiremath SS, editor. Textbook of preventive and community dentistry. Elsevier: India; 2007. p. 326.
14. Vamos C, Quinonez R, Gaston A, Sinton J. Addressing early preventive oral health care among young children: a pilot evaluation of the baby oral health program (bOHP) among dental professionals. J Dent Hyg. 2014;88:202–12.
15. Wennhall I, Martensson EM, Sjunnesson I, Matsson L, Schröder U, Twetman S. Caries-preventive effect of an oral health program for preschool children in a low socio-economic, multicultural area in Sweden: results after one year. Acta Odontol Scand. 2005;63:163–7.
16. Yudkin PL, Moher M. Putting theory into practice: a cluster randomized trial with a small number of clusters. Stat Med. 2001;20:341–9.
17. American Academy of Pediatric Dentistry. Guideline on caries-risk assessment and management for infants, children, and adolescents. Pediatr Dent. 2016;38:142–9.
18. World Health Organization. Oral health surveys: basic methods. 5th ed. Geneva: World Health Organization; 2005. p. 42–7.
19. Nyvad B, Machiulskiene V, Baelum V. Reliability of a new caries diagnostic system differentiating between active and inactive caries lesions. Caries Res. 1999;33:252–60.
20. Ludke RL, Kudel I, Weber DL. Dental health literacy assessment instrument. In: University of Cincinnati; 2008.
21. Ismail, A. The impact of family dental wellness on early childhood caries in Batu Pahat district. [dissertation]: University of Malaya; 2016.
22. Twetman S, Dhar V. Evidence of effectiveness of current therapies to prevent and treat early childhood caries. Pediatr Dent. 2015;37:246–53.
23. Astrom AN, Kiwanuka SN. Examining intention to control preschool children's sugar snacking: a study of carers in Uganda. Int J Paediatr Dent. 2006;16:10–8.
24. Hallet KB, O'Rourke PK. Social and behavioural determinants of early childhood caries. Aust Dent J. 2003;48:27–33.
25. Saied-Moallemi Z, Virtanen JI, Ghofranipour F, Murtomaa H. Influence of mothers' oral health knowledge and attitudes on their children's dental health. Eur arch Paediatr Dent. 2008;9:79–83.
26. Pendrys DG. An anticipatory guidance program may help prevent severe early childhood caries, but more research is needed. J Evid Based Dent Pract. 2011;11:43–5.
27. Ramazani N, Zareban I, Ahmadi R, ZadSirjan S, Daryaeian M. Effect of anticipatory guidance presentation methods on the knowledge and attitude of pregnant women relative to maternal, infant and Toddler's oral health care. J Dent (Tehran). 2014;11:22–30.
28. Stellefson ML, Hanik BW, Chaney BH, Chaney DJ. Challenges for tailored messaging in health education. J Health Educ. 2008;39:303–11.
29. Kreuter MW, Bull FC, Clark EM, Oswald DL. Understanding how people process health information: a comparison of tailored and nontailored weight-loss materials. Health Psychol. 1999;18:487–94.

23

Association between sickle cell disease and the oral health condition of children and adolescents

Carla Figueiredo Brandão[*], Viviane Maia Barreto Oliveira, Ada Rocha Ramony Martins Santos, Taísa Midlej Martins da Silva, Verônica Queiroz Cruz Vilella, Gleice Glenda Prata Pimentel Simas, Laura Regina Santos Carvalho, Raissa Aires Costa Carvalho and Ana Marice Teixeira Ladeia

Abstract

Background: Sickle cell disease (SCD) is the most prevalent monogenic hereditary pathology associated with the presence of hemoglobin SS in the world. It can affect individuals, leading to changes in the face and body, causing a deficiency in dental and bone tissue formation that can ultimately result in a higher level of predisposition to developing dental caries. This study aimed to evaluate the oral condition of children and adolescents with SCD in comparison with the condition of healthy controls.

Methods: This was a cross-sectional study of children and adolescents aged 5 to 18 of both sexes from a hematology center in Bahia, Brazil, and subjects without hemoglobinopathies from a public school of the same state (comparison group). There were 124 individuals, 63 in the comparison group and 61 in the disease group. Interviews, dental and periodontal exams using the DMFT and Periodontal Community Index, respectively, were performed, and the salivary buffer capacity and salivary flow rates of the entire sample population were evaluated. The categorical variables were compared using a chi-square test or Fisher's exact test. For comparison of means, the Student's-t test was used for independent samples that presented symmetrical distribution.

Results: The study showed that the DMFT was 2.08 (2.71) for the SCD group and 1.05 (1.67) for the comparison group ($p = 0.013$). For dmft, the values were 2.3 (2.6) and 0.88 (1.2), respectively, ($p = 0.018$). Exams of the periodontium showed the presence of gingival bleeding and dental calculus, with no statistical significance between groups ($p = 0.984$). When evaluating salivary flow and buffer capacity, no significant differences were observed for the flow rates ($p = 0.485$), but the SCD group presented a lower buffer capacity compared with the comparison group ($p = 0.006$). Individuals who used hydroxyurea had a dmft (2.50) higher than that of the comparison group (2.00), and salivary flow was lower than the normal rate in 70% of the children who did not use this medication.

Conclusion: Children and teenagers with SCD had deficient oral health when compared with the comparison group, presenting a higher level of dental caries and lower buffer capacity.

Keywords: Sickle cell disease, Child, Oral health, Dental caries, Periodontal disease, Saliva

* Correspondence: cfbrandao@hotmail.com
Bahiana School of Medicine and Public Health, Avenida Dom João VI, no. 275, Brotas. ZIP: 40.290-000, Salvador, Bahia, Brazil

Background

Sickle cell disease (SCD) is caused by a mutant Hb S hemoglobin that modifies a normally shaped cell shape into a sickle shape. This mutant cell defines a group of hemoglobinopathies, at least one of which is Hb S hemoglobin. The most frequent SCD variations are sickle cell anemia (or Hb SS), S beta thalassemia and the heterozygous Hb SC and Hb SD [1].

SCD is a multisystemic disease associated with acute illness and progressive organic damage, leading to organ involvement, which may cause changes in development or functioning. Individuals with this pathology may also present changes in their face, mouth, and teeth caused by the deficient formation of dental and bone tissues [2–4], which may, for example, lead to a higher level of predisposition for developing caries diseases [5–7].

The first study of the prevalence of dental caries in patients with SCD was conducted by Okafor et al. in 1986, who observed a higher prevalence in subjects without SCD (54%) compared with those who had the disease (35.13%) [8]. Since then, some studies have been conducted to verify the association between sickle disease and dental caries, with divergent results [5–7, 9–11]. In the literature, few studies are found that associate the presence of dental caries with salivary flow rates and buffer capacity in sickle cell patients [12]; these are essential factors in the development of caries disease [5–7].

These patients also have a higher risk of developing dental caries due to the high prevalence of opacities in the teeth (alterations in enamel and dentin formation and calcification) [2, 8], frequently used medications containing sucrose and many episodes of hospitalization that make it difficult to perform adequate oral hygiene [13].

Another aspect to be studied is the presence of periodontal problems in sickle cell patients, as these patients are more susceptible to infections. Individuals with SCD have a higher level of predisposition to developing periodontal disease due to the presence of these pathogens in the mouth, as well as alterations in their cellular and humoral immune response [14, 15].

From the knowledge of how these diseases manifest, health promotion measures can be adopted and target treatments instituted for this group of patients, respecting their individualities.

This study aimed to evaluate the oral condition of children and teenagers diagnosed with SCD compared with healthy controls and to assess the influence of salivary flow and buffer capacity on predicting oral health.

Methods

This was a descriptive and analytical cross-sectional study conducted with children and teenagers aged 5 to 18 of both sexes, from the Hematology and Hemotherapy Foundation in Bahia (HEMOBA), who formed the sickle cell disease group. They were compared with subjects without hemoglobinopathies, selected from among children enrolled in the State School Francisco da Conceição Menezes (comparison group). To be selected for the SCD group, the following inclusion criteria were to be met: Participants had to have SCD and Hb S diagnosed by Hb electrophoresis and/or high-performance liquid chromatography. For the comparison group, individuals had to be in the same age group, not have SCD and be clinically healthy. In both groups, participants were not to be undergoing orthodontic treatment. This research was approved by the Research Ethics Committee of the Bahiana School of Medicine and Public Health and is referenced as 54.637.816.7.0000.5544. The participants' signature of the term of informed consent/assent ensured the possibility of conducting the study.

Our sample was calculated by estimating that the prevalence of oral disorders in the general population would be 50%; expecting to find a detectable difference of 20% in the prevalence of the group with SCD for a value of $\alpha = 0.05$, a minimum of 48 individuals in each group was necessary.

Data collection

In this research, the dental data were collected in accordance with the methodology used by the SB Brasil Project Field Team 2010 and recommended by the World Health Organization (WHO) [16]. Data consisted of records of the teeth, obtained by using mean dmft indexes for deciduous dentition and DMFT for permanent dentition, and reported as the sum of decayed, missing and filled teeth [17].

The Periodontal Community Index (CPI), an instrument used by the SB Brasil 2010 Project, was used to examine the periodontium according to the field team manual [17], which allowed evaluation of periodontal health relative to hygiene, gingival bleeding and the presence of calculus in children over 12 years of age. In each sextant of the mouth - 16, 11, 26, 36, 31 and 46, six teeth were examined on each of the buccal and lingual surfaces, covering the mesial, middle and distal regions.

When there was no index tooth, the sextant was canceled [17]. This evaluation was performed only in patients older than 12 years; this is an international standard for assessing the conditions of tooth injuries, since it is the youngest age at which the individual has the complete permanent dentition, disregarding eruption of the third molar [18].

Subjects under 18 years of age were not treated; thus, the presence of a periodontal pocket was not investigated since soft tissue alterations could be associated with the eruption of a tooth and not with the presence of pathological periodontal changes [17].

A clinical file was adapted from epidemiological studies conducted by the WHO [16], in the fourth edition of oral health surveys. These basic methods guided the data necessary for characterization of the sample, which were recorded individually among participants and included name, age, and sex. The following information was added: skin color (self-reported), schooling, family income, time of diagnosis of the disease, use of medications, daily oral hygiene and regularity of attendance at dental appointments (provided by the dentist), as well as saliva conditions.

The calibration exercise was carried out in two steps. In the first step, a single investigator conducted theoretical training for recognition of the different oral health conditions according to the SB Brasil 2010 Field Team Manual and to standardize the oral exams and the diagnostic criteria [17]. The next step consisted of the examination of 12 children and adolescents. The exams were performed on two separate occasions with a 4-month interval between sessions. Data analysis involved the calculation of Kappa coefficients for the evaluation of intra-observer agreement. (Kappa = 0.71).

During the examination, the child was seated in a chair, under natural light, and the examiner used a flat mouth mirror, a CPI probe for the oral epidemiological examination, gauze and a wooden spatula [17].

To determine the salivary flow rate and assess the amount of saliva produced by the child in 1 min, a piece of paraffin (Parafilm ®), a 25 mL graduated beaker, a funnel and a stopwatch were used. First, the paraffin was left in the patient's mouth for 1 min; the patient was asked to swallow the accumulated saliva during that period; then Parafilm® was chewed for 5 min [19, 20]. After this, the saliva produced was collected through a funnel into a beaker from the time the stopwatch was started, and the salivary flow was measured directly by reading the total volume of stimulated saliva obtained in the time determined. The final result was expressed in milliliters of stimulated saliva produced per minute (mL/min). The results were interpreted by the amount of saliva produced: normal (above 1.0 mL/min), low (0.7 to 1.0 mL/min), very low (0.1 to 0.7 mL/min), xerostomia (below 0.1 mL min) and hypersalivation (above 2.00 mL/min) [19].

For the buffer capacity, 1.0 mL of the saliva collected from each child was added to 3.0 mL of 0.005% HCl solution. After stirring the tube and waiting for 10 min, this mixture was taken for pH reading in the digital potentiometer DMPH-2, which was previously calibrated using pH 4.0 and 7.0. The buffer capacity was expressed by the potentiometer reading of the final pH of the saliva-acid mixture and evaluated as normal (above 6.0), reduced (5.5) and low (below 4. 0) [19].

Statistical analysis

Statistical analysis was then performed with the descriptive measures. Quantitative variables were represented by their means and standard deviations. Categorical variables were expressed by frequencies and percentages. For comparison of the categorical variables, the Chi-square test was used through bivariate analysis. The Student's t-test for independent samples was used to compare the means. The Statistical Package for the Social Sciences (SPSS Inc., Chicago, IL, United States of America), version 21.0 was used.

Results

A total of 124 children and teenagers were examined, of whom 61 had SCD and 63 were healthy. Their distribution by age, sex, race (self-reported), educational level of the child and mother, as well as family income are described in Table 1, and no difference was observed between groups.

DMFT and dmft data are described in Tables 2 and 3. These indexes were higher for the SCD group than for the comparison group and were statistically significant. The decayed component was found to be more predominant in the permanent and deciduous dentition of the SCD group.

There was no association between SCD and caries disease in this study. Decayed teeth were found in 36 subjects of the SCD group (59%) and in 30 subjects (49.2%) of the comparison group ($p = 0.276$).

The results of the periodontal examination were classified according to their degree of involvement, but no difference was observed between the groups (Table 4).

As regards the salivary examination, the results are described in Table 5. In the majority of the sample, the buffer capacity of saliva was evaluated as being normal. In the SCD group, 83.1% of its subjects had normal salivary pH and 17% had reduced pH. On the other hand, in the comparison group, 98.2% of the participants had a pH within the normal range. Statistically significant differences were found between groups when assessing reduced buffer capacity ($p = 0.006$).

The salivary flow presented no significant difference between the groups since the distribution between them was similar ($p = 0.485$).

A relationship was found between DMFT and buffer capacity in patients with SCD, and there was a significant difference between the groups in the decayed component and DMFT; however, this value was higher in participants in the SCD group who had normal buffer capacity (Table 6).

Table 7 shows the results for individuals with SCD in regard to use of hydroxyurea; 33 (54.1%) of these patients took this medication, and 28 (45.9%) patients

Table 1 Socio-demographic characteristics of the sample

	SCD Group (n = 61)	Comparison Group (n = 63)	p value
Age (years) mean ± SD	12.4(2.9)	11.1 (2.9)	0.014*
Age Range			0.119**
5 to 8 years	6 (9.8)	11 (17.5)	
9 to 12 years	24 (39.3)	31 (49.2)	
13 to 18 years	31 (50.8)	21 (33.3)	
Sex			0.605**
Male	34 (55.7)	38 (60.3)	
Female	27(44.3)	25 (39.7)	
Race			0.066**
Black	18 (29.5)	26 (41.3)	
Mixed	42 (69.9)	32 (50.8)	
Others	1 (1.6)	5 (8)	
Educational Level	(n = 60)	(n = 61)	0.114**
Illiterate	4 (6.7)	3 (4.9)	
Middle school	48 (80.0)	56 (91.8)	
High school	8 (13.3)	2 (3.3)	
Maternal Education	(n = 56)	(n = 56)	0.902**
Illiterate	2 (3.6)	1 (1.8)	
Middle school	28 (50.0)	31 (55.4)	
High school	23 (41.1)	21 (37.5)	
University	3 (5.4)	3 (5.4)	
Income	(n = 57)	(n = 55)	0.081**
No income	8 (14.0)	3 (5.5)	
Up to 1 monthly Brazilian minimum wage	40 (70.2)	35 (63.6)	
Above 2 monthly Brazilian minimum wages	9 (15.8)	17 (30.9)	

* Independent t-test; ** Chi-square test; m = average; SD = standard deviation. Brazilian minimum wage = US$300.00. *p* < 0.05

did not. When assessing the association between DMFT and hydroxyurea, individuals who did not use the medication were observed to have a higher DMFT value. However, in deciduous dentition, dmft values were higher for those who had taken the medication, and the number of filled teeth was also higher, but there was a significant difference (Table 8).

Table 9 presents the findings of salivary conditions in individuals who did and did not use hydroxyurea. The salivary flow was lower than the normal rate in 75% of children and adolescents who used the medication. The buffer capacity was reduced in 18.2% of the medication users.

Discussion

SCD is a disease that has been widely discussed in several ways that are important for understanding it. This recessive and hereditary disease was discovered in African black people; however, today it affects individuals with other racial characteristics because of intermarriage [21]. In this study, there was a higher prevalence of brown individuals, although Bahia is a state with one of largest black populations in Brazil and an extensive mixture of races.

The consequences of SCD to the human body have been explored from multiple aspects. Among these observations, there has been rising concern about its manifestations in some parts of the oral cavity, which causes alterations in different tissues that form teeth and bones, in spite of these manifestations not being pathognomonic signs of the disease [3, 4, 9, 22, 23].

Caries disease is a globally studied pathology; its emergence and development are related to intrinsic factors associated with socioeconomic, cultural and educational aspects that are demonstrated by the degree of impairment of the oral health of the affected population [9, 24, 25]. In this study, all of the abovementioned factors were constantly present in all the subjects; therefore, these could not be considered potential confounding biases.

No association of caries disease with SCD was observed in this study because the presence of decayed teeth was verified in 59% of the individuals in the SCD group, and in 49.2% of the comparison group; that is, there was a difference of 10% between them. The data in this research corroborated the findings of the study by Passos et al. [10], who assessed 190 patients of African descent, with and without SCD; these patients had a mean age of 30, which was higher than in our study (11.7 years). Luna et al. [26] found a prevalence of 47% of caries in 250 children and adolescents with SCD, a lower value than that found in this study.

Table 2 Means of DMFT values of children and adolescents

	SCD Group (n = 61)	Comparison Group (n = 63)	p value
Dental Condition	mean ± SD	mean ± SD	
Decayed	1.5 ± 2.38	0.8 ± 1.23	0.003*
Missing	0.8 ± 0.33	0.98 ± 0.3	0.620*
Filled	0.5 ± 1.0	0.24 ± 0.7	0.004*
DMFT	2. ± 2.7	1.1 ± 1.7	0.013*

*Independent t-test; SD = standard deviation. DMFT - mean of the components D (decayed), M (missing or extracted due to caries) and F (filled or restored) permanent dentition. *p* < 0.05

Table 3 Means of dmft values in children assessed

Dental Condition	SCD Group (n = 23)	Comparison Group (n = 24)	p value
	mean ± DP	mean ± DP	
Decayed	1.3 ± 1.8	0.7 ± 1.12	0.039*
Missing/Extracted	0.65 ± 1.23	0.12 ± 0.34	0.000*
Filled	0.35 ± 0.8	0.2 ± 0.6	0.222*
dmft	2.3 ± 2.6	0.88 ± 1.2	0.018*

*Independent t-test; SD = standard deviation. Dmft - Mean of the components d (decayed), and m (extracted) and f (filled or restored) deciduous dentition. p < 0,05

Nevertheless, some studies have found this association when evaluating different age groups. Luna et al. [9] evaluated 160 children with SCD aged 3 to 12 years of age in Recife and found a higher frequency of dental caries in children with SCD. Similarly, Laurence et al. [5] conducted a retrospective cohort study in Baltimore and Washington with 102 individuals over 18 years, with and without SCD. They also found an association when they assessed the presence of caries disease and socioeconomic factors; they verified that individuals with SCD coming from lower-income families had a greater tendency towards caries disease because they had less access to treatment.

Furthermore, in this study, the DMFT and dmft values found were 2.1 and 2.30, respectively, for individuals with SCD and 1.1 and 0.88 for the comparison group. This result was close to the values in the study by Luna et al. [9] that evaluated only children with SCD and found a DMFT of 1.5 and dmft of 2.2, mainly for deciduous teeth. Furthermore, Fernandes et al. [7] analyzed 56 children and 50 adolescents with SCD and 205 children and 180 adolescents in a control group, both aged 8 to 14, at a hematology center in Minas Gerais, Brazil. In this case, the DMFT value was 1.3 in the SCD group and 1.8 in the control group. For patients with SCD, in general, the condition of their oral health was better.

In our study, in spite of the SCD subjects having worse oral health conditions, the observed results agreed with the SB Brasil 2010 [27] data, which found dmft = 2.43 and DMFT = 2.07.

In a similar manner, Ralstrom et al. [11] evaluated 54 American adolescents of African descent with a mean age of 14 years, who had the Hb SS and Hb SC sickle cell genotypes. The mean DMFT found was 1.94 in the disease group and 2.96 in the control group. There was no significant difference in the frequency values for dental caries between the SCD adolescents and controls, potentially due to high exposure to the fluoride present in the water supply in that region. The data found were similar to those of the present study relative to individuals with SCD. It is worth noting that in Brazil there are public health policies that regulate the fluoridation of the water supply; this is an important measure for the prevention of caries disease [28].

In the study conducted by Singh et al. [6] in India, with 750 patients with SCD and Betalassemia, aged 3 to 15 years, a DMFT of 6.59 was observed for patients with the disease. This value differs from our findings and those of other studies, probably due to different health policies in the regions concerned, possibly making treatment less accessible.

Costa et al. [29], when evaluating the care offered to patients with SCD in Maranhão, Brazil, found that children had fewer filled teeth than did adults and that there was also an increase in number of filled teeth as age increased. Dental treatments were probably due to the lack of specific oral health programs for this population. These patients often present severe systemic health problems that can place their lives at risk. Their oral health care is neglected, and they are denied access to preventive care; thus, only curative treatment programs are available to them [6, 29]. These factors were probably responsible for the increase in caries in the population of this study.

Table 4 Mean and percentage values of individuals according to their periodontal condition

Periodontal Condition	SCD Group (n = 35)	Comparison Group (n = 37)	p value
	n (%)	n (%)	0.984**
Healthy periodontium	1 (2.9)	1 (2.7)	
Gingival bleeding	12 (34.3)	12 (32.4)	
Dental calculus	22 (62.9)	24 (64.9)	

** Chi-square test. p < 0.05

Table 5 Sample distribution according to salivary conditions

	SCD Group n = 59 (%)	Comparison Group n = 55(%)	p value
Salivary Flow			0.485**
Hyposalivation (0.1 to 0.7 mL/min)	19 (32.2)	18 (32.7)	
Low (0.70 to 1.0 mL/min)	17 (28.8)	13 (23.6)	
Normal (> 1.0 mL/min)	23 (39.0)	22 (40.0)	
Hypersalivation (> 2.0 mL/min)	0	2 (3.6)	
Buffer Capacity			0.006**
Normal (pH > 6.0)	49 (83.1)	54 (98.2)	
Reduced (below 5.5)	10 (16.9)	1 (1.8)	

** Chi-square test. $p < 0.05$

The presence of caries disease, a lack of attention to the need, and a worsening of the condition lead to the need for more complex treatments. This need is not only limited to the population studied but also affects the general population with similar socio-demographic characteristics, as was reflected in the data of SB Brasil 2010 [6, 11, 27].

With regard to the periodontal condition, the presence of SCD did not change its oral manifestation. Individuals aged 12 years and older presented a similar situation with the presence of gingival bleeding, and the majority of them had dental calculus. Passos et al. [10] also found no association between sickle cell disease and periodontal disease when evaluating 190 patients, 99 with systemic alteration and 91 controls. Fernandes et al. [7] found that only the adolescents showed the presence of gingival bleeding, but no significant differences were observed between the SCD and control groups. Carvalho et al. [30] evaluated several criteria indicative of periodontal diseases in patients with SCD, patients with the trait of the disease and patients without the disease. They observed that none of these criteria were associated with the patients with SCD, suggesting no association between these two pathologies.

Mahmoud, Ghandour and Atalla [31] evaluated the association between periodontal disease and SCD in 113

Table 6 Comparison of the mean DMFT with the buffer capacity of children and adolescents with SCD

	Normal (n = 49)	Reduced (n = 10)	p value
Dental Condition	mean ± SD	mean ± SD	
Decayed	1.5 ± 1.99	0.5 ± 0.84	0.014*
Missing	0.8 ± 0.33	0.10 ± 0.3	0.877*
Filled	0.6 ± 1.2	0.20 ± 0.42	0.063*
DMFT	2.20 ± 2.4	0.6 ± 1.0	0.002*

* Independent t-test; SD = standard deviation. $p < 0.05$

adolescents aged 12 to 16 and found no statistically significant differences between the groups; but when evaluating the disease group, they were able to verify an increase in the prevalence of gingival inflammation in adolescents with SCD when compared with the control group. Tonguç, Unal and Aspaci [32] also verified a lack of differences in the periodontal health status of 49 children with SCD and 39 systemically healthy children in the control groups. The most important finding of their study was that gingival enlargement was more prevalent in children with SCD. Singh et al. [6], in their study, observed a higher prevalence of periodontal disease in patients with beta thalassemia, followed by those with SCD, and, last, the controls.

Salivary flow is an essential and reliable measure to evaluate pathological alterations [33–35]. Reduced salivary flow may cause greater vulnerability to caries disease and oral infections and to changes in chewing, swallowing, tasting and speaking [36]. When the saliva is stimulated, it may promote positive actions in the oral cavity, such as potentiation of tooth remineralization capacity, removal of substances, neutralization of acids and antimicrobial action [37].

Studies have shown a positive correlation between salivary flow and the buffer capacity of saliva [21, 38]. Few articles were found on the topic of salivary parameters in children and adolescents with SCD. In our study, the observed salivary flow was lower in 61% of sickle cell patients and in 56.3% of patients the comparison group.

Leone et al. [14] carried out a systematic review of 600 articles in the MEDLINE and EMBASE databases on salivary aspects as indicators of caries disease risk and concluded that the salivary buffer capacity presented a weak-to-moderate association with the risk of developing the disease, unlike the flow that showed a strong correlation with its appearance. This study showed a prevalence of 17% for reduced buffer capacity in the SCD group. A decrease in salivary flow was found in both groups, suggesting that the association of these factors may lead to higher predisposition for the development of dental caries. Furthermore, the SCD group had a higher risk of developing caries.

It is interesting to notice that in our study, among individuals with SCD, those with normal saliva buffer capacity had higher DMFT values than those with reduced buffer capacity; this difference was specifically observed relative to the number of decayed teeth. Buffer capacity and salivary flow alone cannot be used as determinant indexes for diagnosis of caries disease since other factors need to be considered to determine the potential of cariogenic activity. Bacterial biofilms, deficient oral hygiene, systemic diseases, previous and/or current use of a fluoridated water supply, the frequency of sugar ingestion and microorganism counts contribute to dental

Table 7 Comparison of the mean DMFT values of children and adolescents with Hb SS relative to the use of hydroxyurea

	Users of Hydroxyurea(n = 33)	Non users of Hydroxyurea(n = 28)	p value
Dental Condition	mean ± SD	mean ± SD	
Decayed	1.12 ± 1.78	1.96 ± 2.91	*0.122
Missing	0.90 ± 0.29	0.07 0.37	*0.718
Filled	0.45 ± 0.90	0.60 ± 1.28	*0.121
DMFT	1.64 ± 2.11	2.61 ± 3.23	*0.024

* Independent T-test; SD = standard deviation. $p < 0.05$

caries development [1, 2, 5, 8–12]. The continuous use of medications may cause xerostomia and thus increase the risk of caries disease development, as they lead to a decrease in salivary flow and cause changes in saliva [36].

Hydroxyurea, which is approved by the US Food and Drug Administration (FDA), is a drug currently used in the treatment of Hb SS [39]. This drug has a strong positive impact on the quality of life of SCD patients by reducing many negative aspects of the disease including vaso-occlusive crises, the need for transfusions, the number of hospitalizations, the length of hospital stays, and acute neurological events; in addition, it has decisively demonstrated a reduction in the number of deaths resulting from neurological events or SCD when compared with the same number of patients in a group not using the drug. [40]

Salvia et al. [41] assessed 69 patients with a mean age of 26 years who had SCD. Among these patients, there were users and non-users of hydroxyurea. When evaluating salivary flow and DMFT, these authors verified that DMFT was higher in patients taking the medication (9.10 ± 6.93) than in those who did not or in the respective controls (7.67 ± 6.06; 7.72 ± 5.91; 7.59 ± 7.14). All groups presented normal salivary flow, ranging from 1.21 ± 0.88 to 1.33 ± 0.73. In our study, 32 individuals used hydroxyurea, and the DMFT and dmft results were lower for children and adolescents using the medication (1.64 ± 2.11; 2.0 ± 2.95). When evaluating the saliva, 75% of those taking the medication had low salivary flow and

18% had reduced buffer capacity. This divergence in results may be related to differences in the methodology.

No other studies about hydroxyurea and its effects on the oral cavity were found in the researched literature, but this study showed that the use of the medication changed the salivary flow and buffer capacity of saliva, which predisposed patients to the development of oral pathologies.

Another aspect that should be discussed in this study was that both groups evaluated were mostly treated mostly in the Sistema Único de Saúde – SUS, a public health care program that offers patients basic care without adopting an effective health promotion plan. At this health center, patients with SCD are offered routine medical appointments, administration of medications, transfusions, and referrals for hospitalization in the most severe cases. However, due to the lack of specialized care in the different areas of dentistry, such as pediatric dentistry, endodontics, prosthesis, periodontics and orthodontics, the patients who demand/require these specific treatments are not always given the appropriate attention.

In Brazil and in other countries it has been observed that in the most severe cases of the disease, the patients who are most affected systemically require hospitalizations for transfusions and treatments. These patients require primary oral health care, such as daily tooth brushing after main meals and careful selection of the type of diet consumed, both of which may lead to a lower level of predisposition for developing oral diseases [5, 8, 10].

There were some limitations to this study. The examiner was not blinded to the dental examination and, therefore, could have introduced examiner's bias. However, this aspect was calibrated for in the field data collection phase, and the clinical criteria were clearly defined; thus, this bias is unlikely to have distorted the data from the exams. A few of the more severely ill SCD patients were unwilling to participate because of the discomfort caused by their disease symptoms. Perhaps this could have minimized the differences between the groups.

Table 8 Comparison of the mean dmft values of children and adolescents with Hb SS relative to the use of hydroxyurea

	Users of Hydroxyurea (n = 14)	Non-users of Hydroxyurea (n = 9)	p value
Dental Condition	m ± SD	m ± SD	
Decayed	1.35 ± 1.94	1.22 ± 1.71	*0.913
Extracted	0.64 ± 1.39	0.66 ± 1.00	*0.934
Filled	0.50 ± 0.94	0.11 ± 0.33	*0.021
dmft	2.50 ± 2.95	2.00 ± 1.93	*0.149

* Independent t-test; SD = standard deviation. $p < 0.05$

Table 9 Sample distribution according to salivary conditions and hydroxyurea

	Users of Hydroxyurea ($n = 33$)	Non users of Hydroxyurea ($n = 26$)	p value
Salivary Flow			0.032**
Hyposalivation (0.1 to 0.7 mL/min)	13 (39.4)	6 (23.1)	
Low (0.7 to 1.0 mL/min)	12 (36.4)	5 (19.2)	
Normal (> 1.0 mL/min)	8 (24.2)	15 (57.7)	
Hypersalivation (> 2.0 mL/min)	0	0	
Buffer Capacity			0.776**
Normal (pH > 6.0)	27 (81.8)	22 (84.6)	
Reduced (below 5.5)	6 (18.2)	4 (15.4)	

** Chi-square test. $p < 0.05$

Conclusion

The children and adolescents with SCD had unfavorable oral conditions when compared with healthy patients, presenting higher dental caries indexes in both deciduous and permanent dentition and lower buffer capacity values. These results suggested that these individuals needed better and continuous oral health care integrated with the clinical aspects of their systemic health.

Abbreviations

CPI: Periodontal Community Index; dmft: mean of the components d (decayed), and m (extracted) and f (filled or restored) deciduous dentition; DMFT: mean of the components D (decayed), M (missing or extracted due to caries) and F (filled or restored) permanent dentition; DNA: deoxyribonucleic acid; Hb SC: Genotype hemoglobin SC; Hb SD: genotype hemoglobin SD; Hb SS: genotype hemoglobin SS; HCL: hydrochloric acid; min: minute; mL: milliliter; SCD: sickle cell disease; WHO: World Health Organization

Acknowledgements

The authors would like to thank the Hematology and Hemotherapy Foundation in Bahia (HEMOBA) and the State School Francisco da Conceição Menezes for allowing this research to be conducted, and Caio Brandão Maciel, who helped with the translation and organization of the manuscript.

Authors' contributions

CFB: prepared the study, collected the data, performed the statistical analysis, put together and revised the manuscript; VMBO: assisted in the preparation of the study, manuscript and data analysis; ARRMS: assisted with data collection; TMMS: assisted with data collection; VQCV: assisted with data collection; GGPPS: assisted with data collection; LRSC: assisted with data collection; RACC: assisted with data collection; AMTL: assisted with the preparation of the study, manuscript and data analysis. All authors approved of the final version of the manuscript.

Competing interests

The authors declare that they have no competing interests.

References

1. Brasil. Ministério da Saúde. Secretaria de Atenção à Saúde. Departamento de Atenção à Saúde. Doença Falciforme: Condutas básicas para tratamento. Brasília (DF), Ministério da Saúde, 2012. (Série B. Textos Básicos de Saúde).
2. Taylor LB, Nowak AJ, Giller RH, Casamassimo PS. Sickle cell anemia: a review of the dental concerns and a retrospective study of dental and bony changes. Spec Care Dentist. 1995;15:38–42.
3. Souza SFC, HLCC C, CPS C, EBAF T. Association of sickle cell haemoglobinopathies with dental and jaw bone abnormalities. Oral Dis. 2017.
4. Carvalho HLCC, Rolim JYS, Thomaz EBAF, Souza SFC. Are dental and jaw changes more prevalent in a Brazilian population with sickle cell anemia? Oral Surg Oral Med Oral Pathol Oral Radiol. 2017;124(1):76–84.
5. Laurence B, George D, Woods D, Shosanya A, Katz RV, Lanzkron S, et al. The association between sickle cell disease and dental caries in African Americans. Spec Care Dentist. 2006;26:95–100.
6. Singh J, Singh N, Kumar A, Kedia NB, Agarwal A. Dental and periodontal health status of Beta thalassemia major and sickle cell anemic patients: a comparative study. J Int Oral Health. 2013;5(5):53–8.
7. Fernandes MLMF, Kawachi I, Fernandes AF, Corrêa-Faria P, Paiva SM, Pordeus IA. Caries prevalence and impact on oral health-related quality of life in children with sickle cell disease: cross-sectional study. BMC Oral Health. 2016;38(2):106–12.
8. Okafor LA, Nonnoo DC, Ojehanon PI, Aikhionbare O. Oral and dental complications of sickle cell disease in Nigerians. Angiology. 1986;37(9): 672–5.
9. Luna AC, Rodrigues MJ, Menezes VA, Marques KM, Santos FA. Caries prevalence and socioeconomic factors in children with sickle cell anemia. Braz Oral Res. 2012;26:43–9.
10. Passos CP, Santos PRB, Aguiar MRC, Cangussu MC, Toralles MB, da Silva MC, et al. Sickle cell disease does not predispose to caries or periodontal disease. Spec Care Dentist. 2012;32:55–60.
11. Ralstrom E, da Fonseca MA, Rhodes M, Amini H. The impact of sickle cell disease on oral health-related quality of life. Pediatr Dent 2014; 36:24–28.
12. Leone CW, Oppenheim FG. Physical and chemical aspects of saliva as indicators of risk for dental caries in humans. J Dent Educ. 2001;65(10): 1054–62.
13. Brasil. Ministério da Saúde. Secretaria de Atenção à Saúde. Departamento de Atenção Especializada. Manual de Educação em Saúde. Brasília (DF): Ministério da Saúde; 2008.
14. Javed F, Correa FOB, Nooh N, Almas K, Romanos GE, Al-Hezaimi K. Orofacial manifestations in patients with sickle cell disease. Am J Med Sci. 2011;345: 234–7.
15. Veiga PC, Schroth RJ, Guedes R, Freire SM, Nogueira-Filho G. Serum cytokine profile among Brazilian children of African descent with periodontal inflammation and sickle cell anemia. Arch Oral Biol. 2013;58:505–10.
16. World Health Organization. Oral health surveys: basic methods. 4th ed. Geneva: World Health Organization; 1997.
17. Brasil. Secretaria de Vigilância à Saúde. Secretaria de Atenção à Saúde. Departamento de Atenção Básica. Coordenação Nacional de Saúde Bucal. SB Brasil 2010: Manual da Equipe de Campo. Brasília (DF). 2009; 37–42.
18. Domingos PAS. Aspectos epidemiológicos da saúde bucal de crianças em um município brasileiro. Arq Odontol. 2010;45(2):82–7.
19. Arai OS, Camargo ALS, Jorge AOC, Rego MA. Avaliação do risco de cárie em crianças através de método convencional e do programa cariograma. JBP J Bras Odontopediatr Odontol Bebê. 2003;6(32):317–24.
20. Garcia LB, Bulla JR, Kotaca CR, Tognim MCB, Cardoso CL. Testes salivares e bacteriológicos para avaliação do risco de cárie. RBAC. 2009;41(1):69–76.
21. Calvo-Gonzalez E, Rocha V. "Está no sangue": a articulação de ideias sobre"raça", aparência e ancestralidade entre famílias de portadores de doença falciforme em Salvador. Bahia Revista de Antropologia. 2010;53(1): 278–320.
22. Acharya S. Oral and dental considerations in management of sickle cell anemia. Int J Clin Pediatr Dent. 2015;8(2):141–4.
23. Botelho DS, Vergne AA, Bittencourt S, Ribeiro EP. Perfil sistêmico e conduta odontológica em pacientes com anemia falciforme. Int J Dent. 2009;8(1):28–35.
24. Berkowitz RJ. Causes, treatment and prevention of early childhood caries: a microbiologic perspective. J Can Dent Assoc. 2003;69(5):304–7.
25. Çolak H, Dulgergil ÇT, Dalil M, Hamidiet MM. Early childhood caries update: a review of causes, diagnoses and treatments. J Nat Sci Biol Med. 2013;4(1): 29–38.

26. Luna A, Gomes M, Granville-Garcia A, Menezes V. Perception of treatment needs and use of dental Services for Children and Adolescents with sickle cell disease. Oral Health Prev Dent. 2018;16(1):51–7. https://doi.org/10.3290/j.ohpd.a39817.

27. Brasil. Ministério da Saúde. Coordenação Nacional de Saúde Bucal. Projeto SB Brasil 2010: Pesquisa Nacional de Saúde Bucal: resultados principais. Brasília (DF), 2011.

28. Ramires I, Buzalaf MAR. A fluoretação da água de abastecimento público e seus benefícios no controle da cárie dentária: cinquenta anos no Brasil. Ciênc Saúde Coletiva. 2007;12(4):1057–65.

29. Costa SPC, Aires BTC, Thomaz EBAF, Souza SFC. Dental care provided to sickle cell anemia patients stratified by age: a population-based study in northeastern Brazil. Eur J Dent. 2016;10(3):356–60.

30. Carvalho HLCC, Thomaz EBAF, Alves CMC, Souza SFC. Are sickle cell anemia and sickle cell trait predictive factors for periodontal disease? A cohort study. J Periodontal Res. 2015:1–15.

31. Mahmoud MO, Ghandour IA, Atalla B. Association between sickle cell anemia and periodontal disease among 12 to 16 year old Sudanese children. Periodontal disease. Oral Health Prev Dent. 2013;11(4):375–81.

32. Tonguç MO, Unal S, Aspaci RB. Gingival enlargement in children with sickle cell disease. J Oral Sci. 2018;60(1):105–14.

33. Moimaz SAS, Garbin CAS, Aguiar ACA, Silva MB. Capacidade Tampão da Saliva Frente a Diversos Estímulos Gustativos. Rev Fac Odontol Lins. 2002; 14(1):19–23.

34. Bretas LP, Rocha ME, Vieira MS, Rodrigues ACP. Fluxo salivar e capacidade tamponante da saliva. Pesqui Bras Odontopediatria Clín Integr. 2008;8(3): 289–93.

35. Cortelli SC, Chaves MGAM, Faria IS, Landucci LF, Oliveira LD, Sherma AP, et al. Avaliação da condição bucal e do risco de cárie de alunos ingressantes em curso de Odontologia. PGR-Pós-Grad rev. 2002;5(1):35–42.

36. World Health Organization. Oral Health Surveys Basic Methods. 5th ed. Brazil: World Health Organization; 2013.

37. Tenovuo J. Antimicrobial agents in saliva — protection for the whole body. J Dent Res. 2002;81(12):807–9.

38. Krasse B. Exame da saliva. In: Risco de cárie: guia prático para controle e assessoramento. Quintessence: São Paulo; 1988.

39. Ware RE, Aygun B. Advances in the use of hydroxyurea. Hematol Am Soc Hematol Educ Program. 2009;2009:62–9.

40. Cançado RD, Lobo C, Angulo IL, Araújo PCI, Jesus JA. Clinical protocol and therapeutic guidelines for the use of hydroxyurea in sickle cell disease. Revista Brasileira de Hematologia e Hematerapia. 2009;31(5):361–6.

41. Salvia ARD, Figueiredo MS, Braga JAP, Pereira DFA, Brighenti FL, Koga-Ito CY. Hydroxyurea therapy in sickle cell anemia patients aids to maintain oral fungal colonization balance. J Oral Pathol Med. 2013;42:570–5. https://doi.org/10.1111/jop.12029.

24

Bactericidal effect of a diode laser on *Enterococcus faecalis* in human primary teeth—an in vitro study

Shanshan Dai[1,2], Gang Xiao[1,2], Ning Dong[1,2], Fei Liu[1,2], Shuyang He[1,2] and Qingyu Guo[1,2*]

Abstract

Background: In recent years, the diode laser (810 nm) has been used for root canal disinfection, which plays an important role in endodontic therapy. This study was undertaken to evaluate the disinfecting ability of a diode laser in experimentally infected root canals of primary teeth.

Methods: Human retained mandibular primary anterior teeth without apical foramen resorption were selected and contaminated with *Enterococcus faecalis* for 21 days. The specimens were randomly divided into four groups: the negative group (no treatment), positive group (5.25% NaOCl), diode laser group (diode laser), and diode-NaOCl group (diode laser combined with NaOCl). The disinfecting abilities of the treatments were measured by the numbers of bacteria, scanning electron microscopy and confocal laser microscopy (live-dead staining).

Results: Eighty teeth were selected. After irradiation and irrigation, the elimination of bacteria and the smear layer in the laser groups and positive group were significantly superior, compared with the negative group ($p < 0.01$). In the diode-NaOCl group, bacterial reduction reached nearly 100% on the surfaces of root canals; live bacteria were rarely observed, even in deeper dentinal tubules.

Conclusion: Use of a diode laser, especially in combination with NaOCl, was effective for disinfecting infected root canals of primary teeth.

Keywords: Diode laser, Primary teeth, Disinfection, *Enterococcus faecalis*

Background

Dental caries and pulpitis are common diseases in children; notably, if the pulpitis cannot be controlled, it can result in primary tooth loss at early ages, affecting chewing, pronunciation, and aesthetics. Root canal therapy of the primary teeth is a commonly used therapeutic method. The main objective of endodontic treatment is to effectively eliminate bacteria and necrotic pulp tissue remnants from the root canal system [1], in order to preserve the teeth. Although most bacterial species are eliminated, some microorganisms may remain viable even after mechanical instrumentation, which may lead to an unfavorable root canal treatment outcome [2]. In addition, a biomechanical preparation cannot completely eliminate the microorganisms present in the root canal system; each technique has unique limitations [3]. Therefore, root canal system disinfection plays an important role in the success of endodontic treatment [4].

Numerous studies have proven that the bactericidal effect of a diode laser (810 nm) is based on thermal properties; furthermore, bacteria cannot develop resistance to laser exposure [5, 6]. A diode laser has been used in several areas of dentistry with promising disinfection outcomes [7–9]. Studies on the efficacy of lasers in endodontic therapy have mostly focused on permanent teeth [10], while studies on primary teeth have been rarely reported. Meanwhile, because of the complicated anatomical structure of the pulpal chamber [11], choosing the most effective disinfection protocol for pulp-infected primary teeth becomes particularly important.

This study evaluated the bactericidal efficacy of 810-nm diode laser irradiation and the combination of diode laser irradiation with 5.25% NaOCl in primary teeth by using

* Correspondence: guoqinyu@mail.xjtu.edu.cn
[1]Key Laboratory of Shaanxi Province for Craniofacial Precision Medicine Research, Xi'an 710004, China
[2]Department of Pediatric Dentistry, Hospital of Stomatology Xi'an Jiaotong University College of Medicine, Xi'an 710004, Shaanxi, China

scanning electron microscopy (SEM), confocal laser microscopy (CLM), and counting colony-forming units (CFUs).

Methods

The protocol of this study was approved by the Research Ethics Committee of Xi'an Jiaotong University, Xi'an, China.

Sample preparation

Retained human mandibular primary incisors without apical foramen resorption that had been extracted were included. The samples were stored temporarily in physiological saline solution at 4 °C. Teeth were decoronated and roots were normalized to 7 mm in length. The root canals were prepared using the crown down technique and stainless-steel K files up to size 30 (Dentsply Maillefer Ballaigues, Switzerland). Specimens were irrigated with 2 mL of 5.25% NaOCl during instrumentation. Teeth were ground longitudinally from the lingual portion with a high-speed diamond bur (MANI, Japan) to expose the inner parts of the root canals, followed by 2 mL of normal saline solution. A self-etching adhesive (3 M Dental Products, USA) was coated on the external surfaces of the roots to avoid microbial contamination. All sections were sterilized in an autoclave at 121 °C for 20 min. The root sections were then incubated in brain-heart infusion (BHI) broth for 24 h at 37 °C to isolate them from bacterial contamination.

Female mold of the half side of the root canal preparation

In a randomly selected sample, the root canal was filled with molten red wax and solidified. A small amount of silicone rubber impression material was fully mixed and placed in plastic molding manufactured in-house (cylindrical, approximately 2.0 cm in diameter and 2.0 cm high). Then, the root was placed in the impression material until the material solidified; then, the root was removed. The female mold of the half side of the root canal was made and soaked in 1% peracetic acid for 30 min for disinfection after each sample was inserted into the mold.

Enterococcus faecalis culture and inoculation

Enterococcus faecalis (ATCC 29212) was inoculated on BHI agar (Land Bridge, China) and incubated anaerobically at 37 °C for 24 h. A single colony was collected and aseptically resuspended in 10 mL of BHI broth. The sterilized specimens in 1 mL of sterile BHI broth were placed in 0.5 mL cultures (10^8 CFU/mL as determined by a spectrophotometer). The specimens were then incubated under anaerobic conditions at 37 °C for 21 days. The medium was exchanged with fresh BHI broth every 2 days to remove

dead bacteria and supply nutrition. All procedures were conducted under sterile conditions. After incubation, the specimens were removed from the tubes, rinsed in 2 mL of sterile saline, and then randomly divided into four groups.

Experimental groups

All infected samples were placed into the female mold created from the silicone rubber impression material.

In the negative group ($n = 20$), there was no treatment.

In the positive group ($n = 20$), the sections were irrigated with 5 mL of 5.25% NaOCl for 60 s.

In the diode laser group ($n = 20$), the specimens were dried and irradiated with the diode laser at an output power of 2.0 W for 5 s and a wavelength of 810 nm in continuous mode (Lambda Dental Laser, LAMBDA Scientifica S.p.A, Italy). An optical fiber 200 μm in diameter was inserted into the root canal 1 mm short of the working length. The irradiation was repeated four times at 10-s intervals.

In the diode-NaOCl group ($n = 20$), the irradiation procedure was the same as in the diode laser group and was repeated four times. During each irradiation, the canals were irrigated with 1.25 mL of 5.25% NaOCl. All samples were rinsed with 2 mL of sterile saline to remove the remaining bacteria and NaOCl.

Bacteriological evaluation

After the disinfection procedures, 10 samples from each group were subjected to CFU-counting evaluations. Five samples among them were split into three equal pieces (namely the coronal, middle, and apical regions of the root canal). Each specimen was placed into a sterile Eppendorf tube with 1 mL of physiological saline solution and sonicated at 7 W for 60 s using an ultrasonic device [12] (P5 Newtron XS, Satelec, France). After mixing, the liquid was diluted in log base 10 steps and 100 μL of each dilution was inoculated onto BHI agar plates, which were then incubated for 24 h at 37 °C under anaerobic conditions. Bacterial CFUs were observed and counted.

Examination by SEM

Another five samples from each group were fixed in 2.5% glutaraldehyde for 24 h. Following dehydration in graded concentrations of ethanol, the specimens were air dried, coated with a layer of platinum (Ion Sputter E-1045, Hitachi, Japan), and observed by SEM (S-4800, Hitachi, Japan).

The coronal, middle, and apical regions were examined. Photographs were taken at various magnifications ranging from 30× to 500,000× by the same operator. Two observers blinded to the group allocations evaluated the remaining smear layers based on a scoring system described by Takeda [13]. A score of 1 represents no smear layer or debris evident in the dentinal tubules; a score of 2 represents a few regions of dentinal tubules covered with a smear layer and debris, with most tubules cleaned and opened; a score of 3 represents that most regions of dentinal tubules were covered with a smear layer and debris with a few tubules cleaned and opened; and a score of 4 represents dentinal tubules completely covered with a smear layer and debris.

Analysis of CLM

The remaining samples were stained with a LIVE/DEAD BacLight Bacterial Viability Kit (L7012, Life, USA) for 15 min, in accordance with the manufacturer's instructions. The stained samples were cut into three equal parts using a low-speed diamond saw (SYJ150, MTI, USA). The specimens were covered with aluminum foil to prevent light exposure and maintained at 4 °C. The samples were then mounted onto glass slides and visualized under an Olympus confocal laser scanning microscope (FV10-ASW, Olympus, Japan) at 20× magnification. Green and red fluorescence were detected using wavelengths of 488 nm and 543 nm, respectively. The digital images were imported into the Image-Pro Plus 6.0 program (MediaCybernetics, USA) to evaluate the efficacy of disinfection by measuring the green-to-red fluorescence area ratio in each portion.

Statistical analysis

The statistical analysis was performed with SPSS 19.0 for Windows (SPSS, China). An analysis of variance (ANOVA) model was used to compare the mean CFUs and fluorescence area ratios among the groups. The smear layer scores were analyzed using the Kruskal–Wallis test to estimate the ultrastructural morphological changes. The level of significance was set at $\alpha = 0.05$.

Results

Eighty teeth were selected and randomized into the four groups equally ($n = 20$ per group).

Bacteriological evaluation

The numbers of recovered bacteria from different parts of specimens from each group are presented in Table 1. The negative group demonstrated the least bactericidal effect, followed by the positive group, diode laser group, and

diode-NaOCl group. In the negative group, 10^5 CFU/mL of bacteria were detected. After irrigation and irradiation, bacterial reductions were significantly greater on the surfaces of the root canals ($p < 0.01$). Disinfection of the root canal portions in the diode laser group was superior to that in the positive group except for the apical part ($p < 0.05$). In addition, the diode-NaOCl group showed that the bacterial reduction reached nearly 100% on the surface of each part of the root canal and there were significant differences between each of the group pairs ($p < 0.01$). In each group, the bacteria were eliminated more effectively in the coronal and middle parts compared with the apical parts ($p < 0.05$).

SEM examination

The kappa value showed excellent reliability and reproducibility between the two observers at 0.89. The calculated smear layer scores from different parts of the specimens from each group are presented in Table 2. A heavy, continuous smear layer was observed on the entirety of the root canal walls in the negative group and the debris and bacteria displayed a smooth surface (Fig. 1A–C). In the positive group, a few shrunken smear layers were discovered and the dentinal tubules were visible but not completely opened (Fig. 1D–F). In the diode laser group, few smear layers were observed and sparse bacteria were detected (Fig. 1G, H) except in the apical part (Fig. 1I). The diode-NaOCl group presented the best disinfection outcome. The smear layer was thoroughly cleaned, the tubules were opened, and almost no bacteria existed on the root canal surface (Fig. 1J–L). The analysis showed that the combination of diode laser irradiation and NaOCl resulted in the lowest score ($p < 0.01$), followed by the diode laser group, positive group, and negative group ($p < 0.05$). Meanwhile, in all experimental groups except for the diode-NaOCl group, the smear layers on the coronal and middle regions were removed more effectively than those on the apical regions ($p < 0.05$).

CLM analysis

CLM analysis allowed us to distinguish viable from nonviable bacteria on root canal walls and in dentinal tubules. To detect the presence of green bacteria (vital) in

Table 1 Bacterial counts (CFU/mL, mean ± SD) and bacterial reductions (BR) in the different groups

	negative group	positive group		diode laser group		diode-NaOCl group	
	Mean ± SD (log10)	Mean ± SD (log10)	RD (%)	Mean ± SD (log10)	RD (%)	Mean ± SD (log10)	RD (%)
Coronal region	5.82 ± 4.74^A	4.51 ± 3.78^B ^{a}	95.12	4.38 ± 3.60^C ^{a}	99.44	3.30 ± 1.78^D ^{a}	99.74
Middle region	5.72 ± 4.83^A	4.49 ± 3.70^B ^{a}	94.13	4.36 ± 3.78^C ^{a}	95.70	3.30 ± 2.70^D ^{a}	99.70
Apical region	5.70 ± 4.80^A	4.51 ± 3.85^B ^{b}	93.25	4.40 ± 3.78^B ^{b}	94.94	3.30 ± 2.70^C ^{b}	99.54
Integrity	5.82 ± 4.15^A	4.58 ± 3.90^B	94.16	4.36 ± 3.85^C	96.47	3.30 ± 2.78^D	99.72

SD, standard deviation; BR, bacterial reduction; CFU, colony-forming units
Data with different uppercase letters (A, B, C, D) indicate significant differences within each group ($p < 0.05$)
Data with different lowercase letters (a, b) indicate a significant difference within each region ($p < 0.05$)

Table 2 Smear layer scores (Mean ± SD) in different groups and three regions of root canal

	negative group	positive group	diode laser group	diode-group
Coronal region	3.71 ± 0.46^A	2.57 ± 0.49^B a	1.86 ± 0.35^C a	1.14 ± 0.35^D a
Middle region	3.86 ± 0.35^A	2.43 ± 0.49^B a	1.71 ± 0.42^C a	1.14 ± 0.35^D a
Apical region	3.71 ± 0.45^A	3.14 ± 0.35^B b	2.43 ± 0.49^B b	1.29 ± 0.45^D a

Data with different uppercase letters (A, B, C, D) indicate significant differences within each group ($p < 0.05$)
Data with different lowercase letters (a, b) indicate significant difference within each region ($p < 0.05$)

the biofilms or red bacteria (non-vital) in the biofilms, the means and standard deviations of the green-to-red fluorescence area ratios were determined for each fragment and are shown in Table 3. From high to low, the area ratios in the groups were as follows: the negative group, positive group, diode laser group, and diode-NaOCl group. In the positive group, the ratio was close to 1.0 except in the apical region where it was greater than 1.0 ($p > 0.01$). In the diode laser group and diode-NaOCl group, the area ratios in each portion were less than 1.0 ($p > 0.01$). The corresponding images are shown in Fig. 2. Regardless of the root portion, the negative group revealed a much greater amount of green (vital) fluorescence than other groups ($p < 0.01$). Conversely, the rest of the groups presented various degrees of green and red (non-vital) fluorescence. In the positive group, the amounts of green and red fluorescence were equal, which showed statistically significant differences with the other groups ($p < 0.01$). The diode laser group showed much more red fluorescence in the dentinal tubules indicative of non-vital bacteria in the biofilms and the merged picture was dominated by red fluorescence ($p < 0.01$). Moreover, the diode-NaOCl group showed little green and mostly red fluorescence and no green fluorescence in the deeper dentinal tubules ($p < 0.01$).

Discussion

Disinfection is one of the key steps in successful root canal treatment. The methods include microbial reduction through mechanical preparation removal of residual pulp tissue and debris, and chemical preparation to maintain teeth. Once tooth reserve failure, it would affects children's chewing, aesthetics, and eruption of permanent teeth.

Enterococcus faecalis is a gram-positive facultative anaerobic organism that can be commonly isolated from failed root canal treatment [14]. Several studies showed that *E. faecalis* bacteria became more resistant in the starvation

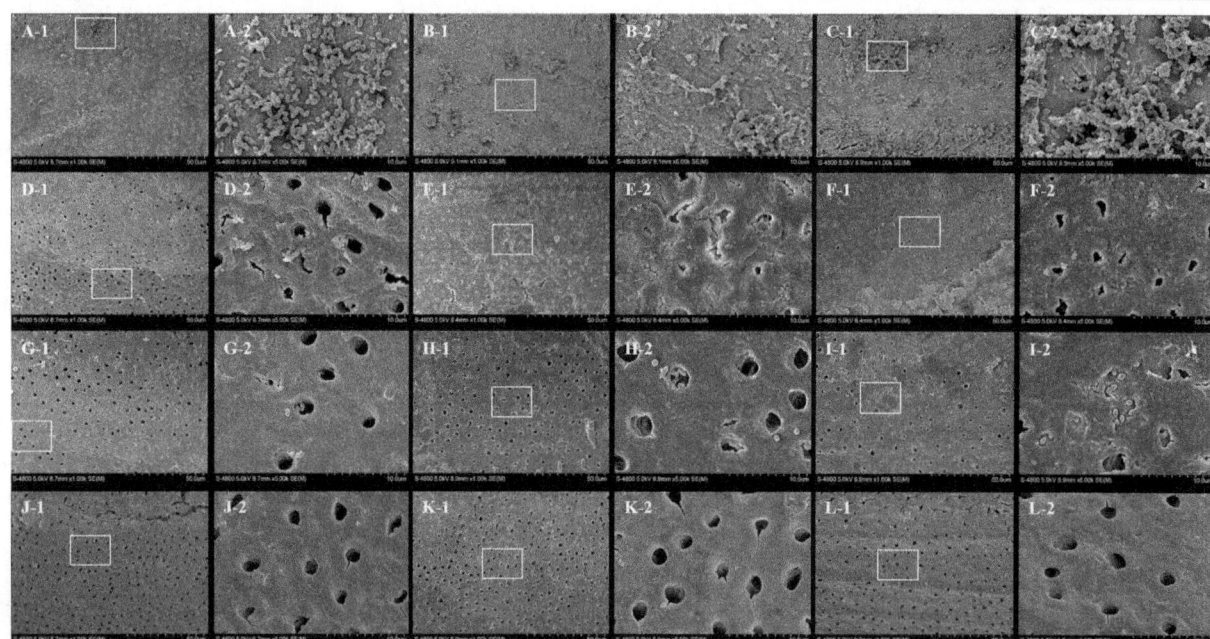

Fig. 1 Scanning electron microscopy (SEM) observation of the smear layer and *Enterococcus faecalis* removed after treatment in each group. Negative group: a heavy smear layer and biofilm-like structures are observed on the surface of the root canal (A–C, A: coronal region; B: middle region; C: apical region). Positive group: a few smear layer-covered areas and tubules are visible but have not completely opened and the remaining biofilm is shrunken (D–F, D: coronal region; E: middle region; F: apical region). Diode laser group: a small amount of smear layer is evidenced on the smooth root canal surface and sparse bacteria are detected (G–I, G: coronal region; H: middle region; I: apical region). Diode-NaOCl group: the smear layer is uniformly clean and the tubules are opened; there are almost no bacteria on the root canal surface (J–L, J: coronal region; K: middle region; L: apical region). Magnification: A~L-1 1000×; A~L-2 5000×

Table 3 The ratio between green and red fluorescence area (Mean ± SD) in different groups

	negative group	positive group	diode laser group	diode-NaOCl group
Coronal region	37.15 ± 2.35[a]	0.93 ± 0.02[b]	0.62 ± 0.01[c]	0.02 ± 0.003[d]
Middle region	14.81 ± 2.73[a]	0.96 ± 0.02[b]	0.64 ± 0.04[c]	0.05 ± 0.004[d]
Apical region	10.98 ± 1.38[a]	1.67 ± 0.04[b]	0.47 ± 0.02[c]	0.12 ± 0.003[d]

Data with different lowercase letters (a, b, c, d) indicate a significant difference within each group ($p < 0.01$)

phase and were difficult to eradicate [14–16]. Additionally, conventional irrigations cannot completely eliminate it. The results from our bacteriological evaluation showed that the diode-NaOCl group demonstrated the lowest amount of bacteria, followed by the diode laser group and positive group. In the diode-NaOCl group, there was a reduction of at least 99.7% in *E. faecalis* on the surface of the root canal. This finding could be attributed to the efficient removal of the smear layer from the dentinal surface by the diode laser, which resulted in improved contact between the NaOCl and bacteria. This finding makes the results of this study noteworthy. Hence, it could be concluded that the bactericidal and permeation effects of NaOCl, which are well known, are enhanced by the use of a diode laser.

In our experiment, the sample was divided into two parts; however, this is difficult with primary teeth [17]. Therefore, we first used a silicone rubber impression material to prepare a mold of the root. The mold could simulate the state of rinse reflux in the apical portion, which provided a better simulation of the root. In comparison with other parts of root canal, removal of the smear layer and elimination of bacteria were significantly greater in the coronal and middle regions than in the apical region. Our results suggested that most residual bacteria are in the apical region following disinfection; this is why we focus on root canal filling in the apical portion [18]. These findings may be due to the structure of the apical portion of the root, which does not facilitate irrigation, and the tip of the laser, which cannot reach

the apical portion. However, in the diode-NaOCl group, there were no statistically significant differences among the three regions. The area ratio of the green-to-red fluorescence was also the lowest among the groups, which suggested the most effective disinfection from the lack of live bacteria. This again proved that a diode laser in combination with NaOCl had greater disinfectant properties in the apical portion.

The diode laser technique has been performed in endodontics treatment for a decade [19]. It is well known that different parameters of lasers and fibers, the output power of the laser, and the duration of application have different effects on disinfection [6]. The thermal effect is the most important point to be considered in laser applications. A temperature rise to a critical level could have deleterious effects on the tissues surrounding the tooth. The temperature increases by approximately 10 °C and a treatment duration of 1 min can cause irreversible injury to periodontal tissues [20]. Gutknecht et al. [21] demonstrated that diode laser irradiation for 5 s, with 10 s of resting time, should be considered to avoid a temperature rise to an undesired level. Schoop et al. [22] also drew similar conclusions that a diode laser showed the lowest temperature increases compared with other laser devices and was suitable for the disinfection of root canals. Therefore, according to the information, we adopt a safe mode of diode laser to perform root canal therapy. Several studies have shown that a 3.0 W diode laser with an 810-nm

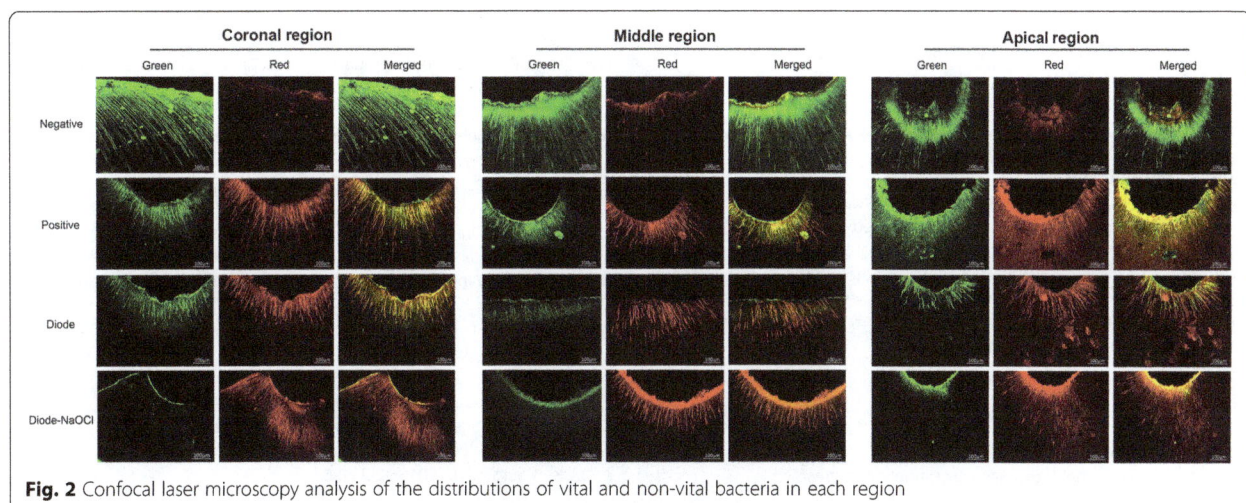

Fig. 2 Confocal laser microscopy analysis of the distributions of vital and non-vital bacteria in each region

wavelength could eliminate bacteria when used on permanent teeth [5]. Because of the different structures and components between permanent and primary teeth, the laser power used for permanent teeth may not be suitable for primary teeth [23]. Our pilot experiment revealed that a 2.0 W diode laser was the most efficient at removing the smear layer on primary teeth while avoiding dentinal melting [24]. In our study, diode laser irradiation was performed with an output of 2.0 W for 5 s followed a 10-s interval or irrigation, in accordance with the method used in the study by Akyuz [25]. However, further studies are required to confirm the biological safety of diode laser application.

Conclusions

In conclusion, both diode laser groups, especially the diode-NaOCl group, showed satisfactory bactericidal effects in experimentally contaminated root canals of primary teeth. The combination of a diode laser and NaOCl could be an ideal protocol to improve the success rate of therapy and reduce negative impacts on children, and can provide helpful guidance for the clinical application of primary root canal disinfection.

Abbreviations
ATCC: American Type Culture Collection; BHI: Brain Heart Infusion; CFUs: Colony-Forming Units; CLM: Confocal Laser Microscopy; E. faecalis: Enterococcus faecalis; NaOCl: Sodium hypochlorite; SEM: Scanning Electron Microscopy

Acknowledgments
We would like to thank Shanghai Tian Ying medical Instrument Co.,Ltd. for providing the diode laser(810 nm).

Funding
The study was funded by Science and Technology Program of Shaanxi Province(2015KTCL03-07).

Authors' contributions
SD participated in the study design, collected the data, performed statistical analyses and interpretation of the data, and drafted the manuscript. GX participated in the study design and data collection. ND assisted in data collection and revised the manuscript. FL participated in the study design and data collection. SH performed statistical analyses and interpretation of the data. QG designed the study and revised the manuscript. All authors read and approved the final manuscript.

Competing interests
The authors declare that they have no competing interests.

References
1. Topcuoglu G, Topcuoglu HS, Akpek F. Evaluation of apically extruded debris during root canal preparation in primary molar teeth using three different rotary systems and hand files. Int J Paediatr Dent. 2016;26(5):357–63.
2. Nair PN, Henry S, Cano V, Vera J. Microbial status of apical root canal system of human mandibular first molars with primary apical periodontitis after "one-visit" endodontic treatment. Oral Surg Oral Med Oral Pathol Oral Radiol Endod. 2005;99(2):231–52.
3. Peters OA, Schonenberger K, Laib A. Effects of four Ni-Ti preparation techniques on root canal geometry assessed by micro computed tomography. Int Endod J. 2001;34(3):221–30.
4. Tennert C, Feldmann K, Haamann E, Al-Ahmad A, Follo M, Wrbas KT, Hellwig E, Altenburger MJ. Effect of photodynamic therapy (PDT) on enterococcus faecalis biofilm in experimental primary and secondary endodontic infections. BMC oral health. 2014;14:132.
5. Asnaashari M, Safavi N. Disinfection of contaminated canals by different laser wavelengths, while Performing Root Canal Therapy. J Lasers Med Sci. 2013;4(1):8–16.
6. de Souza EB, Cai S, Simionato MR, Lage-Marques JL. High-power diode laser in the disinfection in depth of the root canal dentin. Oral Surg Oral Med Oral Pathol Oral Radiol Endod. 2008;106(1):e68–72.
7. Gutknecht N, Franzen R, Schippers M, Lampert F. Bactericidal effect of a 980-nm diode laser in the root canal wall dentin of bovine teeth. J Clin Laser Med Surg. 2004;22(1):9–13.
8. Pearson GJ, Schuckert KH. The role of lasers in dentistry: present and future. Dent update. 2003;30(2):70–74, 76.
9. Wang X, Sun Y, Kimura Y, Kinoshita J, Ishizaki NT, Matsumoto K. Effects of diode laser irradiation on smear layer removal from root canal walls and apical leakage after obturation. Photomed Laser Surg. 2005;23(6):575–81.
10. Mathew J, Emil J, Paulaian B, John B, Raja J, Mathew J. Viability and antibacterial efficacy of four root canal disinfection techniques evaluated using confocal laser scanning microscopy. J Conserv Dent. 2014;17(5):444–8.
11. Gondim JO, Avaca-Crusca JS, Valentini SR, Zanelli CF, Spolidorio DM, Giro EM. Effect of a calcium hydroxide/chlorhexidine paste as intracanal dressing in human primary teeth with necrotic pulp against Porphyromonas gingivalis and enterococcus faecalis. Int J Paediatr Dent. 2012;22(2):116–24.
12. Aires CP, Del Bel Cury AA, Tenuta LM, Klein MI, Koo H, Duarte S, Cury JA. Effect of starch and sucrose on dental biofilm formation and on root dentine demineralization. Caries Res. 2008;42(5):380–6.
13. Takeda FH, Harashima T, Kimura Y, Matsumoto K. A comparative study of the removal of smear layer by three endodontic irrigants and two types of laser. Int Endod J. 1999;32(1):32–9.
14. Pinheiro ET, Gomes BP, Ferraz CC, Sousa EL, Teixeira FB, Souza-Filho FJ. Microorganisms from canals of root-filled teeth with periapical lesions. Int Endod J. 2003;36(1):1–11.
15. George S, Kishen A, Song KP. The role of environmental changes on monospecies biofilm formation on root canal wall by enterococcus faecalis. J Endod. 2005;31(12):867–72.
16. Cheng X, Guan S, Lu H, Zhao C, Chen X, Li N, Bai Q, Tian Y, Yu Q. Evaluation of the bactericidal effect of Nd:YAG, Er:YAG, Er,Cr:YSGG laser radiation, and antimicrobial photodynamic therapy (aPDT) in experimentally infected root canals. Lasers Surg Med. 2012;44(10):824–31.
17. Jiang LM, Verhaagen B, Versluis M, van der Sluis LW. Influence of the oscillation direction of an ultrasonic file on the cleaning efficacy of passive ultrasonic irrigation. J Endod. 2010;36(8):1372–6.
18. Gomes BP, Pinheiro ET, Jacinto RC, Zaia AA, Ferraz CC, Souza-Filho FJ. Microbial analysis of canals of root-filled teeth with periapical lesions using polymerase chain reaction. J Endod. 2008;34(5):537–40.
19. Moritz A, Gutknecht N, Schoop U, Goharkhay K, Doertbudak O, Sperr W. Irradiation of infected root canals with a diode laser in vivo: results of microbiological examinations. Lasers Surg Med. 1997;21(3):221–6.
20. Eriksson AR, Albrektsson T. Temperature threshold levels for heat-induced bone tissue injury: a vital-microscopic study in the rabbit. J Prosthet Dent. 1983;50(1):101–7.
21. Gutknecht N, Franzen R, Meister J, Vanweersch L, Mir M. Temperature evolution on human teeth root surface after diode laser assisted endodontic treatment. Lasers Med Sci. 2005;20(2):99–103.
22. Schoop U, Kluger W, Moritz A, Nedjelik N, Georgopoulos A, Sperr W. Bactericidal effect of different laser systems in the deep layers of dentin. Lasers Surg Med. 2004;35(2):111–6.

23. Zhang S, Chen T, Ge LH. Scanning electron microscopy study of cavity preparation in deciduous teeth using the Er:YAG laser with different powers. Lasers Med Sci. 2012;27(1):141–4.

24. Dai SS, Xiao G, Zhang L, Guo QY. The cleaning effect of diode laser on smear layer on root canals of primary teeth. J Oral Sci Res. 2016;32(07):742–5.

25. Akyuz Ekim SN, Erdemir A. Comparison of different irrigation activation techniques on smear layer removal: an in vitro study. Microsc Res Tech. 2015;78(3):230–9.

25

A prospective clinical study to evaluate the performance of zirconium dioxide dental implants in single-tooth edentulous area

Kai-Hendrik Bormann[1,2]* ⓘ, Nils-Claudius Gellrich[1], Heinz Kniha[3,4], Sabine Schild[5], Dieter Weingart[5] and Michael Gahlert[3,4]

Abstract

Background: Traditionally, dental implants have been made from titanium or titanium alloys. Alternatively, zirconia-based ceramic implants have been developed with similar characteristics of functional strength and osseointegration. Ceramic implants offer advantages in certain settings, e.g. in patients who object to metal dental implants. The aim of this study was to investigate the mid-term (36 months) clinical performance of a ceramic monotype implant in single-tooth edentulous area.

Methods: This was a prospective, open-label, single-arm study in patients requiring implant rehabilitation in single-tooth edentulous area. Ceramic implants (PURE Ceramic Implant, Institut Straumann AG, Basel, Switzerland) with a diameter of 4.1 mm were placed following standard procedure and loaded with provisional and final prostheses after 3 and 6 months, respectively. Implant survival rate and implant success rate were evaluated and crestal bone levels were measured by analysing standardized radiographs during implant surgery and at 6, 12, 24 and 36 months.

Results: Forty-four patients received a study implant, of whom one patient withdrew consent after 3 months. With one implant lost during the first 6 months after surgery, the implant survival rate was 97.7% at 6 months. No further implants were lost over the following 30 months, and 3 patients were lost to follow-up during this time frame. This led to a survival rate of 97.5% at 36 months.
Six months after implant surgery 93.0% of the implants were considered "successful", increasing to 97.6% at 12 months and remaining at this level at 24 months (95.1%) and 36 months (97.5%).
Bone loss was most pronounced in the first half-year after implant surgery (0.88 ± 0.86 mm). By contrast, between 12 and 36 months the mean bone level remained stable (minimal gain of 0.06 [± 0.60] mm). Hence, the overall bone loss from implant surgery to 36 months was 0.97 (± 0.88) mm.

Conclusions: In the follow-up period ceramic implants can achieve favourable clinical outcomes on a par with titanium implants. For instance, these implants can be recommended for patients who object to metal dental implants. However, longer term studies with different edentulous morphology need to confirm the present data.

Keywords: Dental implant, Zirconium dioxide, Ceramic implant, Zirconia, ZrO2, ZLA

* Correspondence: bormann@bormann-praxis.de
[1]Hannover Medical School, Hannover, Germany
[2]Dental Clinic, Bormann Oralchirurgie am Hafen, Hamburg, Germany
Full list of author information is available at the end of the article

Background

For over 40 years, dental implants have been used for the replacement of compromised, lost or missing teeth, following the principles of osseointegration as reported by Brånemark and Adell [1, 2]. While clinical studies have proved the longevity and success of titanium dental implants [3–8], the aesthetics of titanium implants can be challenging, especially in the maxillary incisor area when the dark grey colour of the metal becomes visible. Furthermore, there is a risk of hypersensitivity reaction in patients who are allergic to metals or patients might demand metal-free restorations [9].

Ceramic (zirconia [ZrO_2]) implants were developed to solve the limitations associated with titanium-based alloys. For instance, the ceramic implant is a good option when it comes to aesthetics, as the shade of zirconia is similar to the colour of a tooth. Like titanium, zirconia also has excellent mechanical, biocompatible and osseointegration properties [10–17] with the potential to serve as a successful implant material with high survival and success rates [18, 19] and only small bone losses [20–22]. However, it is difficult to make a consensus regarding the efficacy of ceramic implants due to the variations in ceramic implants and study designs [23].

It has already been shown that certain ceramic implants can achieve clinical outcomes like those of titanium implants after 12 months of follow-up [24]. The present study aims to investigate the safety and clinical performance of this type of ceramic implant concerning survival and success rates, as well as hard and soft tissue parameters after 36 months in the same cohort.

Methods

The study was a prospective 36-month follow-up of an open-label, single-arm study. In the meantime, the study has been extended to 10 years, with planned patient visits at 5 and 10 years after implant surgery. The materials and methods of the study were published previously [24] and are briefly set out below. The study is registered under www.clinicaltrials.gov (study no. NCT02163395).

Patients

Patients were selected according to predefined eligibility criteria. The main inclusion criterion was a single-tooth edentulous area in the mandible (Fédération Dentaire Internationale [FDI] tooth positions 36 to 46) or maxilla (FDI tooth positions 16 to 26), and a natural tooth had to be distally and mesially adjacent to the implant site. The implant positions had to have mainly healed (at least 8 weeks after extraction) and any bone augmentation with autogenous bone had to have been performed at least 3 months prior to implant surgery. Exclusion criteria included different systemic diseases (e.g., uncontrolled

diabetes, mucosal disease, untreated periodontitis, gingivitis, or endodontic lesions), smoking more than 10 cigarettes a day, probing pocket depth of ≥4 mm on a tooth immediately adjacent to the implant site, severe bruxing or clenching habits, inadequate oral hygiene and history of local irradiation therapy. Additional secondary exclusion criteria were applied at or after surgery: lack of implant primary stability, inappropriate implant position for prosthetic requirements, major simultaneous augmentation procedures at surgery, and X-ray not showing the implant from first bone contact to apical tip. The complete list of the eligibility criteria can be found in the first publication of the study [24].

Study device

Ceramic implants (PURE Ceramic Implant, Institut Straumann AG, Basel, Switzerland) with a regular diameter (4.1 mm) were placed in this study. These ceramic implants represent monotype one-piece zirconia implants with already integrated abutments into the implant design, avoiding a microgap between implant and abutment. They are made of yttria-stabilized zirconia (Y-TZP) and are available in 4 different lengths and 2 different abutment heights. The implant is based on the features of the Straumann® Tissue Level Standard Plus and Straumann® Bone Level Implants (Institut Straumann AG, Basel, Switzerland) and has a sandblasted, large-grit, acid-etched surface like the SLA surface present in titanium implants. Further details are provided in the first publication of the study [24].

Surgical and restoration procedure

The implant surgeries were performed by KHB, HK, SS and MG at baseline following standard procedures. Sutures were removed 7 to 14 days after implant surgery, and provisional and final prostheses were placed 11 to 13 weeks and 24 to 28 weeks, respectively, after the implants had been placed. No particular prosthetic procedure was defined in the study protocol. Due to the monotype design of the ceramic implant, lithium disilicate glass–ceramic or zirconium dioxide ceramic crowns were inserted in most cases. Permanent glass ionomer luting cement was used to cement the crowns directly onto the implant abutment. Dental floss was used to remove eventual cement remnants.

The patients attended follow-up visits 12, 24 and 36 months after surgery. Additional follow-up visits are planned 5 and 10 years after implant surgeries. Further details are provided in the first publication of the study [24].

Efficacy evaluations

This is a report of secondary outcomes at 24 and 36-months after implant surgery of:

- Implant survival
- Implant success
- Mean (distal and mesial) bone levels

Implant survival

Implants that were still in place 6, 12, 24 and 36 months after implant surgery were considered as surviving implants.

Implant success

Implant success was defined according to these previously described criteria [25]:

- Absence of pain, foreign body discomfort or dysaesthesia
- Absence of recurrent peri-implant infection with suppuration
- Absence of implant mobility
- Absence of continuous peri-implant radiolucency.

Failed implants were considered as not successful.

Bone levels

Standardized radiographs were taken at baseline (day of implant surgery) as well as 6, 12, 24 and 36 months after implant surgery. Vertical bone level assessment was performed by measuring from the implant shoulder to the first visible bone contact on the implant. Measurements were made at the distal and mesial aspects of each implant, and an average was calculated (Fig. 1). Distortions (changes on the radiographs from the true implant dimensions) were accounted for by normalizing the measurements to the known thread pitch of the implants.

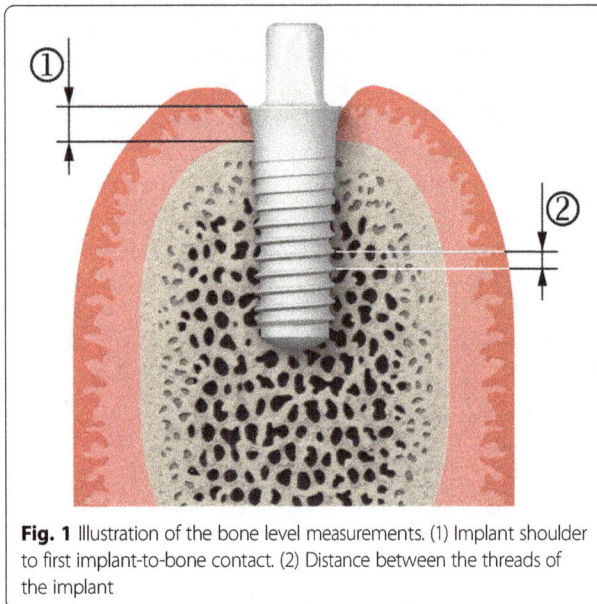

Fig. 1 Illustration of the bone level measurements. (1) Implant shoulder to first implant-to-bone contact. (2) Distance between the threads of the implant

All measurements were analysed by an independent specialist.

Plaque index, sulcus bleeding index and Oral hygiene instructions

Plaque and sulcus bleeding indices were assessed at the implant site and in the adjacent teeth investigating if there was plaque and bleeding, respectively (yes/no).

All patients were given oral hygiene instructions during each study visit. Further details about efficacy evaluations are provided in the first publication of the study [24].

Complications

Adverse events (AEs) and device deficiencies (DDs) monitoring was performed throughout the study. The patients were asked at every visit if they experienced any complication (like pain, bleeding, etc) since the last visit.

Statistical analysis

Data management was performed using DMSys data management software (Version 5.3), Sigmasoft International, and statistical analysis using IBM SPSS statistical software (Version 21, IBM).

In short, descriptive summary statistics were calculated for all documented parameters, including mean values and standard deviations.

For survival and success rates, patients who were lost to follow-up during the 36-month follow-up period were excluded. At each follow-up visit survival and success rates were calculated by dividing implants still in place and patients meeting all the success criteria, respectively, by the patient population at this follow-up visit. 95% confidence intervals (CIs) were calculated using the modified Wald method.

Mean bone level changes were calculated by subtracting the average bone levels at 6, 12, 24 and 36 months from the average bone level at baseline (day of implant surgery). In other words, positive changes represent bone gain between baseline and 6, 12, 24 and 36 months, respectively, whereas negative changes represent bone loss.

The intention to treat (ITT) population includes all patients who received implant treatment and underwent at least one measurement after surgery, regardless of any major protocol deviations or premature termination. The per protocol (PP) population includes all patients who received an implant and completed the 36-month follow-up period without major protocol deviations. The safety analysis set (SAS) includes all patients who received implant treatment.

Further statistical analysis details are provided in the first publication of the study [24].

Results

Patients

In October 2011, the first patient was enrolled. Four years later (in October 2015), the last patient completed the 36-month study period.

Forty-six patients were screened, of whom 44 (17 males and 27 females) subsequently received the study implant and were analysed according to the ITT data set. Patients were on average 48 ± 14 years old (median: 49 years, range: 18 to 78 years). Most of the implants were placed in the maxilla (40 implants; 90.9%), whereas only 4 implants (9.1%) were placed in the mandible (Fig. 2). Bone augmentation was necessary in 31.8% of the cases (14 out of 44 sites); all of them in the aesthetic zone and at the time of surgery. All were considered as non-major augmentations.

Of these 44 patients, 5 terminated the study early and were therefore excluded from the PP analysis. They were either lost to follow-up (3 patients; after 6, 12 and 24 months, respectively), withdrew consent (1 patient; after 3 months) or experienced an AE leading to the implant loss (1 patient; after 6 months). A further 8 patients were excluded from the PP analysis due to major protocol deviations. One patient, who terminated the study early, experienced a major protocol deviation, as a provisional crown had not been placed.

In addition, time window deviations were observed for many patients. These were considered "minor protocol deviations", with no consequences for the data set allocation.

Hence, in total, 13 patients in the ITT population had to be excluded from the PP population, and efficacy analysis according to PP analysis was possible in 31 patients.

Clinical performance evaluations

Implant survival and success

The implant survival and success rates were derived from the ITT data set, with patients who were lost to follow-up being excluded from the analysis. The only implant loss during the 36-month follow-up period occurred before final implant loading. Three patients were lost between 6 and 36 months. These led to a survival rate of 97.7%, with 95% CIs of 86.9% to > 99.9% within the first 6 months after implant surgery and stayed at this level until 36 months (Fig. 3).

During the 36-month follow-up period, a total of 4 implants were considered as "not successful". One patient lost the implant before month 6. At 6 months, 2 patients experienced a mucositis, one of whom also showed continuous radiolucency around the implants. At 24 months, one patient was considered as "not successful" as he/she experienced a mucositis and also pain, foreign body discomfort or dysesthesia. At 12 and 36 months, the only implant considered as "not successful" was the lost implant. Hence, the success rate is equal to the survival rate at these two visits. Overall, the implant success rate was greater than 90% throughout the 36-month follow-up period and, at 12, 24 and 36 months, greater than 95% (Fig. 3).

Bone levels

Bones levels were derived from the ITT data set. Missing data were not calculated. Over the 36 months 54.1% of implant sites ($n = 20$) showed bone loss of less than 1.0 mm or bone gain (Fig. 4). Bone loss in general was most pronounced in the first half-year after implant surgery (0.88 ± 0.86 mm). By contrast, between 12 and 36 months the mean bone level remained stable (minimal gain of 0.06 [± 0.60] mm). Hence, the overall bone loss between implant surgery and 36 months was 0.97 (± 0.88) mm. The bone levels at 6, 12, 24 and 36 months were significantly different from baseline at implant surgery (Fig. 5). The ranges of bone losses were 0.1 to 4.4 mm, – 0.2 to 4.6 mm, – 0.2 to 4.7 mm and – 0.8 to 3.0 mm 6, 12, 24 and 36 after the implant surgery, respectively. Note, negative bone losses representing bone gains.

Plaque index

Plaque was observed in 17 (38.6%) patients during the study, mostly at screening (10 occurrences [58.8%]), at

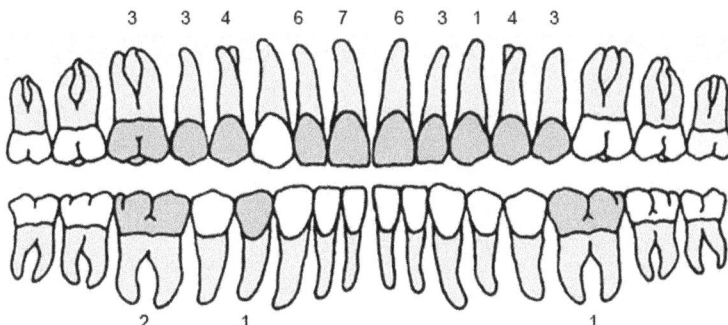

Fig. 2 Distribution of implants placed in the study. Number of implants placed at each tooth position. $N = 44$. N: Total number of implants placed

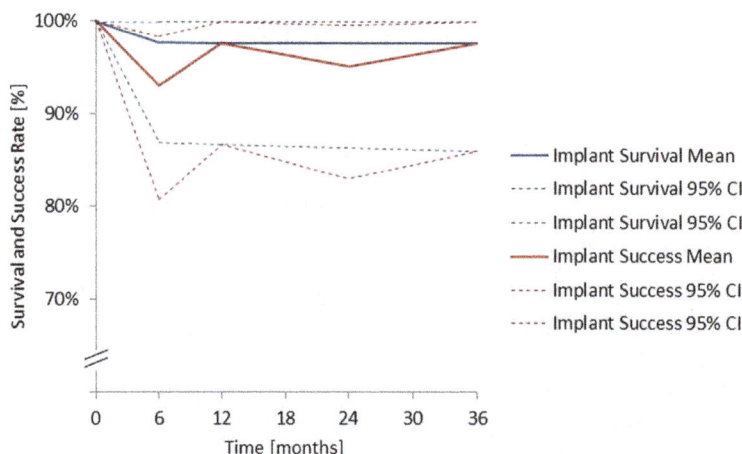

Fig. 3 Survival and success rate analysis. Scaling of the Y-axis 70% to 100%. ITT population (*n* = 44). n (0 m) = 44; n (6 m) = 43; n (12 m) = 42; n (24 m) = 41; n (36 m) = 40. Patients lost to follow-up during the 36-month follow-up period were excluded. CI: Confidence interval; ITT: Intention to treat; m: Months; n: Number

month 36 (8 occurrences [47.1%]) and at month 12 (7 occurrences [41.2%]). Until month 24 plaque occurrence was only recorded for the adjacent tooth or teeth, whereas at month 36, 3 of the 8 occurrences were reported for the implant site (Fig. 6).

Sulcus bleeding index
Bleeding was detected in 15 (34.1%) patients during the study, mostly at month 36 (8 occurrences [53.3%]), at month 12 (7 occurrences [46.7%]) and at month 24 (6 occurrences [40.0%]). Bleeding occurred either at the implant site, the adjacent teeth or at both locations (Fig. 6).

Complications
In total, the following 27 (39.7%) AEs out of the 68 AEs that occurred over the 36-month follow-up period were deemed to be related to the study device or study

treatment: pain (*n* = 18), bleeding, swelling, inflammation/infection (*n* = 6) and unfulfilled implant success criteria (*n* = 3). None (0%) of the 7 SAEs were deemed to be related to the study device or study treatment.

Discussion
The prospective, open-label, single-arm study investigated ceramic implants for replacing a single missing tooth. The implant survival and success rates 36 months after implant surgery were both 97.5%. The mean bone loss was most pronounced in the first half-year after implant surgery (0.88 mm) and remained relatively stable between 12 and 36 months, which resulted in an overall bone loss of 0.97 mm at 36 months.

The survival and success rates of 97.5% 36 months after implant surgery described here are comparable with the published literature on ceramic and titanium

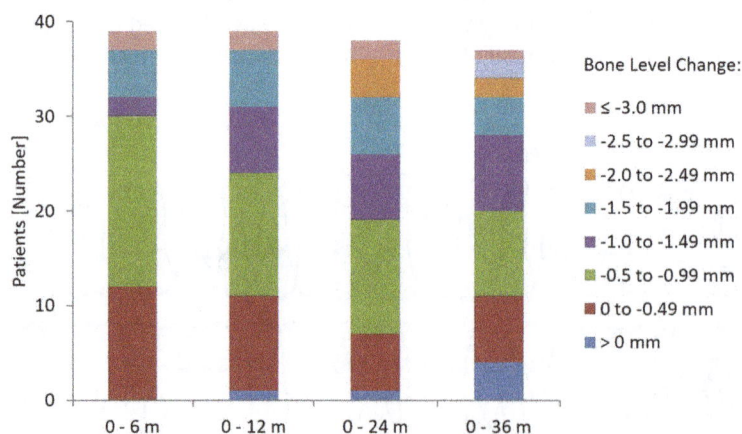

Fig. 4 Categorized bone level changes. ITT population (*n* = 44). n (0–6 m) = 39; n (0–12 m) = 39; n (0–24 m) = 38; n (0–36 m) = 37. Missing values were excluded from the analysis. ITT: Intention to treat; m: Months; n: Number

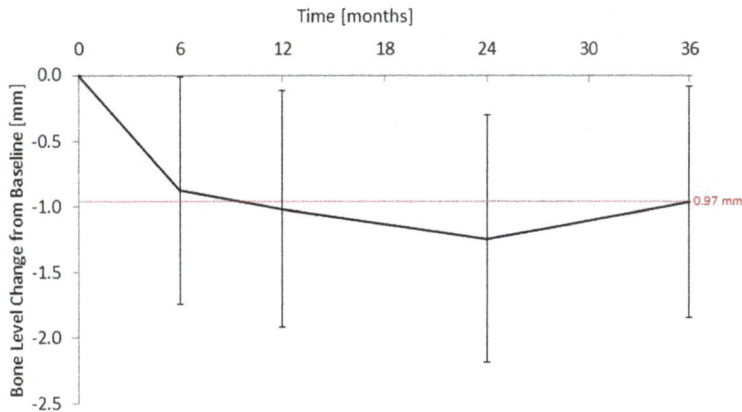

Fig. 5 Bone levels (mean ± SD) from implant surgery to 36-month follow up visit. ITT population ($n = 44$). n (0–6 m) = 39; n (0–12 m) = 39; n (0–24 m) = 38; n (0–36 m) = 37. Missing values were excluded from the analysis. ITT: Intention to treat; m: Months; n: Number; SD: Standard deviation

implants [26, 27], confirming the good clinical performance of ceramic implant. This within the limits of this study, as a single-arm study design was selected for this study.

In a recent systematic review that included 14 studies using zirconia implants, an overall survival rate of 92% (95% CIs: 87% to 95%) after one year of functional loading was calculated [26]. Only 4 of these 14 studies examined a monotype ceramic implant system separately, and these had an average observational period of at least 2 years. The survival rate in these 4 studies after an average of 2 to 5.9 years was between 77.3 and 100% [22, 28, 29]. The authors state that the heterogeneity of the selected studies may be behind the differences in survival rates. On the one hand the examined zirconia implants varied considerably in implant design and surface characteristics while, on the other, the studies differed in their surgical protocols and prosthetic superstructures [26].

In a systematic review that analysed 46 studies with a mean follow-up of at least 5 years in function after the insertion of titanium implants, the overall survival rate of titanium implants supporting single crowns was 97.2% (95% CIs: 96.3% to 97.9%) after 5 years [27], which

is comparable to the survival rate evaluated in the current study. This strengthens the results of several animal studies showing that zirconia implants undergo osseointegration similar to [10, 14, 15, 30–36], or even better than [16], titanium implants, and confirms the biocompatibility of zirconia as a dental implant material [37]. Furthermore, various in vivo and in vitro studies investigating soft tissue response around zirconia discovered similar [38] or even superior healing response, less inflammatory infiltrate and reduced plaque adhesion on zirconium oxide discs compared to pure titanium [39–42]. Excellent gingival conditions around monotype ceramic implants were described by Kniha [43]. In addition, like titanium, zirconia is known to have excellent mechanical properties [11, 13, 17].

In contrast to other ceramic implants, the body of the study device features the ZLA surface, a sandblasted, large-grit, acid-etched surface like the SLA surface of titanium implants [24]. Gahlert compared the removal torque of zirconia implants with either machined or sandblasted surfaces placed in mini-pig jaws [44]. The results revealed that a sandblasted surface can display greater stability in bone than machined surfaces, leading

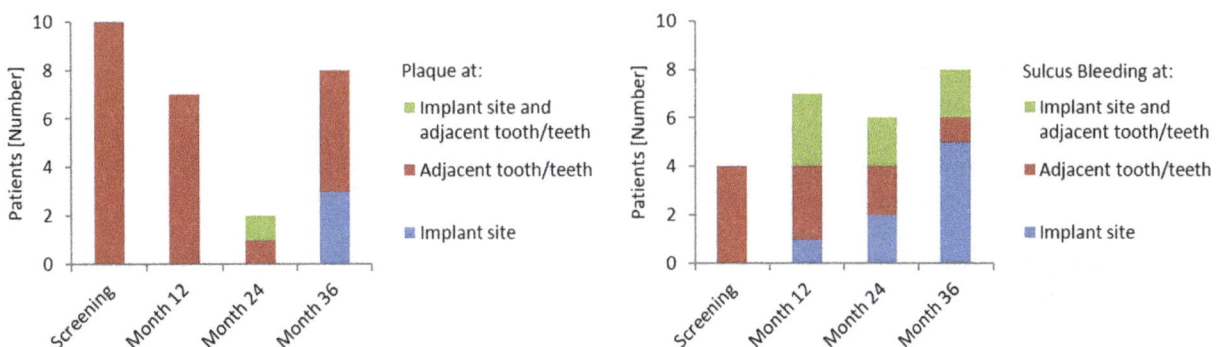

Fig. 6 Number of patients with plaque and sulcus bleeding. ITT population ($n = 44$). ITT: Intention to treat; n: Number

to the conclusion that roughening the zirconia implants improves bone anchoring. Oliva compared zirconia implants with 3 different surfaces in a large study: uncoated, coated and acid-etched. Each group consisted of at least 240 implants [28]. The uncoated implants were roughened by mechanical grinding, while the coated implants were roughened, given a bioactive ceramic coating and subsequently sintered. The survival rate for the acid-etched implants was highest, at 97.6% (n: 333, mean: 3.1 years, range: 1 to 4 years), followed by the coated implants, at 93.6% (n: 249, mean: 3.6 years, range: 2 to 5 years) and the uncoated implants, at 92.8% (n: 249, mean: 3.5 years, range: 2 to 5 years).

In the current study bone loss was 0.97 (± 0.88) mm from implant surgery to month 36, which was similar to [22], or slightly less than [29, 45], results reported in other studies with zirconia implants. The first European Workshop on Periodontology [46] considered a bone loss of less than 1.9 mm after 36 months as "successful." Hence, the bone loss in the current study may be considered as such, all the more so as most of the implants were placed in the maxilla (90.9%) [24]. Marginal bone loss during the first year of loading has been shown to be more pronounced for implants inserted in the maxilla than for those placed in the mandible [29, 45]. The reported bone loss in two studies on zirconia implants (1.63 mm overall and 1.21 mm for single implants after 48 months, and 1.29 mm after 24 months, respectively) [45] was slightly greater than that observed in the current study. As in the study by Borgonovo [45], in this study also bone loss occurred mainly during the first year and stabilized thereafter. Borgonovo assumed that the relatively large bone loss in the first year could be related to bone maturing after surgery and adapting to withstand functional forces [45]. Furthermore, simultaneous augmentation procedures might result in bone loss during the first year of this study – this might be an explanation for bone losses greater than 3 mm after 6, 12 and 24 months at two implants. In this study, the bone loss of 1.02 (± 0.90) mm during the first 12 months after surgery was below the limit of 1.5 mm and considered to be "successful" [46]. As in the study by Borgonovo [45], even a small bone gain was also observed in this study during the follow-up period. In contrast to the previously reported results, in this study bone gain occurred at a later stage (between month 24 and month 36). Borgonovo assumed that bone gain occurred because of new bone trabeculae forming as a result of bone maturation [45].

Most of the AEs that occurred during the 36 months of this study and that were considered to be "related" to the study treatment were experienced during surgery (visit 2), within one week of surgery, or shortly after/in relation to another study intervention. Hence, these AEs can be considered as expected complications following the insertion of dental implants, confirming that there is no safety issue associated with the placement of the ceramic implants.

Conclusion

The results demonstrate that ceramic implants achieve favourable clinical outcomes in the follow-up; so are survival and success rates as well as bone losses comparable to titanium and other ceramic implants. These implants offer a reliable and successful treatment alternative, especially useful for patients who object to metal and request metal-free implants. However, longer term studies with different edentulous morphology need to confirm the present data.

Abbreviations
AE: Adverse event; CI: Confidence interval; DD: Device deficiency; FDI: Fédération Dentaire Internationale; ITT: Intention to treat; m: Months; n: Number; PP: Per protocol; SAS: Safety analysis set; SD: Standard deviation; Y-TZP: Yttria-stabilized zirconia; ZrO$_2$: Zirconia

Acknowledgments
Not applicable.

Funding
This study was funded by Institut Straumann AG, Basel, Switzerland.

Authors' contributions
KHB: carried out surgical procedures, data acquisition and data interpretation (advisor), and took part in drafting the manuscript and critically revised it for important intellectual content. HK: carried out surgical procedures, data acquisition and data interpretation, and revised the manuscript critically for important intellectual content. SS: carried out surgical procedures, data acquisition and data interpretation, and revised the manuscript critically for important intellectual content. MG: carried out surgical procedures, data acquisition and data interpretation, and revised the manuscript critically for important intellectual content. All authors read and approved the final manuscript.

Competing interests
All authors except DW are involved in training and education activities for Institut Straumann AG, Basel, Switzerland. The authors declare that they have no further competing interests. Institut Straumann AG manufactures the implants. Therefore, Institut Straumann AG gains financially, if the PURE Ceramic Implants would be more widely used.

Author details
[1]Hannover Medical School, Hannover, Germany. [2]Dental Clinic, Bormann Oralchirurgie am Hafen, Hamburg, Germany. [3]Dental Clinic Kniha Gahlert, Munich, Germany. [4]High Tech Research Center, University Hospital Basel, Basel, Switzerland. [5]Klinikum Stuttgart, Katharinenhospital, Stuttgart, Germany.

References

1. Branemark PI, Hansson BO, Adell R, Breine U, Lindstrom J, Hallen O, et al. Osseointegrated implants in the treatment of the edentulous jaw. Experience from a 10-year period. Scand J Plast Reconstr Surg Suppl. 1977;16:1–132.

2. Adell R, Lekholm U, Rockler B, Branemark PI. A 15-year study of osseointegrated implants in the treatment of the edentulous jaw. Int J Oral Surg. 1981;10:387–416.

3. Jemt T. Single implants in the anterior maxilla after 15 years of follow-up: comparison with central implants in the edentulous maxilla. Int J Prosthodont. 2008;21:400–8.

4. Mijiritsky E, Lorean A, Mazor Z, Levin L. Implant tooth-supported removable partial denture with at least 15-year long-term follow-up. Clin Implant Dent Relat Res. 2015;17:917–22.

5. Astrand P, Ahlqvist J, Gunne J, Nilson H: Implant treatment of patients with edentulous jaws: a 20-year follow-up. Clin Implant Dent Relat Res 2008, 10: 207–217.

6. Krebs M, Schmenger K, Neumann K, Weigl P, Moser W, Nentwig GH. Long-term evaluation of ANKYLOS(R) dental implants, part i: 20-year life table analysis of a longitudinal study of more than 12,500 implants. Clin Implant Dent Relat Res. 2015;17(Suppl 1):e275–86.

7. Dhima M, Paulusova V, Lohse C, Salinas TJ, Carr AB. Practice-based evidence from 29-year outcome analysis of management of the edentulous jaw using osseointegrated dental implants. J Prosthodont. 2014;23:173–81.

8. Chappuis V, Buser R, Bragger U, Bornstein MM, Salvi GE, Buser D. Long-term outcomes of dental implants with a titanium plasma-sprayed surface: a 20-year prospective case series study in partially edentulous patients. Clin Implant Dent Relat Res. 2013;15:780–90.

9. Sicilia A, Cuesta S, Coma G, Arregui I, Guisasola C, Ruiz E, et al. Titanium allergy in dental implant patients: a clinical study on 1500 consecutive patients. Clin Oral Implants Res. 2008;19:823–35.

10. Depprich R, Zipprich H, Ommerborn M, Mahn E, Lammers L, Handschel J, et al. Osseointegration of zirconia implants: an SEM observation of the bone-implant interface. Head Face Med. 2008;4:25.

11. Luthardt RG, Holzhuter M, Sandkuhl O, Herold V, Schnapp JD, Kuhlisch E, et al. Reliability and properties of ground Y-TZP-zirconia ceramics. J Dent Res. 2002;81:487–91.

12. Moller B, Terheyden H, Acil Y, Purcz NM, Hertrampf K, Tabakov A, et al. A comparison of biocompatibility and osseointegration of ceramic and titanium implants: an in vivo and in vitro study. Int J Oral Maxillofac Surg. 2012;41:638–45.

13. Ozkurt Z, Kazazoglu E. Zirconia dental implants: a literature review. J Oral Implantol. 2011;37:367–76.

14. Scarano A, Di CF, Quaranta M, Piattelli A. Bone response to zirconia ceramic implants: an experimental study in rabbits. J Oral Implantol. 2003;29:8–12.

15. Kohal RJ, Weng D, Bachle M, Strub JR. Loaded custom-made zirconia and titanium implants show similar osseointegration: an animal experiment. J Periodontol. 2004;75:1262–8.

16. Schultze-Mosgau S, Schliephake H, Radespiel-Troger M, Neukam FW. Osseointegration of endodontic endosseous cones: zirconium oxide vs titanium. Oral Surg Oral Med Oral Pathol Oral Radiol Endod. 2000;89:91–8.

17. Zhang Y, Pajares A, Lawn BR. Fatigue and damage tolerance of Y-TZP ceramics in layered biomechanical systems. J Biomed Mater Res B Appl Biomater. 2004;71:166–71.

18. Kohal RJ, Knauf M, Larsson B, Sahlin H, Butz F. One-piece zirconia oral implants: one-year results from a prospective cohort study. 1. Single tooth replacement. J Clin Periodontol. 2012;39:590–7.

19. Andreiotelli M, Wenz HJ, Kohal RJ. Are ceramic implants a viable alternative to titanium implants? A systematic literature review. Clin Oral Implants Res. 2009;20(Suppl 4):32–47.

20. Borgonovo AE, Fabbri A, Vavassori V, Censi R, Maiorana C. Multiple teeth replacement with endosseous one-piece yttrium-stabilized zirconia dental implants. Med Oral Patol Oral Cir Bucal. 2012;17:e981–7.

21. Cannizzaro G, Torchio C, Felice P, Leone M, Esposito M. Immediate occlusal versus non-occlusal loading of single zirconia implants. A multicentre pragmatic randomised clinical trial. Eur J Oral Implantol. 2010;3:111–20.

22. Roehling S, Woelfler H, Hicklin S, Kniha H, Gahlert M. A retrospective clinical study with regard to survival and success rates of zirconia implants up to and after 7 years of loading. Clin Implant Dent Relat Res. 2016;18: 545–58.

23. Vohra F, Al-Kheraif AA, Ab Ghani SM, Abu Hassan MI, Alnassar T, Javed F. Crestal bone loss and periimplant inflammatory parameters around zirconia implants: a systematic review. J Prosthet Dent. 2015;114:351 7.

24. Gahlert M, Kniha H, Weingart D, Schild S, Gellrich NC, Bormann KH. A prospective clinical study to evaluate the performance of zirconium dioxide dental implants in single-tooth gaps. Clin Oral Implants Res. 2016;27: e176–84.

25. Buser D, Weber HP, Lang NP. Tissue integration of non-submerged implants. 1-year results of a prospective study with 100 ITI hollow-cylinder and hollow-screw implants. Clin Oral Implants Res. 1990;1:33–40.

26. Hashim D, Cionca N, Courvoisier DS, Mombelli A. A systematic review of the clinical survival of zirconia implants. Clin Oral Investig. 2016;20:1403–17.

27. Jung RE, Zembic A, Pjetursson BE, Zwahlen M, Thoma DS. Systematic review of the survival rate and the incidence of biological, technical, and aesthetic complications of single crowns on implants reported in longitudinal studies with a mean follow-up of 5 years. Clin Oral Implants Res. 2012; 23(Suppl 6):2–21.

28. Oliva J, Oliva X, Oliva JD. Five-year success rate of 831 consecutively placed zirconia dental implants in humans: a comparison of three different rough surfaces. Int J Oral Maxillofac Implants. 2010;25:336–44.

29. Payer M, Arnetzl V, Kirmeier R, Koller M, Arnetzl G, Jakse N. Immediate provisional restoration of single-piece zirconia implants: a prospective case series - results after 24 months of clinical function. Clin Oral Implants Res. 2013;24:569–75.

30. Dubruille JH, Viguier E, Le NG, Dubruille MT, Auriol M, Le CY. Evaluation of combinations of titanium, zirconia, and alumina implants with 2 bone fillers in the dog. Int J Oral Maxillofac Implants. 1999;14:271–7.

31. Hoffmann O, Angelov N, Gallez F, Jung RE, Weber FE. The zirconia implant-bone interface: a preliminary histologic evaluation in rabbits. Int J Oral Maxillofac Implants. 2008;23:691–5.

32. Gahlert M, Roehling S, Sprecher CM, Kniha H, Milz S, Bormann K. In vivo performance of zirconia and titanium implants: a histomorphometric study in mini pig maxillae. Clin Oral Implants Res. 2012;23:281–6.

33. Wenz HJ, Bartsch J, Wolfart S, Kern M. Osseointegration and clinical success of zirconia dental implants: a systematic review. Int J Prosthodont. 2008; 21:27–36.

34. Kohal RJ, Wolkewitz M, Hinze M, Han JS, Bachle M, Butz F. Biomechanical and histological behavior of zirconia implants: an experiment in the rat. Clin Oral Implants Res. 2009;20:333–9.

35. Assal PA. The osseointegration of zirconia dental implants. Schweiz Monatsschr Zahnmed. 2013;123:644–54.

36. Ichikawa Y, Akagawa Y, Nikai H, Tsuru H. Tissue compatibility and stability of a new zirconia ceramic in vivo. J Prosthet Dent. 1992;68:322–6.

37. Akagawa Y, Ichikawa Y, Nikai H, Tsuru H. Interface histology of unloaded and early loaded partially stabilized zirconia endosseous implant in initial bone healing. J Prosthet Dent. 1993;69:599–604.

38. Pae A, Lee H, Kim HS, Kwon YD, Woo YH. Attachment and growth behaviour of human gingival fibroblasts on titanium and zirconia ceramic surfaces. Biomed Mater. 2009;4:025005.

39. Rimondini L, Cerroni L, Carrassi A, Torricelli P. Bacterial colonization of zirconia ceramic surfaces: an in vitro and in vivo study. Int J Oral Maxillofac Implants. 2002;17:793–8.

40. Scarano A, Piattelli M, Caputi S, Favero GA, Piattelli A. Bacterial adhesion on commercially pure titanium and zirconium oxide disks: an in vivo human study. J Periodontol. 2004;75:292–6.

41. Degidi M, Artese L, Scarano A, Perrotti V, Gehrke P, Piattelli A. Inflammatory infiltrate, microvessel density, nitric oxide synthase expression, vascular endothelial growth factor expression, and proliferative activity in peri-implant soft tissues around titanium and zirconium oxide healing caps. J Periodontol. 2006;77:73–80.

42. Grossner-Schreiber B, Herzog M, Hedderich J, Duck A, Hannig M, Griepentrog M. Focal adhesion contact formation by fibroblasts cultured on surface-modified dental implants: an in vitro study. Clin Oral Implants Res. 2006;17:736–45.

43. Kniha K, Gahlert M, Hicklin S, Bragger U, Kniha H, Milz S. Evaluation of hard and soft tissue dimensions around zirconium oxide implant-supported crowns: a 1-year retrospective study. J Periodontol. 2016;87:511–8.

44. Gahlert M, Gudehus T, Eichhorn S, Steinhauser E, Kniha H, Erhardt W. Biomechanical and histomorphometric comparison between zirconia implants with varying surface textures and a titanium implant in the maxilla of miniature pigs. Clin Oral Implants Res. 2007;18:662–8.

45. Borgonovo AE, Censi R, Vavassori V, Dolci M, Calvo-Guirado JL, Delgado Ruiz RA, et al. Evaluation of the success criteria for zirconia dental implants: a four-year clinical and radiological study. Int J Dent. 2013;2013:463073.

Association between tooth loss and cognitive impairment in community-dwelling older Japanese adults

Sho Saito[1], Takashi Ohi[1,2*] , Takahisa Murakami[3], Takamasa Komiyama[1], Yoshitada Miyoshi[1], Kosei Endo[1], Michihiro Satoh[3], Kei Asayama[4,5], Ryusuke Inoue[6], Masahiro Kikuya[7], Hirohito Metoki[3], Yutaka Imai[5], Takayoshi Ohkubo[4] and Yoshinori Hattori[1]

Abstract

Background: Numerous prospective studies have investigated the association between the number of remaining teeth and dementia or cognitive decline. However, no agreement has emerged on the association between tooth loss and cognitive impairment, possibly due to past studies differing in target groups and methodologies. We aimed to investigate the association between tooth loss, as evaluated through clinical oral examinations, and the development of cognitive impairment in community-dwelling older adults while considering baseline cognitive function.

Methods: This 4-year prospective cohort study followed 140 older adults (69.3% female) without cognitive impairment aged ≥65 years (mean age: 70.9 ± 4.3 years) living in the town of Ohasama, Iwate Prefecture, Japan. Cognitive function was evaluated with the Mini-Mental State Examination (MMSE) in baseline and follow-up surveys. Based on a baseline oral examination, the participants were divided into those with 0–9 teeth and those with ≥10 teeth. To investigate the association between tooth loss and cognitive impairment, we applied a multiple logistic regression analysis adjusted for age, sex, hypertension, diabetes, cerebrovascular/cardiovascular disease, hypercholesterolemia, depressive symptoms, body mass index, smoking status, drinking status, duration of education, and baseline MMSE score.

Results: In the 4 years after the baseline survey, 27 participants (19.3%) developed cognitive impairment (i.e., MMSE scores of ≤24). Multiple logistic regression analysis indicated that participants with 0–9 teeth were more likely to develop cognitive impairment than those with ≥10 teeth were (odds ratio: 3.31; 95% confidence interval: 1.07–10.2). Age, male gender, and baseline MMSE scores were also significantly associated with cognitive impairment.

Conclusions: Tooth loss was independently associated with the development of cognitive impairment within 4 years among community-dwelling older adults. This finding corroborates the hypothesis that tooth loss may be a predictor or risk factor for cognitive decline.

Keywords: Cognitive impairment, Cohort study, Community-dwelling, Elderly, Tooth loss

* Correspondence: tohi@dent.tohoku.ac.jp
[1]Division of Aging and Geriatric Dentistry, Department of Oral Function and Morphology, Tohoku University Graduate School of Dentistry, 4-1 Seiryo-machi, Aoba-ku, Sendai, Miyagi 980-8575, Japan
[2]Japanese Red Cross Ishinomaki Hospital, Ishinomaki, Japan
Full list of author information is available at the end of the article

Background

Dementia is the leading reason for older people needing long-term care in Japan. It is also a major social problem because the need for long-term care not only reduces the patient's quality of life but also places psychological and financial burdens on the family and other caregivers. According to World Health Organization estimates, the number of people with dementia worldwide reached around 50 million in 2017 and is increasing by nearly 10 million new cases annually [1]. Because no effective treatment for dementia has been established, the modifiable predictors and risk factors must be identified in order to reduce the incidence of dementia.

Numerous prospective studies [2–13] have reported an association between oral health, particularly the number of remaining teeth, and dementia or cognitive decline in old age. Conversely, some reports [14–18] found no such association. Recent systematic reviews [19–21] have reached no consensus position on the question. The inconsistencies between studies may arise from differences in target groups and methodologies. Some studies have analyzed specific occupational groups or nursing home residents [3–5, 9, 12, 14]. Several studies have determined the number of remaining teeth through subject-administered questionnaires [7–10, 15, 18], whereas some others have used clinical oral examinations [2, 11, 13, 16, 17]. Furthermore, although baseline cognitive function is closely related to subsequent cognitive decline, only two studies [8, 11] have examined baseline cognitive function as a confounding factor.

We therefore aimed to elucidate the association between tooth loss, as evaluated through oral examinations, and the subsequent development of cognitive impairment in community-dwelling older adults while considering baseline cognitive function.

Methods

Study design and population

This study was performed as a component of the Ohasama Study, a prospective cohort study on hypertension/cardiovascular disease that has followed general inhabitants of Ohasama, a rural town in northern Japan's Iwate Prefecture, since 1986 [22, 23]. Figure 1 shows the study flow diagram. From 2005 to 2012, 448 inhabitants aged ≥65 years participated in the baseline survey. Of them, we excluded 40 participants with missing data and 82 participants who exhibited cognitive decline on cognitive function tests. The remaining 326 inhabitants were included as participants. Of them, 150 (46%) participated in the follow-up survey between 2009 and 2016. After excluding 10 participants with incomplete follow-up survey data, we included 140 participants in the final analysis as the "follow-up group." The mean (± standard deviation) follow-up period was 4.0 ±

0.1 years. We included 176 people who did not participate in the follow-up survey in our "drop-out group."

This study was approved by the Institutional Review Board of the Tohoku University Graduate School of Pharmaceutical Science and conformed to the principles of the Declaration of Helsinki. Written informed consent to participate was obtained from all participants.

Measurements

Tooth loss at the time of the baseline survey was evaluated via count of the number of remaining teeth by specially trained dentists. The median number of remaining teeth was 10, so the participants were divided into those with 0–9 teeth and those with ≥10 teeth. We defined having 0–9 teeth as "multiple tooth loss."

Cognitive function was evaluated with the Mini-Mental State Examination (MMSE) [24] in the baseline and follow-up surveys. Participants with a total score of ≤24 (full score: 30 points) were defined as having cognitive impairment. This cut-off reportedly achieves 83% sensitivity and 93% specificity in diagnosing dementia in Japanese patients [25]. We defined hypertension as a home blood pressure of ≥135/85 mmHg [26], use of antihypertensive medications, or a history of hypertension; diabetes mellitus as a non-fasting glucose concentration of ≥200 mg/dL [27], a glycated hemoglobin concentration of ≥6.5%, use of anti-diabetes medications, or a history of diabetes mellitus; cerebrovascular/cardiovascular disease as a history of atrial fibrillation, heart disease, or cerebrovascular disease; and hypercholesterolemia as a total cholesterol level of ≥220 mg/dL, use of anti-hypercholesterolemia medications, or a history of hypercholesterolemia. Depressive symptoms were evaluated with the Zung Self-Rating Depression Scale (SDS) [28]. The maximum SDS score is 80, and participants with scores of ≥40 were defined as having depressive symptoms. Body mass index (BMI) was calculated as weight in kilograms divided by height in meters squared. Participants were categorized as being current smokers/drinkers or not being current smokers/drinkers. Duration of education was categorized as being either less than 10 years or at least 10 years.

Statistical analysis

Bivariate analyses were performed with Student's t-test or the Wilcoxon rank sum test for continuous variables and the chi-squared test for categorical variables. A multiple logistic regression analysis was used to calculate adjusted odds ratios (ORs) and their 95% confidence intervals (CIs) for the development of cognitive impairment within 4 years of the baseline survey. Because few participants developed cognitive impairment, we applied logistic regression with penalized maximum likelihood

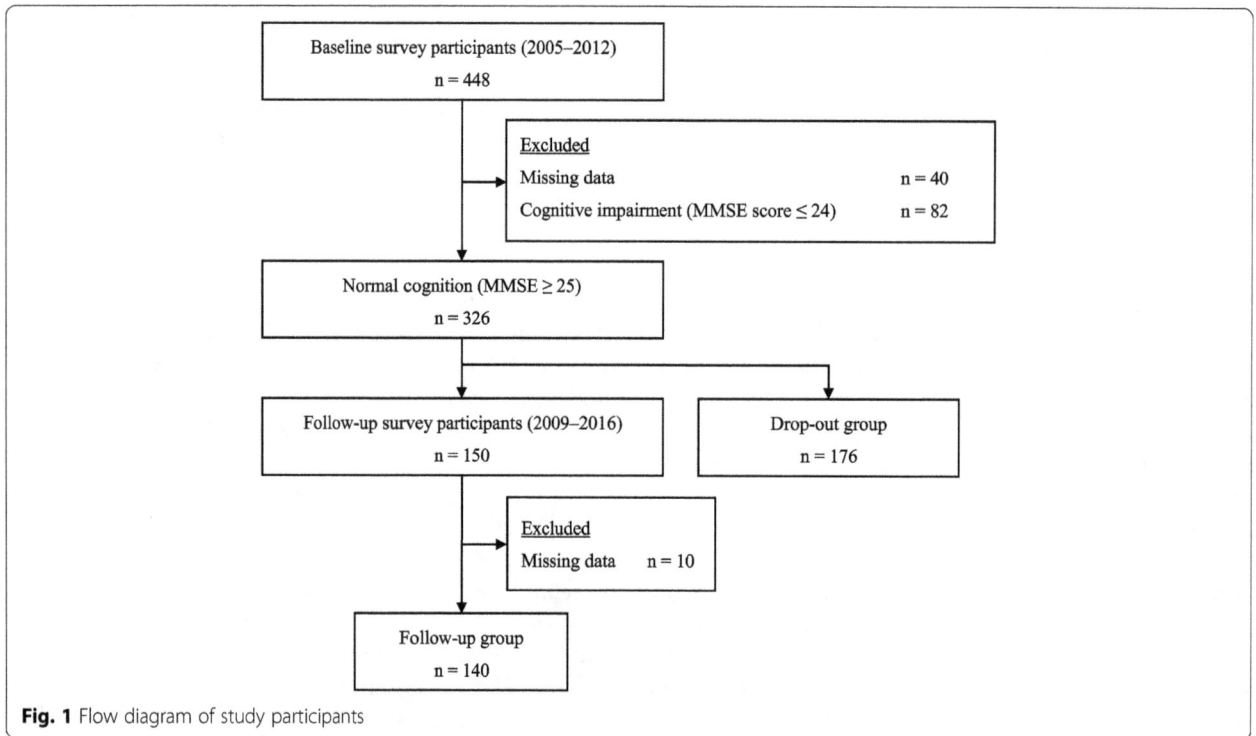

Fig. 1 Flow diagram of study participants

estimation for rare events analysis [29]. The statistical significance threshold was $p < 0.05$ for all tests. Statistical analyses were performed with JMP Pro 12 (SAS Institute, Cary, NC, USA) and Stata 14 (StataCorp LLC, College Station, TX, USA).

Results

The baseline characteristics of the follow-up and drop-out groups are shown in Table 1. The drop-out participants were significantly older and more likely to have hypertension than the follow-up group participants were, but the two groups did not significantly differ in sex, duration of education, BMIs, baseline MMSE scores, or frequencies of multiple tooth loss, current smoker status, current drinker status, diabetes mellitus, cerebro-vascular/cardiovascular disease, hypercholesterolemia, or depressive symptoms. Of the follow-up participants, 27 (19.3%) had cognitive impairment at the follow-up

Table 1 Characteristics of the follow-up and drop-out groups

	Follow-up ($n = 140$)	Drop-out ($n = 176$)	P-value
Age (mean ± SD)	70.9 ± 4.3	73.2 ± 4.8	< 0.0001
Male (%)	30.7	29.0	0.7
Hypertension (%)	53.6	66.5	0.02
Diabetes (%)	11.4	17.6	0.1
Cerebrovascular/cardiovascular disease (%)	12.9	15.3	0.5
Hypercholesterolemia (%)	60.7	54.0	0.2
Depressive symptoms (%)	10.7	10.2	0.9
BMI (mean ± SD)	23.6 ± 3.2	23.9 ± 2.8	0.4
Current smoker (%)	7.1	5.7	0.6
Current drinker (%)	39.3	32.4	0.2
< 10 years of education (%)	73.6	76.7	0.5
Baseline MMSE score (mean ± SD)	27.7 ± 1.6	27.8 ± 1.5	0.4
Multiple tooth loss (%)	50.7	46.6	0.5

P-values were determined with Student's t-test or the Wilcoxon rank sum test for continuous variables and the chi-squared test for categorical variables. Multiple tooth loss was defined as having 0–9 remaining teeth
BMI body mass index, MMSE Mini-Mental State Examination, SD standard deviation

survey. Table 2 compares the baseline characteristics of individuals who retained normal cognition and those who developed cognitive impairment by the follow-up survey. Compared to the participants with normal cognition, those with cognitive impairment were significantly older, had significantly lower baseline MMSE scores, and were significantly more likely to be male and to exhibit multiple tooth loss.

Table 3 shows the ORs and 95% CIs for developing cognitive impairment. In the age- and sex-adjusted model, multiple tooth loss was associated with an increased likelihood of developing cognitive impairment (OR: 3.39; 95% CI: 1.29–8.88). This association remained (OR: 3.31; 95% CI: 1.07–10.2) even after adjusting for age, sex, hypertension, diabetes, cerebrovascular/cardiovascular disease, hypercholesterolemia, depressive symptoms, BMI, smoking status, drinking status, duration of education, and baseline MMSE score. Greater ages, male gender, and lower baseline MMSE scores were also significantly associated with developing cognitive impairment. We did not find an interaction between age and tooth loss ($p = 0.925$).

Discussion

In the present study, we examined whether multiple tooth loss, as evaluated with professional clinical oral examinations, is associated with developing cognitive impairment in community-dwelling older adults. We found that the presence of multiple tooth loss significantly increased the risk of developing cognitive impairment within 4 years independently of age, sex, hypertension, diabetes, cerebrovascular/cardiovascular disease, hypercholesterolemia, depressive symptoms, BMI, smoking

status, drinking status, duration of education, and baseline MMSE score. This finding suggests that maintaining healthy dentition reduces the risk of cognitive impairment.

This study is one of the few longitudinal studies [2, 11, 13, 16, 17] to investigate the association between tooth loss, as evaluated with oral examinations, and cognitive impairment in community-dwelling older adults. A survey of community-dwelling older adults in South Korea [2] reported that a paucity of remaining teeth was related to the onset of dementia within 2.4 years. A 5-year prospective cohort study of Japanese community residents [11] reported that tooth loss predicted the development of mild memory impairment, and another 5-year cohort study of older adults in Japan [13] found that tooth loss was associated with an increased risk of developing all-cause dementia and Alzheimer's disease. Our observation of a significant association between tooth loss and cognitive dysfunction corroborates these previous studies' results. However, some studies [16, 17] found no association between tooth loss and cognitive decline. These studies differ from the others in that the participants were all older women [17] or in that the participants included middle-aged people as well as older ones [16].

In this study, we included the baseline MMSE score as a confounding factor in the multivariate analysis in order to consider the possible effect of mild cognitive decline that went undetected in screening tests. However, multiple tooth loss remained associated with cognitive impairment even after adjusting for baseline MMSE scores. Only two previous studies [8, 11] have adjusted for baseline cognitive function. A cohort study of older Japanese adults [8] found that having few teeth without

Table 2 Baseline characteristics of individuals with normal cognition and those who developed cognitive impairment

	Normal cognition ($n = 113$)	Cognitive impairment ($n = 27$)	P-value
Age (mean ± SD)	70.5 ± 4.2	72.3 ± 4.5	0.04
Male (%)	26.6	48.2	0.03
Hypertension (%)	52.2	59.3	0.5
Diabetes (%)	9.7	18.5	0.2
Cerebrovascular/cardiovascular disease (%)	11.5	18.5	0.3
Hypercholesterolemia (%)	61.1	59.3	0.9
Depressive symptoms (%)	8.9	18.5	0.1
BMI (mean ± SD)	23.4 ± 3.0	24.3 ± 4.0	0.2
Current smoker (%)	7.1	7.4	0.9
Current drinker (%)	41.6	29.6	0.3
< 10 years of education (%)	71.7	81.5	0.3
Baseline MMSE score (mean ± SD)	28.0 ± 1.6	26.4 ± 1.2	< 0.0001
Multiple tooth loss (%)	46.0	70.4	0.02

P-values were determined with Student's t-test or the Wilcoxon rank sum test for continuous variables and the chi-squared test for categorical variables. Multiple tooth loss was defined as having 0–9 remaining teeth

BMI body mass index, MMSE Mini-Mental State Examination, SD standard deviation

Table 3 Multiple logistic regression model for development of cognitive impairment

	Age- and sex-adjusted model		Fully adjusted model[a]	
	OR (95% CI)	P-value	OR (95% CI)	P-value
Age	1.07 (0.98–1.18)	0.1	1.14 (1.01–1.29)	0.03
Male gender	3.34 (1.32–8.46)	0.01	4.60 (1.25–16.7)	0.02
Hypertension			1.28 (0.44–3.70)	0.6
Diabetes			3.77 (0.79–18.0)	0.1
Cerebrovascular/cardiovascular disease			2.62 (0.68–10.1)	0.2
Hypercholesterolemia			1.68 (0.56–5.00)	0.3
Depressive symptoms			2.50 (0.54–11.4)	0.2
BMI			1.04 (0.87–1.25)	0.6
Current smoker			0.48 (0.69–3.42)	0.5
Current drinker			0.50 (0.14–1.72)	0.3
Duration of education			1.31 (0.33–5.14)	0.7
Baseline MMSE score			0.48 (0.31–0.74)	0.001
Multiple tooth loss	3.39 (1.29–8.88)	0.013	3.31 (1.07–10.2)	0.037

The objective variable for the multiple logistic regression analysis was whether cognitive function declined within 4 years, and the explanatory variable was whether multiple tooth loss was present. Multiple tooth loss was defined as having 0–9 remaining teeth
[a]Adjusted for age, sex, hypertension, diabetes, cerebrovascular/cardiovascular disease, hypercholesterolemia, depressive symptoms, BMI, current smoker status, current drinker status, duration of education, and baseline MMSE score
BMI body mass index, *CI* confidence interval, *MMSE* Mini-Mental State Examination, *OR* odds ratio, *SD* standard deviation

dentures was associated with an increased risk of dementia independently of forgetfulness. A 5-year prospective cohort study of Japanese community residents [11] found that tooth loss was associated with developing mild memory impairment even after adjusting for baseline MMSE scores.

Several mechanisms may explain the association between tooth loss and cognitive impairment. First, the association may depend on chronic inflammation arising from periodontal disease, which is a major cause of tooth loss in later life. Previous studies showed that periodontal disease was the most common reason for tooth extraction in patients older than 45 years [30, 31]. Therefore, chronic exposure to periodontal disease–related inflammation is presumably a more serious problem in older adults with multiple tooth loss than in those without multiple tooth loss. Clinical attachment loss [32] and alveolar bone resorption [33], both of which indicate the cumulative history of periodontal disease, are associated with cognitive impairment. Systemic inflammatory reactions arising from periodontal disease are a hypothesized risk factor for Alzheimer's disease [34–36].

Second, the association may depend on changes in food intake and nutritional status due to tooth loss. Poor nutritional status and nutrient deficiencies are reportedly associated with cognitive decline and Alzheimer's disease [37–39]. A nationwide survey in the United States [40] found that individuals with fewer than 28 teeth had significantly lower intakes of carrots, tossed salads, and dietary fiber and had lower serum concentrations of β-carotene, folic acid, and vitamin C relative to individuals who were fully dentate. A survey of older Japanese adults [41] found that tooth loss was associated with decreased intakes of vegetables, fish, and shellfish. Therefore, macronutrient and micronutrient deficiencies resulting from decreased masticatory performance may contribute to cognitive impairment in older adults with missing teeth.

Third, the association may arise from deteriorations in masticatory performance reducing brain stimulation. Mastication-related trigeminal nerve sensory inputs reportedly increase cerebral blood flow [42], which in turn promotes arousal and activates a broad region that includes the sensory motor cortex, supplementary motor cortex, insular cortex, thalamus, and cerebellum [43]. Alzheimer's disease model rats fed soft foods exhibit deficiencies in memory and learning abilities relative to rats fed hard foods [44], and rats with extracted molars exhibit reduced acetylcholine release in the cerebral cortex and deficiencies in spatial memory [45]. Therefore, masticatory dysfunction due to tooth loss may adversely affect brain function and thereby promote cognitive impairment.

Besides tooth loss, the factors significantly associated with cognitive impairment were advanced age, male gender, and low baseline MMSE scores. However, unlike tooth loss, these additional factors are unmodifiable. Practicing proper oral health to maintain healthy dentition may reduce the risk of future cognitive impairment. Furthermore, maintaining masticatory performance through prostheses and balanced nutritional intakes may reduce the negative impact of tooth loss on cognitive function. A 4-year prospective cohort study of individuals aged ≥65 years in Japan's Aichi Prefecture [8] found that those with few teeth and no dentures had an increased risk of dementia relative to those with ≥20 teeth, but the risk of dementia was not significantly elevated in individuals with few teeth who used dentures. Intervention studies are needed to clarify whether restoring masticatory function and balancing nutritional intakes can prevent cognitive impairment.

This study has several limitations. First, the follow-up rate was not high (46%), and the follow-up pool might have been biased towards individuals who were healthier and had greater health awareness. Therefore, the possibility of selection bias should be considered when generalizing the present findings. However, this bias will not affect the internal validity of the relationship between tooth loss and the onset of cognitive impairment. Further, the follow-up and drop-out groups did not differ in any baseline characteristics except for age and hypertension rates. As for oral health, the participants' average baseline number of teeth, measured from 2005 to 2012, was approximately five fewer than the average number in age-matched older Japanese adults recorded in national survey data from 2011 [46]. This suggests that our participants might not have been in good oral health. In addition, we may have lacked the participation of elderly people who were developing severe cognitive impairment during the 4 year follow-up; therefore, there is a possibility that the association between tooth loss and cognitive impairment was underestimated. Second, we did not evaluate dementia onset as an outcome. Instead, we screened for dementia with the MMSE, but this test is an indicator of cognitive function used worldwide in research and clinical practice. Its reliability for diagnosing dementia has been shown for Japanese patients [25]. Third, the timecourse of tooth loss was not taken into account. A previous prospective study showed that the rates of tooth loss and periodontal disease progression predicted subsequent cognitive decline [4]. Fourth, there is the problem of reverse causality. A previous study reported that cognitive decline was associated with increased odds of complete tooth loss, infrequent toothbrushing, and higher plaque levels [47]. Decline in cognitive function might increase the risk of tooth loss through poor oral hygiene because of reductions in oral health consciousness. In the present study, participants with cognitive decline at the baseline survey were excluded and the baseline MMSE scores were included as a confounding factor in the multivariate analyses to avoid the effect of reverse causality; however, there is the possibility that some participants who lost their teeth due to the influence of mild cognitive decline that was not detected in our evaluation were included.

Finally, we could not adjust for all possible confounding factors. For example, low socioeconomic status, absence of spouse, unhealthy lifestyles, and certain genes are potentially associated with cognitive decline, but we could not collect data on these factors (although duration of education is a potential proxy for socioeconomic status). However, we did control for many potential confounders, including medical history, based on measurements from medical examinations, and our findings were robust.

Conclusions

This prospective cohort study of community-dwelling older adults indicated that multiple tooth loss was associated with the development of cognitive impairment. This finding supports the hypothesis that tooth loss is a predictor or risk factor for cognitive decline. Both tooth loss and cognitive impairment are chronically accumulated over time. Further studies should be conducted to confirm the true nature of the impacts of tooth loss on cognitive impairment.

Abbreviations

BMI: body mass index; CI: confidence interval; MMSE: Mini-Mental State Examination; OR: odds ratio; SDS: Zung Self-Rating Depression Scale

Acknowledgements

The authors are grateful to Dr. Mikio Hirano (Department of Community Medical Support, Tohoku University, Sendai, Japan) and Dr. Aya Hosokawa (Center for Gerontology and Social Science, National Center for Geriatrics and Gerontology, Aichi, Japan) for advice on measuring MMSE scores and to Dr. Jun Aida (Center for Epidemiology, Biostatistics and Clinical Research, Tohoku University Graduate School of Dentistry, Sendai, Japan) for advice on data analysis and other considerations.

Funding

This study was partly supported by Grants-in-Aid for Scientific Research (C) (15 K11146 and 16 K11850) and Grants-in-Aid for Young Scientists (B) (22792106, 23792202, 25861821, and 25862072) from the Ministry of Education, Culture, Sports, Science and Technology of Japan and by a Health Labour Sciences Research Grant (H26-Junkankitou [Seisaku]-Ippan-001) from the Ministry of Health, Labour and Welfare of Japan. This study's funding sources played no part in the design, methods, participant recruitment, data collection, analysis, or preparation of this paper.

Authors' contributions

SS, TO, TK, YI, TO, and YH generated the study concept and design. SS, TO, YM, TK, KE, MS, KA, RI, MK, HM, YI, TO, and YH acquired and organized the data. SS, TO, TM, TK, YM, and KE analyzed and interpreted the data. SS, TO, TM, TK, and YH wrote the first draft of the manuscript. SS, TO, TM, TK, YM, KE, TO, and YH contributed critical revisions and important intellectual content to the manuscript. All authors read and approved the final manuscript.

Competing interests

The authors declare that they have no competing interests.

Author details

[1]Division of Aging and Geriatric Dentistry, Department of Oral Function and Morphology, Tohoku University Graduate School of Dentistry, 4-1 Seiryo-machi, Aoba-ku, Sendai, Miyagi 980-8575, Japan. [2]Japanese Red Cross Ishinomaki Hospital, Ishinomaki, Japan. [3]Division of Public Health, Hygiene and Epidemiology, Faculty of Medicine, Tohoku Medical and Pharmaceutical University, Sendai, Japan. [4]Department of Hygiene and Public Health, Teikyo University School of Medicine, Tokyo, Japan. [5]Department of Planning for Drug Development and Clinical Evaluation, Tohoku University Graduate School of Pharmaceutical Sciences, Sendai, Japan. [6]Department of Medical Informatics, Tohoku University Graduate School of Medicine, Sendai, Japan. [7]Department of Preventive Medicine and Epidemiology, Tohoku Medical Megabank Organization, Tohoku University, Sendai, Japan.

References

1. World Health Organization. Dementia fact sheet. 2017. http://www.who.int/mediacentre/factsheets/fs362/en. Accessed 7 Aug 2018.
2. Kim JM, Stewart R, Prince M, Kim SW, Yang SJ, Shin IS, et al. Dental health, nutritional status and recent-onset dementia in a Korean community population. Int J Geriatr Psychiatry. 2007;22:850–5.
3. Stein PS, Desrosiers M, Donegam SJ, Yepes JF, Kryscio RJ. Tooth loss, dementia and neuropathology in the Nun study. J Am Dent Assoc. 2007;138:1314–22.
4. Kaye EK, Valencia A, Baba N, Spiro A III, Dietrich T, Garcia RI. Tooth loss and periodontal disease predict poor cognitive function in older men. J Am Geriatr Soc. 2010;58:713–8.
5. Stein PS, Kryscio RJ, Desrosiers M, Donegan SJ, Gibbs MB. Tooth loss, apolipoprotein E, and decline in delayed word recall. J Dent Res. 2010;89:473–7.
6. Arrive E, Letenneur L, Matharan F, Laporte C, Helmer C, Barberger-Gateau P, et al. Oral health condition of French elderly and risk of dementia: a longitudinal cohort study. Community Dent Oral Epidemiol. 2012;40:230–8.
7. Paganini-Hill WSC, Atchison A. Dentition, dental health habits, and dementia: The Leisure World Cohort Study. J Am Geriatr Soc. 2012;60:1556–63.
8. Yamamoto T, Kondo K, Hirai H, Nakade M, Aida J, Hirata Y. Association between self-reported dental health status and onset of dementia: a 4-year prospective cohort study of older Japanese adults from the Aichi Gerontological evaluation study (AGES) project. Psychosom Med. 2012;74:241–8.
9. Batty GD, Li Q, Huxley R, Zoungas S, Taylor BA, Neal B, et al. Oral disease in relation to future risk of dementia and cognitive decline: prospective cohort study based on the action in diabetes and vascular disease: Preterax and Diamicron modified-release controlled evaluation (ADVANCE) trial. Eur Psychiatry. 2013;28:49–52.
10. Reyes-Ortiz CA, Luque JS, Eriksson CK, Soto L. Self-reported tooth loss and cognitive function: data from the Hispanic established populations for epidemiologic studies of the elderly (Hispanic EPESE). Colombia Medica. 2013;44:139–45.
11. Okamoto N, Morikawa M, Tomioka K, Yanagi M, Amano N, Kurumatani N. Association between tooth loss and the development of mild memory impairment in the elderly: the Fujiwara-kyo study. J Alzheimer's Disease. 2015;44:777–86.
12. Zhu J, Li X, Zhu F, Chen L, Zhang C, McGrath C, et al. Multiple tooth loss is associated with vascular cognitive impairment in subjects with acute ischemic stroke. J Periodont Res. 2015;50:683–8.
13. Takeuchi K, Ohara T, Furuta M, Takeshita T, Shibata Y, Hata J, et al. Tooth loss and risk of dementia in the community: the Hisayama study. J Am Geriatr Soc. 2017;65:e95–e100.
14. Shimazaki Y, Soh I, Saito T, Yamashita Y, Koga T, Miyazaki H, et al. Influence of dentition status on physical disability, mental impairment, and mortality in institutionalized elderly people. J Dent Res. 2001;80:340–5.
15. Hansson P, Eriksson Sörman D, Bergdahl J, Bergdahl M, Nyberg L, Adolfsson R, et al. Dental status is unrelated to risk of dementia: a 20-year prospective study. J Am Geriatr Soc. 2014;62:979–81.
16. Naorungroj S, Schoenbach VJ, Wruck L, Mosley TH, Gottesman RF, Alonso A, et al. Tooth loss, periodontal disease, and cognitive decline in the atherosclerosis risk in communities (ARIC) study. Community Dent Oral Epidemiol. 2015;43:47–57.
17. Stewart R, Stenman U, Hakeberg M, Hagglin C, Gustafson D, Skoog I. Associations between oral health and risk of dementia in a 37-year follow-up study: the prospective population study of women in Gothenburg. J Am Geriatr Soc. 2015;15:100–5.
18. Tsakos G, Watt RG, Rouxel PL, Oliveira C, Demakakos P. Tooth loss associated with physical and cognitive decline in older adults. J Am Geriatr Soc. 2015;63:91–9.
19. Cerutti-Kopplin D, Feine J, Padilha DM, de Souza RF, Ahmadi M, Rompré P, et al. Tooth loss increases the risk of diminished cognitive function: a systematic review and meta-analysis. JDR Clin Trans Res. 2016;1:10–9.
20. Wu B, Fillenbaum GG, Plassman BL, Guo L. Association between oral health and cognitive status: a systematic review. J Am Geriatr Soc. 2016;64:739–51.
21. Tonsekar PP, Jiang SS, Yue G. Periodontal disease, tooth loss and dementia: is there a link? A systematic review. Gerodontology. 2017;34:151–63.
22. Imai Y, Nagai K, Sakuma M, Sakuma H, Nakatsuka H, Satoh H, et al. Ambulatory blood pressure of adults in Ohasama. Japan Hypertention. 1993;22:900–12.
23. Ohkubo T, Asayama K, Kikuya M, Metoki H, Hoshi H, Hashimoto J, et al. How many times should blood pressure be measured at home for better prediction of stroke risk? Ten-year follow-up results from the Ohasama study. J Hypertens. 2004;22:1099–104.
24. Folstein MF, Folstein SE, McHugh PR. "Mini-mental state". A practical method for grading the cognitive state of patients for the clinician. J Psychiatr Res. 1975;12:189–98.
25. Mori E, Mitani Y, Yamadori A. Usefulness of a Japanese version of the minimental state test in neurological patients (in Japanese). Shinnkei Shinrigaku. 1985;1:2–10.
26. Tsuji I, Imai Y, Nagai K, Ohkubo T, Watanabe N, Minami N, et al. Proposal of reference values for home blood pressure measurement: prognostic criteria based on a prospective observation of the general population in Ohasama. Japan Am J Hypertens. 1997;10:409–18.
27. The Committee of the Japan Diabetes Society on the Diagnostic Criteria of Diabetes Mellitus, Seino Y, Nanjo K, Tajima N, Kadowaki T, Kashiwagi A, et al. Report of the Committee on the Classification and Diagnostic Criteria of Diabetes Mellitus. J Diabetes Investig. 2010;1:212–28.
28. Zung WWK. Depression in the normal aged. Psychosomatics. 1967;8:287–92.
29. Williams R. Analyzing Rare Events with Logistic Regression. 2018. https://www3.nd.edu/~rwilliam/stats3/RareEvents.pdf. Accessed 7 Aug 2018.
30. Aida J, Ando Y, Akhter R, Aoyama H, Masui M, Morita M. Reasons for permanent tooth extractions in Japan. J Epidemiol. 2006;16:214–9.
31. Trovik TA, Klock KS, Haugejorden O. Trends in reasons for tooth extractions in Norway from 1968 to 1998. Acta Odontol Scand. 2000;58:89–96.
32. Gil-Montoya JA, Sanchez-Lara I, Carnero-Pardo C, Fornieles F, Montes J, Vilchez R, et al. Is periodontitis a risk factor for cognitive impairment and dementia? A case-control study. J Periodontol. 2015;86:244–53.
33. Shin HS, Shin MS, Ahn YB, Choi BY, Nam JH, Kim HD. Periodontitis is associated with cognitive impairment in elderly Koreans: results from the Yangpyeong cohort study. J Am Geriatr Soc. 2016;64:162–7.
34. Watts A, Crimmins EM, Gatz M. Inflammation as a potential mediator for the association between periodontal disease and Alzheimer's disease. Neuropsychiatr Dis Treat. 2008;4:865–76.
35. Holmes C, Cunningham C, Zotova E, Woolford J, Dean C, Kerr S, et al. Systemic inflammation and disease progression in Alzheimer disease. Neurology. 2009;73:768–74.
36. Sparks Stein P, Steffen MJ, Smith C, Jicha G, Ebersole JL, Abner E, et al. Serum antibodies to periodontal pathogens are a risk factor for Alzheimer's disease. Alzheimers Dement. 2012;8:196–203.
37. Larrieu S, Letenneur L, Helmer C, Dartigues JF, Barberger-Gateau P. Nutritional factors and risk of incident dementia in the PAQUID longitudinal cohort. J Nutr Health Aging. 2004;8:150–4.
38. Harrison FE. A critical review of vitamin C for the prevention of age-related cognitive decline and Alzheimer's disease. J Alzheimers Dis. 2012;29:711–26.
39. Miller JW, Harvey DJ, Beckett LA, Green R, Farias ST, Reed BR, et al. Vitamin D status and rates of cognitive decline in a multiethnic cohort of older adults. JAMA Neurol. 2015;72:1295–303.
40. Nowjack-Raymer RE, Sheiham A. Numbers of natural teeth, diet, and nutritional status in US adults. J Dent Res. 2007;86:1171–5.
41. Yoshihara A, Watanabe R, Nishimuta M, Hanada N, Miyazaki H. The relationship between dietary intake and the number of teeth in elderly Japanese subjects. Gerodontology. 2005;22:211–8.

42. Momose T, Nishikawa J, Watanabe T, Sasaki Y, Senda M, Kubota K, et al. Effect of mastication on regional cerebral blood flow in humans examined by positron-emission tomography with ^{15}O-labelled water and magnetic resonance imaging. Arch Oral Biol. 1997;42:57–61.

43. Onozuka M, Fujita M, Watanabe K, Hirano Y, Niwa M, Nishiyama K, et al. Mapping brain region activity during chewing: a functional magnetic resonance imaging study. J Dent Res. 2002;81:743–6.

44. Kushida S, Kimoto K, Hori N, Toyoda M, Karasawa N, Yamamoto T, et al. Soft-diet feeding decreases dopamine release and impairs aversion learning in Alzheimer model rats. Neurosci Lett. 2008;439:208–11.

45. Kato T, Usami T, Noda Y, Hasegawa M, Ueda M, Nabeshima T. The effect of the loss of molar teeth on spatial memory and acetylcholine release from the parietal cortex in aged rats. Behav Brain Res. 1997;83:239–42.

46. Japanese Ministry of Health, Labour and Welfare. The survey of dental disease in 2011. 2012. http://www.mhlw.go.jp/toukei/list/dl/62-23-02.pdf. Accessed 7 Aug 2018. [in Japanese].

47. Naorungroj S, Slade GD, Beck JD, Mosley TH, Gottesman RF, Alonso A, et al. Cognitive decline and oral health in middle-aged adults in the ARIC study. J Dent Res. 2015;92:795–801.

Permissions

All chapters in this book were first published in OH, by BioMed Central; hereby published with permission under the Creative Commons Attribution License or equivalent. Every chapter published in this book has been scrutinized by our experts. Their significance has been extensively debated. The topics covered herein carry significant findings which will fuel the growth of the discipline. They may even be implemented as practical applications or may be referred to as a beginning point for another development.

The contributors of this book come from diverse backgrounds, making this book a truly international effort. This book will bring forth new frontiers with its revolutionizing research information and detailed analysis of the nascent developments around the world.

We would like to thank all the contributing authors for lending their expertise to make the book truly unique. They have played a crucial role in the development of this book. Without their invaluable contributions this book wouldn't have been possible. They have made vital efforts to compile up to date information on the varied aspects of this subject to make this book a valuable addition to the collection of many professionals and students.

This book was conceptualized with the vision of imparting up-to-date information and advanced data in this field. To ensure the same, a matchless editorial board was set up. Every individual on the board went through rigorous rounds of assessment to prove their worth. After which they invested a large part of their time researching and compiling the most relevant data for our readers.

The editorial board has been involved in producing this book since its inception. They have spent rigorous hours researching and exploring the diverse topics which have resulted in the successful publishing of this book. They have passed on their knowledge of decades through this book. To expedite this challenging task, the publisher supported the team at every step. A small team of assistant editors was also appointed to further simplify the editing procedure and attain best results for the readers.

Apart from the editorial board, the designing team has also invested a significant amount of their time in understanding the subject and creating the most relevant covers. They scrutinized every image to scout for the most suitable representation of the subject and create an appropriate cover for the book.

The publishing team has been an ardent support to the editorial, designing and production team. Their endless efforts to recruit the best for this project, has resulted in the accomplishment of this book. They are a veteran in the field of academics and their pool of knowledge is as vast as their experience in printing. Their expertise and guidance has proved useful at every step. Their uncompromising quality standards have made this book an exceptional effort. Their encouragement from time to time has been an inspiration for everyone.

The publisher and the editorial board hope that this book will prove to be a valuable piece of knowledge for researchers, students, practitioners and scholars across the globe.

List of Contributors

Reinhilde Jacobs and Michael M. Bornstein
OMFS IMPATH Research Group, Department of Imaging and Pathology, Faculty of Medicine, University of Leuven, Kapucijnenvoer 33, 3000 Leuven, Belgium

Reinhilde Jacobs
Department of Oral and Maxillofacial Surgery, University Hospitals Leuven, Leuven, Belgium

Marina Codari
Unit of Radiology, IRCCS Policlinico San Donato, San Donato Milanese, Italy

Bassam Hassan
Department of Oral Function and Restorative Dentistry, Academic Centre for Dentistry Amsterdam (ACTA), Research Institute MOVE, 1081 LA Amsterdam, The Netherlands

Michael M. Bornstein
Applied Oral Sciences, Faculty of Dentistry, The University of Hong Kong, Hong Kong SAR, China

Anne N. Åstrøm
Oral health Centre of Expertise in Western Norway, Bergen, Hordaland, Norway

Anne N. Åstrøm, Stein Atle Lie and Ferda Gülcan
Department of Clinical Dentistry, Faculty of Medicine, University of Bergen, N-5020 Bergen, Norway

Youn-Hee Choi
Department of Preventive Dentistry, School of Dentistry, Kyungpook National University, Daegu, Republic of Korea

Takayuki Kosaka and Takahiro Ono
Department of Prosthodontics, Gerontology and Oral Rehabilitation, Osaka University Graduate School of Dentistry, Suita-Osaka, Japan

Miki Ojima, Shinichi Sekine and Atsuo Amano
Department of Preventive Dentistry, Osaka University Graduate School of Dentistry, 1-8 Yamadaoka, Suita-Osaka 565-0871, Japan

Yoshihiro Kokubo, Makoto Watanabe and Yoshihiro Miyamoto
Department of Preventive Cardiology, National Cerebral and Cardiovascular Center, Suita-Osaka, Japan

Takahiro Ono
Division of Comprehensive Prosthodontics, Niigata University Graduate School of Medical and Dental Sciences, Niigata, Japan

Wenjian Zhang
Department of Diagnostic and Biomedical Sciences, University of Texas School of Dentistry at Houston, 7500 Cambridge Street, Houston, TX 77054, USA

Keagan Foss
University of Texas School of Dentistry at Houston, 7500 Cambridge Street, Houston, TX 77054, USA

Bing-Yan Wang
Department of Periodontics and Dental Hygiene, University of Texas School of Dentistry at Houston, 7500 Cambridge Street, Houston, TX 77054, USA

Ji-Soo Song
Department of Pediatric Dentistry, Seoul National University Dental Hospital, 101, Daehakno, Jongno-gu, 03080 Seoul, Republic of Korea

Hong-Keun Hyun, Teo Jeon Shin and Young-Jae Kim
Department of Pediatric Dentistry, Dental Research Institute, School of Dentistry, Seoul National University, Seoul National University Dental Hospital, 101, Daehakno, Jongno-gu, 03080 Seoul, Republic of Korea

Morenike O. Folayan, Kikelomo A. Kolawole, Nneka K. Onyejaka, Hakeem O. Agbaje, Nneka M. Chukwumah and Titus A. Oyedele
Department of Child Dental Health, Obafemi Awolowo University, Ile-Ife, Nigeria

Vinodh Bhoopathi
Department of Pediatric Dentistry and Community Oral Health Sciences, Temple University Maurice H. Kornberg School of Dentistry, 3223 N Broad Street, Philadelphia, PA 19140, USA

Ajay Joshi
Pediatric Dentistry Department, Indiana University School of Dentistry, 1121 W. Michigan Street, Indianapolis, IN 46202, USA

Romer Ocanto
Department of Pediatric Dentistry, Nova Southeastern University College of Dental Medicine, 3200 S University Drive, Fort Lauderdale, FL 33328, USA

Robin J. Jacobs
Department of Family and Community Medicine – Research Programs, Baylor College of Medicine, 3701 Kirby Drive, Suite 600, Houston, TX 77098, USA

Qingfei Meng
Department of Stomatology, Xuzhou Central Hospital, Xuzhou 221009, Jiangsu Province, China

Qingfei Meng, Qian Ma, Tianda Wang and Yaming Chen
College of Stomatology, Nanjing Medical University, 136 Hanzhong Road, Nanjing 210029, Jiangsu Province, China

Emad A. Albdour, Eman Shaheen, Myrthel Vranckx, Constantinus Politis and Reinhilde Jacobs
OMFS IMPATH research group, Department of Imaging and Pathology, Faculty of Medicine, University of Leuven and Oral and Maxillofacial Surgery, University Hospitals Leuven, Leuven, Belgium

Emad A. Albdour
Department of Prosthodontics, Royal Medical Services, Jordanian Armed Forces, Amman, Jordan

Francesco Guido Mangano
Department of Medicine and Surgery, Dental School, University of Varese, Varese, Italy

Reinhilde Jacobs
Department of Dental Medicine, Karolinska Institutet, Stockholm, Sweden

Susan Al Bardaweel and Mayssoon Dashash
Department of Paediatric Dentistry, Faculty of Dentistry, Damascus University, Damascus city, Syria

Akio Tada
Department of Health Science, Hyogo University, 2301 Shinzaike Hiraoka-cho, Kakogawa, Hyogo 675-0195, Japan

Hiroko Miura
Department of International Health and Collaboration, National Institute of Public Health, 2-3-6, Minami, Wako, Saitama 351-0197, Japan

Supa Pengpid
ASEAN Institute for Health Development, Mahidol University, Salaya, Thailand

Supa Pengpid and Karl Peltzer
Department of Research and Innovation, University of Limpopo, Turfloop, South Africa

Karl Peltzer
HIV/AIDS/STIs and TB (HAST) Research Programme, Human Sciences Research Council, Private Bag X41, Pretoria 0001, South Africa

Ancuta Banu
Department 2, Discipline of Maxillofacial Surgery, Faculty of Dentistry, "Victor Babes" University of Medicine and Pharmacy Timişoara, 5 Take Ionescu Bvd, 300062 Timisoara, Romania

Costela Şerban,   Marius Pricop and Horatiu Urechescu
Department 3 Functional Sciences, "Victor Babes" University of Medicine and Pharmacy Timişoara, 14 Spl. Tudor Vladimirescu, 300172 Timişoara, Romania

Brigitha Vlaicu
Department 14 Microbiology, "Victor Babes" University of Medicine and Pharmacy Timişoara, 16 Victor Babes Bvd, 300226 Timişoara, Romania

Márk Antal and Emese Battancs
Faculty of Dentistry, Department of Aesthetic and Operative Dentistry, University of Szeged, 6720 Tisza Lajos körút, Szeged 64, Hungary

Márta Bocskai and László Kovács
Faculty of Medicine, Department of Rheumatology and Immunology, University of Szeged, 6725 Kálvária sugárút, Szeged 57, Hungary

Gábor Braunitzer
Laboratory for Perception and Cognition and Clinical Neuroscience, Nyírő Gyula Hospital, 1135 Lehel utca, Budapest 59, Hungary

Elham M. Senan and Ahmed A. Madfa
Restorative and Prosthodontic Department, College of Dentistry, University of Science and Technology, Sanáa, Yemen

Hatem A. Alhadainy
Department of Dentistry, University of Alberta, Edmonton, Canada

Thuraia M. Genaid
Department of Conservative Dentistry, Faculty of Dentistry, Tanta University, Tanta, Egypt

Ahmed A. Madfa
Department of Conservative Dentistry, Faculty of Dentistry, Thamar University, Dhamar, Yemen

Hatem A. Alhadainy
Department of Endodontics, Faculty of Dentistry, Tanta University, Tanta, Egypt

Katja Goetz, Wiebke Winkelmann and Jost Steinhäuser
Institute of Family Medicine, University Hospital Schleswig-Holstein, Campus Luebeck, Ratzeburger Allee 160, 23538 Luebeck, Germany

Ana Luiza Sarno Castro
Department of Health, State University of Feira de Santana, Transnordestina, s/n, Novo Horizonte, Feira de Santana, Bahia CEP 44036-900, Brazil

Maria Isabel Pereira Vianna
Department of Public Oral Health, School of Dentistry, Federal University of Bahia, Araújo Pinho, 62, Canela, Salvador, Bahia CEP 40110040, Brazil

Carlos Maurício Cardeal Mendes
Postgraduate Studies in Interactive Processes of Organs and Systems, Health Science Institute, Federal University of Bahia, Avenida Reitor Miguel Calmon, 1272, Salvador, Bahia CEP 40231300, Brazil

Elham Kateeb and Elizabeth Momany
Public Policy Center, the University of Iowa, Iowa City, IA, USA

Elham Kateeb
Department of Periodontology and Preventive Dentistry, Al-Quds University, College of Dentistry, University Main St., Jerusalem, State of Palestine

C. Welte-Jzyk and M. Daubländer
Department of Oral and Maxillofacial Surgery, University Medical Centre of the Johannes Gutenberg University of Mainz, Mainz, Germany

D. B. Pfau
Mannheim Institute of Public Health (MIPH), Social and Preventive Medicine, University of Heidelberg, Heidelberg, Germany

A. Hartmann
Private Practice Dr. Seiler and colleagues, Filderstadt, Germany

Trine Lise Lundekvam Berge, Gunvor Bentung Lygre and Lars Björkman
Dental Biomaterials Adverse Reaction Unit, Uni Research Health, Bergen, Norway

Trine Lise Lundekvam Berge
Oral Health Centre of Expertise in Western Norway, Bergen, Hordaland, Norway

Stein Atle Lie and Lars Björkman
Department of Clinical Dentistry, University of Bergen, Bergen, Norway

Ana Luiza Sarno Castro
Department of Health, State University of Feira de Santana, Transnordestina, s/n, Novo Horizonte, Feira de Santana, Bahia CEP 44036-900, Brazil

Maria Isabel Pereira Vianna
Department of Public Oral Health, School of Dentistry, Federal University of Bahia, Araújo Pinho, 62, Canela, Salvador, Bahia CEP 40110040, Brazil

Carlos Maurício Cardeal Mendes
Postgraduate Studies in Interactive Processes of Organs and Systems, Health Science Institute, Federal University of Bahia, Avenida Reitor Miguel Calmon, 1272, Salvador, Bahia CEP 40231300, Brazil

Azhani Ismail, Ishak A. Razak and Norintan Ab-Murat
Department of Community Oral Health and Clinical Prevention, Faculty of Dentistry, University of Malaya, 50603 Kuala Lumpur, Malaysia

Azhani Ismail
Klang Dental Clinic, Jalan Tengku Kelana, 41000 Klang, Selangor, Malaysia

Ishak A. Razak
Faculty of Dentistry, MAHSA University, 42610 Bandar Saujana Putra, Selangor, Malaysia

Carla Figueiredo Brandão, Viviane Maia Barreto Oliveira, Ada Rocha Ramony Martins Santos, Taísa Midlej Martins da Silva, Verônica Queiroz Cruz Vilella, Gleice Glenda Prata Pimentel Simas, Laura Regina Santos Carvalho, Raissa Aires Costa Carvalho and Ana Marice Teixeira Ladeia
Bahiana School of Medicine and Public Health, Avenida Dom João VI, no. 275, Brotas. ZIP: 40.290-000, Salvador, Bahia, Brazil

Shanshan Dai, Gang Xiao, Ning Dong, Fei Liu, Shuyang He and Qingyu Guo
Key Laboratory of Shaanxi Province for Craniofacial Precision Medicine Research, Xi'an 710004, China Department of Pediatric Dentistry, Hospital of Stomatology Xi'an Jiaotong University College of Medicine, Xi'an 710004, Shaanxi, China

Kai-Hendrik Bormann and Nils-Claudius Gellrich
Hannover Medical School, Hannover, Germany

Heinz Kniha and Michael Gahlert
High Tech Research Center, University Hospital Basel, Basel, Switzerland

Sabine Schild and Dieter Weingart
Klinikum Stuttgart, Katharinenhospital, Stuttgart, Germany

Sho Saito, Takashi Ohi, Takamasa Komiyama, Yoshitada Miyoshi, Kosei Endo and Yoshinori Hattori
Division of Aging and Geriatric Dentistry, Department of Oral Function and Morphology, Tohoku University Graduate School of Dentistry, 4-1 Seiryo-machi, Aoba-ku, Sendai, Miyagi 980-8575, Japan

Takashi Ohi
Japanese Red Cross Ishinomaki Hospital, Ishinomaki, Japan

Takahisa Murakami, Michihiro Satoh and Hirohito Metoki
Division of Public Health, Hygiene and Epidemiology, Faculty of Medicine, Tohoku Medical and Pharmaceutical University, Sendai, Japan

Takayoshi Ohkubo
Department of Hygiene and Public Health, Teikyo University School of Medicine, Tokyo, Japan

Kei Asayama, Yutaka Imai and Kei Asayama
Department of Planning for Drug Development and Clinical Evaluation, Tohoku University Graduate School of Pharmaceutical Sciences, Sendai, Japan

Ryusuke Inoue
Department of Medical Informatics, Tohoku University Graduate School of Medicine, Sendai, Japan

Masahiro Kikuya
Department of Preventive Medicine and Epidemiology, Tohoku Medical Megabank Organization, Tohoku University, Sendai, Japan

Index